Michael Schiewe

AF710905

FISH IMMUNOLOGY

FISH IMMUNOLOGY

Papers presented at an International Meeting held at Sandy Hook, New Jersey, U.S.A., 8–12 September 1985

Edited by

JOANNE S. STOLEN

Sandy Hook Laboratory, Highlands, NJ 07732 (U.S.A.)

DOUGLAS P. ANDERSON

U.S. Fish and Wildlife Service, National Fish Health Research Laboratory, Box 700, Kearneysville, WV 25430 (U.S.A.)

and

WILLEM B. VAN MUISWINKEL

Department of Experimental Animal Morphology and Cell Biology, Agricultural University, P.O. Box 338, 6700 AH Wageningen (The Netherlands)

This volume is reprinted from the journal *Veterinary Immunology and Immunopathology,* vol. 12.

ELSEVIER Amsterdam – Oxford – New York – Tokyo 1986

ELSEVIER SCIENCE PUBLISHERS B.V.
Sara Burgerhartstraat 25
P.O. Box 211, 1000 AE Amsterdam, The Netherlands

Distribution for the United States and Canada:

ELSEVIER SCIENCE PUBLISHING COMPANY INC.
52, Vanderbilt Avenue
New York, N.Y. 10017, U.S.A.

Library of Congress Cataloging-in-Publication Data

Fish immunology.

(Developments in aquaculture and fisheries science ; 16)
Bibliography: p.
Includes index.
1. Fishes--Immunology--Congresses. I. Stolen, Joanne S. II. Anderson, Douglas P. III. Muiswinkel, Willem B. van. IV. Series.
QL639.1.F558 1986 597'.02'9 86-16561
ISBN 0-444-42667-1

ISBN 0-444-42667-1

© Elsevier Science Publishers B.V., 1986

All rights reserved. No part of this publication may be reproduced, stored in a retrieval system or transmitted in any form or by any means, electronic, mechanical, photocopying, recording or otherwise, without the prior written permission of the publisher, Elsevier Science Publishers B.V./Science & Technology Division, P.O. Box 330, 1000 AH Amsterdam, The Netherlands.

Special regulations for readers in the USA – This publication has been registered with the Copyright Clearance Centre Inc. (CCC) Salem, Massachusetts. Information can be obtained from the CCC about conditions under which photocopies of parts of this publication may be made in the USA. All other copyright questions, including photocopying outside of the USA, should be referred to the publisher.

Printed in The Netherlands

CONTENTS

FISH IMMUNOLOGY at SANDY HOOK

Fish immunology has greatly expanded in technical scope and practical application during the last decade. Recent research results detailing the immune systems of fish have phylogenetic significance for veterinary and clinical immunologists, scientists studying environmental and pollution problems, as well as fundamental information for aquaculturists and fish farmers. It is becoming increasingly clear that fish immune systems function with similarities analogous to mammalian counterparts with a few interesting exceptions due to optimal adaptation to the aquatic environment. The cell interactions, molecular signals and the structure of immunoglobulin molecules and complement components have been conserved throughout vertebrate evolution.

Immunogens against fish disease agents are now commercially available to fish farmers, and in many cases, the immune status of their animals may influence profitability in these large operations. To maximize effectiveness of immunization programs, fish culturists must draw on basic immunological principles included in this book. Not only is it desirable to learn how to best prepare the fish to respond to the bacterins and vaccines, but also necessary how to optimize the formulations for these immunogens. The internal physiological condition of the fish must be ready to process antigens, and give an immune response without the interference of external, detrimental environmental conditions. Pollutants and contaminants may have the potential to modulate or suppress the fishes' abilities to respond quickly when exposed to immunogens that otherwise would stimulate the production of protective antibody or other forms of cell-mediated immunity.

The 47 scientific papers in this volume were presented at an international meeting on fish immunology held by the bay on the Sandy Hook peninsula in New Jersey, USA, September 8-12, 1985. The participants represented 18 different countries and were affiliated with government, academic, or private research organizations. We all had a delightful time.

JOANNE S. STOLEN
DOUGLAS P. ANDERSON
WILLEM B. VAN MUISWINKEL

ACKNOWLEDGEMENTS

The organizers wish to thank the Committee Members, Session Chairpersons and in particular the organizational assistant, Vicky J. Kaspar.

The support by the National Marine Fisheries Service, Fish and Wildlife Service, American Fisheries Society, National Science Foundation, U.S. Dept. of the Army, Food and Drug Administration, Sandy Hook Laboratory, Gateway National Recreation Area, Macalester Bicknell, T.H.F. Publications, Aqua Health, Bio Med, Domsea Farms and Agricultural University (Wageningen) is also gratefully acknowledged.

Veterinary Immunology and Immunopathology, 12 (1986) 1—6
Elsevier Science Publishers B.V., Amsterdam — Printed in The Netherlands

THE USE OF ARTIFICIAL GYNOGENESIS IN STUDIES ON THE IMMUNE SYSTEM OF CARP (*CYPRINUS CARPIO* L.)

W.B. VAN MUISWINKEL, A.J. TIGCHELAAR, E.G.M. HARMSEN and P.M. RIJNDERS
Department of Exp. Animal Morphology & Cell Biology, Agricultural University, P.O. Box 338, 6700 AH Wageningen (The Netherlands)

ABSTRACT

Van Muiswinkel, W.B., Tigchelaar, A.J., Harmsen, E.G.M. and Rijnders, P.M., 1986. The use of artificial gynogenesis in studies on the immune system of carp (*Cyprinus carpio* L.). Vet. Immunol. Immunopathol., 12: 1-6.

Gynogenetic carp were obtained by using γ-irradiated sperm for fertilization followed by a cold shock. The gynogenetic fish and normal siblings of the same parents were analysed for 3 genetic markers: scale pattern, transferrin (Tf) and allograft rejection. Gynogenetic offspring showed only the maternal scale pattern (scattered). In the majority of the gynogenetic fish a heterozygous Tf pattern identical to the mother was observed. Animals homozygous for Tf were rare in this group. A typical paternal Tf band was only seen in normal siblings. An exchange of skin grafts between normal animals was always followed by rejection (median survival time, 12 days at 23 ^{o}C). However, the rejection was delayed in the gynogenetic group (MST, 19,6 days). There were even signs of acceptance in some animals. This approach can be used for the identification of 2nd and 3rd generation gynogenetic fish, which are homozygous for certain MHC haplotypes.

INTRODUCTION

There are at least 4 basic measures to reduce or control fish diseases: 1) treatment with drugs (e.g. antibiotics); 2) eradication of diseased animals followed by disinfection; 3)vaccination at early life stages; 4) improvement of genetic resistance. Most data are available on the first 3 possibilities (Hayes, 1984; De Kinkelin and Michel, 1984; Lamers, 1985). There is not much known in fish about the last approach. In principle, the genetic variability inherent to host-defense mechanisms can be used for selecting disease resistant strains. The major types of defense mechanisms against infection are: mechanical barriers (e.g. skin), phagocytic cells, non-specific factors (e.g. interferon) and the complement and immune systems. It is known from studies in mammals, birds and amphibians that the immune system is under the control of a group of closely linked genes called the major histocompatibility complex or MHC (Götze, 1977; Flaherty and Cohen, 1982). The MHC not only regulates the production of strong transplantation antigens, but also plays an important role in the regulation of the immune response.

0165-2427/86/$03.50 © 1986 Elsevier Science Publishers B.V.

Inbred animals, homozygous for certain genotypes, will be extremely valuable for studies on the genetic aspects of disease resistance. The technique of gynogenetic reproduction, which is uniquely suited for ectothermic vertebrates (amphibians and fish), can be used for obtaining animal populations in which allelic diversity at any gene locus is greatly reduced (Roux and Volpe, 1975; Cherfas, 1981). In this paper the first attempts are described to obtain gynogenetic carp, which are homozygous for certain MHC haplotypes.

In addition to the MHC, another genetic marker called transferrin (Tf) was analysed in this study. The blood protein Tf may also play a role in disease resistance by binding endogenous iron and making it unavailable for bacterial use (Suzumoto et al., 1977).

MATERIALS AND METHODS

Animals and gynogenesis

Common carp (*Cyprinus carpio* L.) were kept at 23 ^{o}C in recirculating aquarium systems. The animals were fed with pelleted dry food (K30, Trouw, Putten). Eggs and sperm were obtained by the standard methods of artificial propagation. The technique of gynogenesis was carried out as described by Nagy et al. (1978). Non-irradiated sperm was used for normal reproduction (control fish). Fertilization and treatment of the developing eggs were carried out at 23 ^{o}C by the method of Woynarovich (1962). To induce gynogenesis, a cold shock at 0 ^{o}C was given for 60 min, starting 15 min after fertilization. Treatment with tannic acid occurred immediately after warming up the eggs.

Genetic markers

1. Scale type. The male carp (W1) used for breeding was scaled (Ss) and the female fish (W11) was scattered (ss).

2. Transferrin (Tf). For this purpose blood samples were taken from the caudal vein of 7-8 month old fish and their parents. Blood was allowed to clot at room temperature and serum, obtained by centrifugation, was stored at -20 ^{o}C before use. Serum proteins were separated by means of vertical polyacrylamide gel electrophoresis (PAGE) at room temperature with a 0,066 M tris-borate solution (pH 9.0) as electrode buffer. A 4% polyacrylamide gel with a 10% separation gel gave best results. The PAGE was done in the absence of SDS. Tf could be detected by specific staining with Nitroso-R-salt (Mueller et al., 1962). The routine gel staining for protein was carried out with Coomassie Blue.

3. Transplantation. For grafting only scattered fish were used. Square pieces (3-5 mm^2) of dorsal skin were reciprocally exchanged between pairs of MS222 anaesthesized fish. The donor skin (allograft) was usually darker than

the surrounding acceptor skin on the lateral side of the fish. The acceptor skin was detached from the underlaying connective tissue to form a square pocket. The donor skin was put into this pocket in order to protect it from mechanical damage. After 2 days the overlaying acceptor skin was removed and the allograft was examined every other day. The survival end point of the allograft was defined as the number of days after transplantation at which all pigment cells (melanophores) were destroyed. The median survival time (MST) of the grafts in the 2 fish groups was calculated from the survival end points.

RESULTS and DISCUSSION

All gynogenetic offspring showed the maternal scattered phenotype which indicates the efficacy of sperm inactivation. The control offspring were scaled (48%) or scattered (52%).

Analysis of the serum electrophoretic pattern (figure 1) shows that in both parents 2 major Tf bands can be observed. Male and female have 1 Tf band in

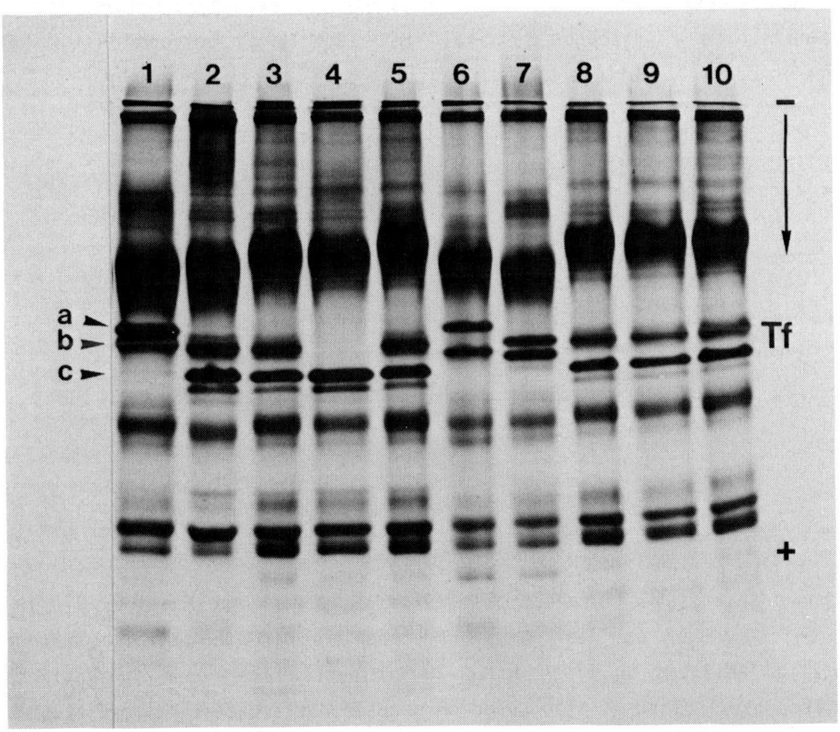

Fig. 1. PAGE pattern of carp serum proteins. The position of the transferrin bands is marked by Tf. Serum samples of the parents are shown in lane 1 (♂) and 2 (♀). Gynogenetic offspring of these fish were used in lanes 3-5 and 8-10. Sera from unrelated fish are shown in lanes 6 and 7 for comparison.

common which migrates at intermediate speed (band b). The sire has 1 slow band (band a) which is absent from the dam. On the other hand, the dam shows 1 fast band (band c). In normal offspring (not shown in figure 1) all possible combinations of these bands were found (3 ab, 9 bb, 6 ac and 7 bc) as can be expected when both Tf alleles are codominantly expressed. The gynogenetic offspring never showed the paternal a band. The majority of these animals (13 out of 14) were identical to the mother (bc type). Interestingly enough, 1 animal (lane 4) showed only the fast c band. This can be regarded as an indication for homozygosity. In this experiment the Tf homozygotes were relatively rare. However, in a review article by Purdom (1984) much higher percentages of homozygous Tf genotypes in carp were mentioned. On the other hand, there are indications from studies in coho salmon, that certain Tf genotypes are more susceptible to bacterial diseases than others (Suzumoto et al., 1977). It is possible, that a strong selection against unfavorable homozygous Tf genotypes has taken place in our gynogenetic carp during their first weeks of life.

The skin transplantation experiment demonstrated a clear difference between normal and gynogenetic fish (Table 1). The allografts exchanged between gynogenetic carp showed a prolonged survival (MST 19.6 days) compared with the same grafts in control siblings (MST 12 days).

TABLE 1.
Number of rejected skin allografts in normal control and gynogenetic offspring of carp (23 ^{o}C).

Experimental group	Days after grafting					
	6-9	10-13	14-17	18-21	22-25	26-28
Control (n=52)	16	28	8			
Gynogenetic (n=24)		5	6	8	5	1

It is known that fish can reject allografts (Hildemann and Haas, 1960). In mammals, this type of cellular immune response is directed against strong transplantation antigens or class I MHC determinants. There are indications that this response in fish is also based on genetic differences. Kallman (1962) was able to show that transplants (fins, hearts and spleens) were accepted if host and donor were of the same clone of <u>Mollienesia formosa</u>. This teleost is reproducing in nature by gynogenesis. A prolonged survival time of scale grafts was observed in gynogenetic goldfish and carp by Nagy et al. (1983). This is in agreement with our observations after skin grafting. Acceptance of skin grafts did not occur in our first generation of artificial gynogenetic carp. It cannot be excluded, that the occurrence of identical MHC haplotypes is low as a result of a relatively high crossover frequency during meiosis. Another, more probable, explanation is the presence of minor histocompatibility genes localized at other chromosomes than the MHC.

It is suggested by Cherfas (1981) that 2 to 3 generations of gynogenesis or 8 to 10 generations of conventional inbreeding are required to obtain highly inbred strains. The data mentioned above and the results of recent *in vitro* tests (mixed leucocyte reaction) provide us with evidence for the existance of an MHC in fish. Moreover, the technique of gynogenesis can be used for the production of carp homozygous for certain MHC haplotypes in the near future. These animals will be used for future studies on the role of the MHC in immune responses of fish and for the selection of disease resistant strains.

ACKNOWLEDGMENTS

The authors wish to thank Prof. N. Cohen (University of Rochester, N.Y., USA) for introducing the skin transplantation technique in our laboratory and the staff of the Fish Culture Experimental Station, Polish Academy of Sciences, Gołysz, for advice on carp propagation and gynogenesis. We are also grateful to Dr T.C. Fletcher and Dr G. Lobb for valuable suggestions on the manuscript, to Mr S.H. Leenstra and Mr P. van Kleef for biotechnical support, to Mrs. H.W. Vertregt-Fonhof for typing this paper.

REFERENCES

Cherfas, N.B., 1981. Gynogenesis in fishes. In: V.S. Kirpichnikov (Ed.), Genetic Bases of Fish Selection, Springer Verlag, Berlin, pp. 255-273.

Flaherty, L. and Cohen, N., 1982. The major histocompatibility complex. In: L.N. Ruben and M.E. Gershwin (Eds.), Immune Regulation, Evolutionary and Biological Significance. Dekker, Inc., N.Y., pp. 1-27.

Götze, D., (Editor), 1977. The Major Histocompatibility System in Man and Animals, Springer Verlag, Berlin.

Hayes, J., (Editor), 1984. Animal Health, 1984 Yearbook of Agriculture, U.S. Government Printing Office, Washington, D.C., 646 pp.

Hildemann, W.H. and Haas, R., 1960. Comparative studies of homotransplantation in fishes. J. Cell. Comp. Physiol., 34: 227-233.

Kallman, K.D., 1962. Gynogenesis in the teleost, *Mollienesia formosa* (Girard), with a discussion of the detection of parthogenesis in vertebrates by tissue transplantation. J. Genet., 58: 7-24.

Kinkelin de, P. and Michel, C., (Editors), 1984. Symposium on Fish Vaccination. O.I.E., Paris, 222 pp.

Lamers, C.H.J., 1985. The reaction of the immune system of fish to vaccination. Ph.D. Thesis, Agricultural University, Wageningen, The Netherlands.

Mueller, J.O., Smithies, O. and Irwin, M.R., 1962. Transferrin variation in *Columbidae*. Genetics Princeton, 47: 1385-1392.

Nagy, A., Rajki, K., Horvàth, L. and Csànyi, V., 1978. Investigation on carp, *Cyprinus carpio* L. gynogenesis. J. Fish Biol., 13: 215-224.

Nagy, A., Monostory, Z. and Csányi,V., 1983. Rapid development of the clonal state in successive gynogenetic generations of carp (Cyprinus carpio). Copeia, 745-749.

Purdom, C.E., 1984. Atypical modes of reproduction in fish. In: J.R. Clarke (Ed.), Oxford Reviews of Reproductive Biology, Vol. 6. Oxford University Press, pp. 303-340.

Roux, K.H. and Volpe, E.P., 1975. Evidence for a major histocompatibility complex in the leopard frog. Immunogenetics, 2: 577-589.

Suzumoto, B.K., Schreck, C.B. and McIntyre, J.D., 1977. Relative resistances of three transferrin genotypes of coho salmon (Oncorynchus kisutch) and their hematological responses to bacterial kidney disease. J. Fish Res. Board Can., 34: 1-8.

Woynarovich, E., 1962. Hatching of carp eggs in "Zuger" glasses and breeding of carp larvae until an age of 10 days. Bamidgeh, 14: 38-46.

Veterinary Immunology and Immunopathology, 12 (1986) 7—12
Elsevier Science Publishers B.V., Amsterdam — Printed in The Netherlands

STRUCTURAL DIVERSITY OF CHANNEL CATFISH IMMUNOGLOBULINS

CRAIG J. LOBB

Department of Microbiology, University of Mississippi Medical Center,
Jackson, MS 39211, USA

ABSTRACT

Lobb, C.J., 1986. Structural diversity of channel catfish immunoglobulins. Vet. Immunol. Immunopathol., 12: 7-12.

This paper describes a number of observations which show that the covalent structure of catfish Ig is heterogeneous and secondly that different Ig L chain classes are present.

INTRODUCTION

The ability of fish to form antibodies in response to a variety of antigens such as proteins, viruses, and bacteria has been clearly shown (reviewed by Marchalonis, 1977). The study of the elicited antibodies to these various antigens has found that the predominant antibody form found in teleosts is a ∿700,000 tetrameric immunoglobulin (Ig). The tetramer is composed of four monomers; each monomer containing equimolar amounts of heavy (H) and light (L) chains (2H:2L). Based upon the mass and carbohydrate content of teleost H chains, fish Ig is often considered to be IgM (reviewed by Nisonoff et al., 1975); although there is no primary structural evidence as yet to support this designation. The tetramer of fish has been thought to be composed of a single class of H chains and a single class of L chains. The advent of monoclonal antibody technology and certain advances in the separation and analysis of proteins has allowed some of these general concepts to be re-examined. This paper reviews some of the recent work done with the Ig of the channel catfish and describes a number of observations which show that the covalent structure of catfish Ig is heterogeneous and secondly that different Ig L chain classes are present.

COVALENT STRUCTURE OF CATFISH ANTIBODIES

Two general approaches have been taken to purify the tetrameric Ig of catfish (Lobb and Clem, 1983, Lobb, 1985). The first approach has been the purification of naturally occurring serum Ig by the combined usage of anion exchange chromatography on DEAE-cellulose and gel filtration chromatography on agarose A-5M. The coupled use of anion exchange and gel filtration chromatography is standard for the separation of many serum proteins, including the serum Igs of higher animals. The historical difficulty of adequately separating large proteins by gel filtration, such as the ∿700,000 dalton tetrameric Ig of fish, has been overcome with several newer gel filtration matrices which have

0165-2427/86/$03.50 © 1986 Elsevier Science Publishers B.V.

exclusion limits $>1x10^6$ daltons. The second approach used to purify the catfish tetramer has been the induction and isolation of catfish antibodies to the hapten DNP. This method is direct and yields purified proteins which can be used for structural studies or antibody binding studies. Both of these general approaches have been exploited to purify the catfish tetramer so its basic structure could be studied.

Several conclusions can now be made regarding the structure of catfish Ig. The channel catfish antibody and Ig, when analyzed by gel filtration in non-denaturing solvents, elutes in a homogeneous peak expected to contain ∿600,000 to ∿750,000 dalton material. There is no evidence at present to suggest that catfish produce low molecular weight antibodies similar to those found in other fish (reviewed by Lobb and Clem, 1981). If the unreduced catfish tetramer is analyzed for mass heterogeneity in denaturing solvents, such as SDS or guanidine-HCl, the catfish Ig exhibits an unusual noncovalent architecture. The antibody, rather than migrating as a homogeneous protein with an expected mass of ∿700,000 daltons, dissociates into eight discrete subpopulations when analyzed by SDS-gels (Fig. 1). This dissociation is not observed with mammalian IgM. The dissociation of catfish Ig is due to the interaction of the protein and SDS which results in the dissociation of the tetramer into only those species which contain covalently associated H and L chains. The molecular masses of the eight subpopulations are ∿750,000, ∿660,000, ∿570,000, ∿480,000, ∿390,000, ∿290,000, ∿190,000, and ∿90,000 respectively. Thus, the eight subpopulations differ in size from one another by ∿90,000 daltons. This mass difference between the subpopulations would be expected if each subpopulation had a different number of heavy-light chain pairs or halfmers. This hypothesis has subsequently been confirmed. Therefore, the covalent tetramer (subpopulation indicated as 8 on Fig. 1) is composed of eight covalently-linked halfmers, subpopulation 7 is composed of seven covalently-linked halfmer, etc. (Lobb and Clem, 1983).

In terms of understanding how these subpopulations might be represented in the tetrameric Ig population, Fig 2 depicts various tetrameric immunoglobulin molecules which differ in their disulfide linkages. In these molecules the disulfide linkage between a single H chain and a single L chain forms the covalent halfmer. This bond has been conserved in these molecules because there has been little evidence to suggest that free H chains or free L chains dissociate from the tetrameric population in denaturing, non-reducing solvents. However, the other disulfide bonds which could serve to link the covalent halfmer to form a tetramer have been changed. Each of the depicted molecules would be expected to dissociate into the indicated subpopulations if the non-covalent associations were disrupted. The key feature that is evident is

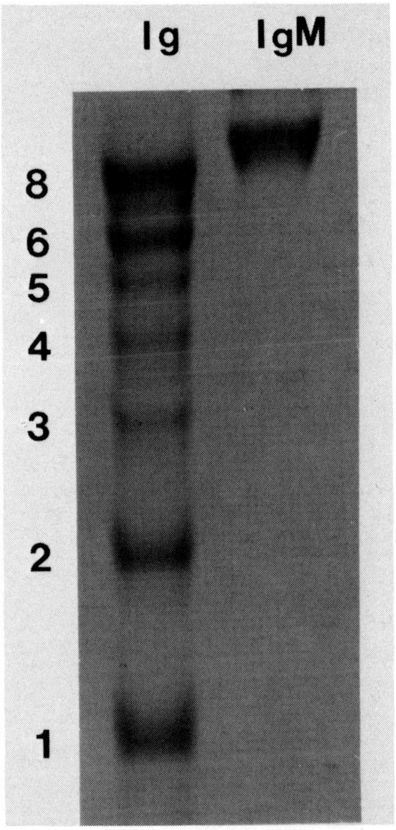

Fig. 1. SDS-polyacrylamide gel analysis of unreduced catfish immunoglobulin (Ig) and human IgM (∿900,000 daltons). The numerical designations 1-8 indicate the number of covalently-linked H-L chain units represented in each subpopulation. Subpopulation 7 can be seen between 6 and 8.

the suggested variability of the disulfide bonds which would likely bridge either the H chains within the basic monomeric unit (interheavy chain bonds) or those bonds which would join one monomeric subunit to another monomeric subunit (intersubunit bonds). For example, in the molecule designated 4 + 2 + 2 there are four intersubunit bonds and one interheavy chain bond. If this molecule were dissociated into the covalently-linked subspecies, this molecule would be composed of one subspecies of subpopulation 4 (four covalently-linked halfmers) and two subspecies of subpopulation 2 (two covalently-linked halfmers). At this time it is not known if any of these possible disulfide linkages actually exist. Nonetheless, it is clear that the catfish tetramer must exhibit considerable variability in the disulfide linkages between covalent halfmers in order to show the mass heterogeneity observed in these populations.

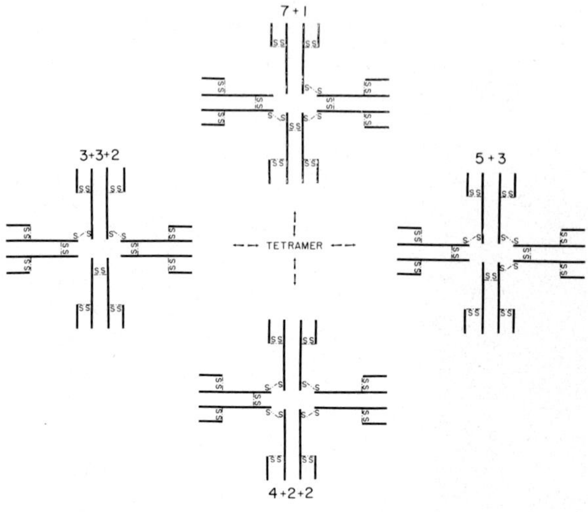

Fig. 2. Various hypothetical catfish tetrameric immunoglobulin molecules. The various tetramers would dissociate into the indicated subpopulations if these molecules were subjected to non-reductive denaturation in dissociative solvents such as SDS or guanidine-HCl.

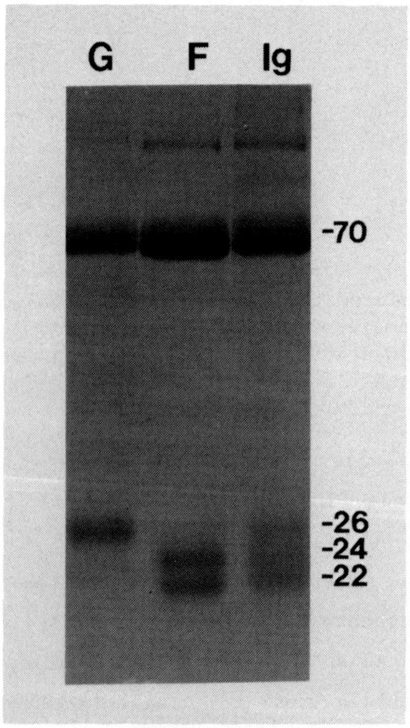

Fig. 3. SDS-polyacrylamide gel analysis of reduced catfish immunoglobulin. G and F are affinity-purified catfish immunoglobulin isolated from immunoabsorbant columns coupled with mAb 1G7 and 3F12, respectively. Ig is catfish immunoglobulin isolated by anion exchange and gel filtration chromatography. The molecular weights in kilodaltons of the component heavy and light chains are indicated based upon their relative mobility to known molecular weight standards.

Recent work has shown that there is no demonstrable change in the relative amounts of various subpopulations during the temporal immune response of catfish to the hapten, DNP (Lobb, 1985). Purified anti-DNP antibody populations were obtained from individual catfish at intervals ranging from 3 months to one year or longer post-immunization. When the antibody population was examined by SDS-gels there was no observable difference in the relative amounts of the subpopulations. Thus this unusual covalent structure is apparently a stable characteristic of this protein.

DIFFERENT LIGHT CHAIN CLASSES IN CATFISH ANTIBODIES

The heterogeneity of the tetrameric Ig population in catfish prompted the development of a battery of different monoclonal antibodies (mAb) to catfish Ig. This direction has proven to be extremely worthwhile in determining if antigenically distinct populations of catfish Ig exist. In this regard two mAbs designated 3F12 and 1G7 had been derived (Lobb and Clem, 1982). These two antibodies have been found to recognize different Ig L chains in the catfish. To review the basic findings regarding the L chains in catfish (Lobb _et al._, 1984), several things need to be discussed. The first is that there are three different molecular weight species of L chains observed when catfish Ig is reduced and analyzed by SDS-polyacrylamide gels. Fig. 3 represents a typical analysis of catfish Ig. The H chains migrate in a single band with a molecular mass of ∿70,000 daltons. The L chains migrate in three different positions with a relative mass of ∿26,000, ∿24,000, and ∿22,000 daltons. Secondly, when the Ig of catfish is purified by affinity chromatography using the immobilized mAbs 3F12 and 1G7, the Ig L chains are differentially represented. In Fig. 3 it can be observed that the catfish Ig defined by mAb 3F12 (F) only bears the ∿24,000 and ∿22,000 L chains. In contrast the Ig defined by mAb 1G7 (G) bears only L chains with a molecular mass of ∿26,000 daltons.

Peptide mapping studies have subsequently shown that the different L chains identified by these two mAbs are structurally distinct. It has also been shown that the antigenic differences between the two L chains represent isotypic rather than allotypic variability. Individual fish have been examined for the presence of both L chains and all fish so far examined have had both. Approximately 60% of the serum Ig L chains are defined by mAb 3F12 whereas ∿40% of the serum Ig L chains are defined by mAb 1G7. The different L chains have been provisionally designated class F and G (based upon reactivities of mAb 3F12 and 1G7, respectively). Amino acid sequencing studies are now required to confirm whether these proteins can be strictly paralleled to the k and λ chains of higher vertebrates.

CONCLUDING REMARKS

The Ig of catfish is represented by different populations of molecules which differ in their covalent structure as well as their component L chains. Ongoing studies to characterize other mAbs to catfish Ig are also identifying other distinct populations of catfish Ig. In this regard it now seems clear that there are distinct forms of catfish H chains. At present three monoclonal antibodies have been defined which recognize different H chain types. The completed characterization of these antigenically different forms of H chains will hopefully continue to add to our understanding of the humoral and secretory immune system of fish. In closing, it now seems that phylogenetic diversification of Ig has occurred at the level of teleost fish. Although it would be premature at this point to suggest that these different Ig forms have different biological functions, clearly the logical extension of these studies will be to determine if such properties can be shown to exist.

ACKNOWLEDGMENTS

This work has been supported in part by NIH grant 1 R23 AI 19412 and USDA grants 82-CRSR-2-1057 and 84-CRSR-2-2403.

REFERENCES

Lobb, C.J. and Clem, L.W., 1981. The metabolic relationships of the immunoglobulins in fish serum, cutaneous mucus, and bile. J. Immunol., 127: 1525-1529.

Lobb, C.J. and Clem, L.W., 1982. Fish lymphocytes differ in the expression of surface immunoglobulin. Dev. Comp. Immunol., 6: 473-479.

Lobb, C.J. and Clem, L.W., 1983. Distinctive subpopulations of catfish serum antibody and immunoglobulin. Mol. Immunol., 20: 811-818.

Lobb, C.J. and Clem, L.W., 1984. Immunoglobulin light chain classes in a teleost fish. J. Immunol., 132: 1917-1923.

Lobb, C.J., 1985. Covalent structure and affinity of channel catfish anti-dinitrophenyl antibodies. Mol. Immunol., 22: 993-999.

Marchalonis, J.J., 1977. Immunity in Evolution. Harvard University Press, Cambridge, 316 pp.

Nisonoff, A., Hopper, J.E. and Spring, S.B., 1975. The Antibody Molecule. Academic Press, New York, 542 pp.

Veterinary Immunology and Immunopathology, 12 (1986) 13—20
Elsevier Science Publishers B.V., Amsterdam — Printed in The Netherlands

CONSERVATION AMONG THE IMMUNOGLOBULINS OF CARCHARHINE SHARKS AND PHYLOGENETIC CONSERVATION OF VARIABLE REGION DETERMINANTS

I. L. ROSENSHEIN, S.F. SCHLUTER and J.J. MARCHALONIS

Department of Biochemistry, Medical University of South Carolina, 171 Ashley Avenue, Charleston, South Carolina 29425 (U.S.A.)

ABSTRACT

Rosenshein, I.L., Schluter S.F. and Marchalonis, J.J., 1986. Conservation among the immunoglobulins of carcharhine sharks and phylogenetic conservation of variable region determinants. Vet. Immunol. Immunopathol., 12: 13-20.

To study primitive vertebrate recognition molecules we have purified the immunoglobulins of three species of carcharhine sharks. The tiger (Galeocerdo cuvieri), the sandbar (Carcharhinus plumbeus) and the galapagos sharks (Carcharhinus galapagensis) possess 18S high molecular weight and 7S low molecular weight immunoglobulin forms. Both within and between species these forms closely resemble each other in polypeptide chain composition, heavy chain mass, carbohydrate content, amino acid composition, antigenic character and amino terminal sequence. These carcharhine species are separated by at least 30 million years of evolutionary time and it is remarkable that so little diversification of immunoglobulin structure has occurred during their evolution. By several criteria carcharhine immunoglobulins most closely resemble mammalian IgM. Studies of serological cross-reactions indicate that some immunoglobulin determinants have been conserved over a broad phylogenetic range of vertebrate classes; most notably J_H and V_Ha-related markers are shared between forms as diverse as sharks and mammals.

INTRODUCTION

Although the immunoglobulin family is one of the most thoroughly studied groups of proteins to date, little detailed molecular information on antibody structure and antibody genes exists for species more primitive than mammals. Consequently, the precise mechanisms of the evolution of immunoglobulin variable and constant regions within the vertebrates remain unclear. To redress this problem we have undertaken a study of the immunoglobulins from sharks. Sharks were chosen because elasmobranchs represent a relatively primitive stage of animal development which nevertheless have been shown (Marchalonis and Edelman, 1965; Clem et al, 1967; Clem and Small, 1967; Suran et al, 1967; Frommel et al, 1971) to possess immunoglobulins which are clearly related to the well characterized immunoglobulin of man and mouse. To date the immunoglobulins from a diverse but small number of species such as the smooth dogfish, horned, lemon, nurse and leopard sharks have been studied. Like mammalian immunoglobulin the basic shark immunoglobulin monomer consists of two heavy and two light chains covalently linked together by disulfide bonds. Two forms exist, a 7S monomer and an 18S pentamer, but immunochemical and physicochemical similarities indicate that they are of the same immunoglobulin class. Based on physicochemical parameters such as heavy chain mass,

0165-2427/86/$03.50 © 1986 Elsevier Science Publishers B.V.

carbohydrate content and amino acid composition, shark immunoglobulin most clearly resembles mammalian IgM.

Our approach has been two-fold. Firstly, we have characterized the immunoglobulins from three species of the same elasmobranch family, the carcharhine sharks. Our studies indicate that very little diversification of immunoglobulin structure has occurred during carcharhine evolution. Secondly, we were interested in whether and to what extent immunoglobulin determinants, in particular heavy chain variable region determinants, are conserved in chordate evolution. Using serological probes against shark immunoglobulins and defined V_H framework regions we show that some determinants are conserved on immunoglobulins from species as phylogenetically diverse and broadly separated as lampreys and humans.

MATERIALS AND METHODS

Sandbar sharks and tiger sharks were taken by us off the coast of South Carolina and exsanguinated by severing the caudal vessels. One large male galapagos shark was caught off the coast of the Ascension Island.

The intact immunoglobulin forms and the individual heavy and light chains were purified as described by Rosenshein and Marchalonis (1985). Enzyme-linked immunosorbent assays (ELISA) were performed in polystyrene microtitre plates as described (Rosenshein and Marchalonis, 1985). Immuno-blot transfer analyses were performed using the Bio-Rad (Bio-Rad Laboratories, Richmond, CA) Trans-Blot apparatus as described (Rosenshein et al, 1985). Sequence analyses were performed on a Beckman 890C automatic protein sequencer as described (Rosenshein and Marchalonis, 1985).

RESULTS AND DISCUSSION

The Immunoglobulins of Carcharhine Sharks are Highly Conserved

The immunoglobulins from three species of carcharhine sharks, the tiger (*Galeocerdo cuvieri*) the sandbar (*Carcharhinus plumbeus*) and the galapagos shark (*Carcharhinus galapagensis*), were purified by a series of salt precipitations followed by gel filtration. Like all immunoglobulins, these shark forms are composed of equi-molar amounts of heavy and light chains (Rosenshein, 1985) (1 monomer = 2 heavy + 2 light). These were individually purified using gel filtration in 6 M guanidinium hydrochloride. For all three species two forms of immunoglobulins were found, a 7S low molecular weight form and an 18S high molecular weight form (Rosenshein, 1985).

These two forms are very similar to each other (see below) and appear to belong to the same immunoglobulin class. By several criteria the immunoglobulins of carcharhine sharks most closely resemble mammalian IgM. Thus, the shark immunoglobulins form pentamers, the molecular weight of the heavy chains is 70,000 and the total carbohydrate content of the heavy chain is 10-15%.

We have extensively characterized both the intact forms and the isolated heavy and light chains of these carcharhine immunoglobulins. In sharp contrast to mammalian immunoglobulins, a prominent feature of the shark immunoglobulins is their marked lack of structural diversity. This observation applies not only to comparisons of the 7S and 18S forms from the same species, but also equally as well to all the immunoglobulin forms from the three shark species studied here. The molecular weights, (as estimated by gel filtration in 6M guanidinium hydrochloride) of the heavy and light chains were identical, being 70,000 and 22,500 respectively (Rosenshein, 1985). The carbohydrate composition of the heavy chains was overall quite similar. Total carbohydrate contents ranged from 9.5% to 18% (compared to 13.6% and 3.2% for human mu and gamma chains respectively), glucosamine was the predominant monosaccharide and the mannose/galactose ratio was very nearly one in all cases (Rosenshein, 1985). Comparisons of the heavy chains by statistical analyses (Marchalonis and Weltman, 1971) of their amino acid contents reveals a very small degree of compositional variability; these polypeptides have virtually the same amino acid compositions (Rosenshein, 1985). Separate analyses of the light chains yields the same conclusion. Two other important points are also evident from amino acid composition analyses. Although clearly different types of molecules, the heavy and light chains are related to each other and also to heavy and light chains of higher vertebrate immunoglobulins (Rosenshein, 1985).

TABLE 1

Percentage cross-reactivity[1] of carcharhine immunoglobulin polypeptide chains with rabbit antisera to galapagos shark heavy and light chains.

		heavy chain[2]	light chain[3]
C. galapagensis	18S IgM	95	91
C. galapagensis	7S IgM	100	100
C. plumbeus	18S IgM	78	100
C. plumbeus	7S IgM	87	88
G. cuvieri	18S IgM	42	84
G. cuvieri	7S IgM	56	84
D. centroura	18S IgM	16	N.D.[4]

[1]Percentage binding = $\frac{\Sigma\text{O.D. of R}\alpha\text{ shark IgM vs test antigen} - \Sigma\text{O.D. of NRS vs test antigen}}{\Sigma\text{O.D. of R}\alpha\text{ shark IgM vs shark IgM} - \Sigma\text{O.D. of NRS vs shark IgM}}$.

[2]Percentage reactivity of isolated heavy chains with rabbit antisera to 7S heavy chain of the galapagos shark.

[3]Percentage reactivity of isolated shark light chains with rabbit antisera to 7S light chain of the galapagos shark.

[4]N.D., not determined.

The results outlined above characterize the carcharhine immunoglobulins in general physicochemical terms. We have also used two methods which provide a much more sensitive indication of protein heterogeneity. Table 1 shows the results of immuno-

TABLE 2

Summary of V_H(FRI) sequence comparisons and serological cross reactions of various vertebrate immunoglobulins.

Species	1	2	3	4	5	6	7	8	9	10	11	12	13	14	15	16	17	18	19	20	Reactivity with rabbit[1] antisera to C. galapagensis 7S IgM	Reactivity with rabbit[1] antisera to V_Ha allotypes
C. galapagensis	E	V	V	L	T	E	I	Q	A	E	Y	G	K	P	G	V	S	L	K	L	+	+
	E											G			G	V	I	L	V			
G. cuvieri	S	V	V	L	T	Q	P	V	A	E	T	V	V	P	V	G	L	V	I		+	+
	E										T											
C. plumbeus	D	V	V	L	T	Q	P	E	A	E	N	G	R	P	V	()	L	K	L		+	+
H. francisci[2]	D	V	V	L	T	Q	P	E	A	E	T	G	K	P	G	G	S	L	R	L	ND	ND
G. cirratum[2]	E	V	T	L	T	Z	P	Z	A	Z	D	S	Z	P	G	G	A	L	T	L	ND	ND
		V																				
T. semifasciata[2]	E	I	V	L	T	E	P	E	A	E											ND	ND
	D																					
D. centroura	E	V	V	L	T	Q	P	A													+	+
Toad[2]	D	V	Q	L	D	Q	S	E	P	V	P	S	K	P	G	Z	S	H	K	G	+	+
										G												
Turkey[2]	A	V	Q	L	D	Q	S	G	G	A	V	Q	G	P	G	V	Q	L	R	L	+	+
MOPC 104E[2]	E	V	Q	L	Q	Q	S	G	P	E	L	V	K	P	G	A	S	V	K	M	+	+
Hu V_H III[2]	E	V	Q	L	L	E	S	G	G	G	L	V	Q	P	G	G	S	L	R	L	+	+
Rabbit V_Ha3	E	-	S	L	E	E	S	G	G	D	L	V	K	P	G	A	S	L	T	L	+	+
Trout IgM									ND												+	+
Lamprey Ig									ND												+	ND

1 Determined by reactivity in ELISA and by immuno-blot transfer analyses.
2 Sequence data from Kabat et al.
ND Not known.
() Indicates a residue with marked heterogeneity.
\- Indicates deletion used to maximize homology.

chemical analyses by ELISA of the heavy and light chains using rabbit antisera raised against the isolated heavy and light chains of the 7S galapagos shark Ig. The results are expressed as the percentage of the reactivity obtained against the homologous antigen. It can be seen that the anti-light chain sera reacts equally as well with the different light chain types as it does with the galapagos light chain, indicating that the light chains are antigenically closely related. The same results were obtained with the heavy chains except that somewhat reduced activity was seen against those from the tiger shark. This is consistent with immune diffusion analyses (Rosenshein, 1985) where reactions of complete identity occur between sandbar and galapagos immunoglobulins but there is slight spurring of the tiger shark precipitin lines. Considering that the tiger shark species occurs in the fossil record some 30 million years before the appearance of the closely related sandbar and galapagos species, it is a little surprising that only relatively small antigenic differences are found. Direct assessment of heterogeneity is obtained by sequence comparisons. We have sequenced the first framework of the heavy and light chains using pooled preparations and the results are presented in Table 2. It attests to the limited diversity present in the different immunoglobulin forms that in most instances only a single predominant residue was obtained for each position. Only the 7S heavy chain sequences are shown but the 18S sequences are very similar (Rosenshein, 1985). A very high degree of sequence homology is apparent when comparing these sequences. A similar degree of homology is also observed with comparisons of light chain first framework sequences (Rosenshein, 1985).

Considering all the physicochemical and immunochemical results just outlined, it is apparent that there is very little to discriminate between carcharhine immunoglobulins. During the evolution of these primitive vertebrates, the immunoglobulins have remained a highly conserved family of proteins. This might also reflect that only a limited gene repertoire is expressed within the carcharhine sharks, a suggestion supported by iso-electric focusing experiments in which sandbar, tiger and galapagos shark light chain preparations gave virtually identical spectrotype patterns (Rosenshein, 1985).

We also have some evidence that not only carcharhine shark immunoglobulins but immunoglobulin from elasmobranchs in general show a high degree of evolutionary conservatism. In Table 1 it can be seen that the anti-heavy chain sera reacted appreciably with immunoglobulin from stingray, an elasmobranch distantly related to carcharhine sharks. In Table 2 a high degree of sequence homology is noted for heavy chains from a variety of elasmobranch species, including the stingray. And in Southern Blot analyses of tiger shark DNA using a variable region gene probe from a very ancient elasmobranch species, the horned shark, extensive cross hybridization was obtained (Rosenshein et al, 1985).

<u>Some immunoglobulin determinants, particulary V_H determinants, have been highly conserved during evolution.</u>

To assess the degree of conservation of immunoglobulin determinants we have used two approaches. Firstly we have performed amino acid sequence comparisons. This is perhaps the most direct and unequivocal means of determining protein relatedness. Shown in Table 2 are heavy chain framework one sequences for a representative sample of "primitive" and "advanced" vertebrates. A very high degree of sequence homology is evident. There is virtually no position in which significant homology is not found and for positions 2,4,14 and 15 the homology is nearly absolute.

Our second approach has been to screen immunoglobulins for reactivity with a number of serological probes. Reactivity was assessed using ELISA and immuno-blot transfer techniques. The first type of reagent we used was rabbit antisera to carcharhine shark immunoglobulin. Since shark immunoglobulins are a relatively undiversified group of molecules, we reasoned that this might be a good general reagent for detecting conserved immunoglobulin determinants. Table 2 summarizes our results and shows that this indeed proved to be the case. Definite reactions were observed with immunoglobulins from very "primitive" species such as stingray and lamprey as well as with immunoglobulins from higher vertebrates such as toad, turkey, trout and even human and mouse (Rosenshein, et al, 1985). These results show that some immunoglobulin determinants have been conserved on immunoglobulin molecules during the evolution of the vertebrates.

TABLE 3

Survey by ELISA of cross-reactions detected by rabbit antisera to a synthetic J_H peptide[1].

	Anti-J_{Hsyn}	Anti-HA_p[2]
MOPC 104E	2.0	0.2
McE	0.69	0.06
C.galapagensis 7S IgM	1.3	0.18

[1] Data given are the absorbancy values after 30 min at a 1/50 dilution.
[2] Synthetic peptide derived from influenza hemagglutinin protein sequence.

In order to more precisely identify these conserved determinants we have also used serological probes of defined specificity. These were directed against defined immunoglobulin framework regions and were rabbit anti-rabbit V_Ha allotype sera and rabbit anti-J_H sera. Rabbit V_Ha allotypes are conformational determinants which are determined by particular clustered residues in the first and third frameworks of the heavy chains (Mage et al, 1984). The anti-J_H sera were raised against a 16 mer synthetic peptide comprising the five C-terminal residues of the D region and the entire J_H1 sequence of the mouse myeloma proteins MOPC-104E or TEPC-15. The reactivity of the anti-allotype sera are summarized in Table 2. Positive reactivity using anti-allotype sera was obtained with immunoglobulins from the carcharhine sharks, stingray, toad, turkey, trout, mouse and humans (Rosenshein and Marchalonis, 1985). In rabbits the V_Ha allotypes are heavy chain markers. This is also the case for the shark immunoglobulins since the antisera reacted with isolated heavy chains but not light chains (Rosenshein and Marchalonis, 1985). The activity of the anti-J_H sera is summarized in Table 3. Shown as a negative control is the activity of antisera raised against a synthetic influenza hemagglutinin peptide. The anti-J_H sera reacts strongly with MOPC-104E as expected since this immunoglobulin contains the prototypic sequence. But also the antisera reacts very well with shark IgM. Indeed, this reactivity is higher than with a human myeloma protein expressing J_H2 sequence (McE). Thus it is clear that the V_H determinants as defined by these antisera show broad phylogenetic conservation.

It is generally believed that immunoglobulins of all species arose by duplication of a common precursor ancestral gene leading to heavy and light chains. Our observations concerning the phylogenetic conservation of immunoglobulin determinants support this concept. When considering immunoglobulin evolution it needs to be considered that variable and constant regions have evolved separately. Thus, in certain "primitive" species such as sharks there appears to have been very little diversity generated in immunoglobulin structure during evolution. This may indicate that constant region mediated effector functions are limited in sharks or, more probably, that shark IgM molecules are similar to mammalian IgM and possess multiple effector functions (eg. complement fixation, opsonisation, neutralization, etc.). But in response to a need for more effector functions and/or specialization of effector functions, the immunoglobulin constant regions of higher vertebrates have evolved into a highly diverse group as reflected, for instance, in a larger number of immunoglobulin classes and subclasses. Although one constant region determinant has been reported to show phylogenetic conservation (Parsons and Herzenberg, 1981) and it seems probable that our anti-shark reagent also sees some conserved constant region determinants, in general antibodies against constant region markers do not show a broad range of cross species reactivity. In contrast we, and others (Eshhar et al, 1983), have shown that immunoglobulin variable framework region structures show remarkable evolutionary conservation. The primary function of antibodies is to bind antigen. The binding site is formed by the variable regions and the precise protein conformation required for activity is set by the framework segments (Ohno et al, 1984). It appears that the same structural-functional constraints apply to the binding regions of immunoglobulins from all vertebrate classes and this has resulted in the phylogenetic conservation of certain critical variable region structures.

ACKNOWLEDGEMENTS

This work was supported in part by NSF grant number DCB-8419880 and NIH grant number GM 30672.

REFERENCES

Clem, L.W. and Small, P.A. 1967. Phylogeny of immunoglobulin structure and function. I. Immunoglobulins of the lemon shark. J. Exp. Med. 125: 893-920.

Clem, L.W., DeBoutaud, F. and Sigel, M.M. 1967. Phylogeny of immunoglobulin structure and function. II. Immunoglobulins of the nurse shark. J. Immunol. 99: 1226-1235

Eshhar, Z., Gigi, O. and Ben-Neriah, Y. 1983. Monoclonal anti-V_H antibodies recognize a common V_H determinant expressed on immunoglobulin heavy chains from various species. Eur. J. Immunol. 13: 533-540.

Frommel, D., Litman, G.W., Finstad, J. and Good, R.A. 1971. The evolution of the immune response. XI. The immunoglobulins of the horned shark, Heterodontus francisci, purification, characterization and structural requirement for antibody activity. J. Immunol. 106: 1234-1243.

Kabat, E.A., Wu, T.T., Bilofsky, H., Reid-Miller, M. and Perry, H. 1983. Sequence of proteins of immunological interest. U.S. Dept. of Health and Human Services, Public Health Service, National Institutes of Health, Bethesda.

Marchalonis, J.J. and Edelman, G.M. 1965. Phylogenic origins of antibody structure. I. Multichain structure of immunoglobulins in the smooth dogfish (Mustelus canis). J. Exp. Med. 122: 601-617.

Marchalonis, J.J. and Weltman, J.K. 1971. Relatedness among proteins: A new method of estimation and its application to immunoglobulins. Comp. Biochem. Physiol. 36B: 609-625.

Ohno, S., Matsunaga, and Lee, A.D. 1984. The invariably present tryptophan loop as the core of all divergent antigen-binding pockets. Scand. J. Immunol. 20: 377-388.

Parsons, M. and Herzenberg, 1981. A monoclonal mouse antiallotype antibody reacts with certain human and other vertebrate immunoglobulins: genetic and phylogenetic findings. Immunogenet. 12: 207-219.

Rosenshein, I.L. 1985. Doctoral Dissertation. Medical University of South Carolina, Charleston.

Rosenshein, I.L. and Marchalonis, J.J. 1985. Broad phylogenetic expression of heavy chain determinants detected by rabbit antisera to V_Ha allotypes. Mol. Immunol. 22: 1177-1183.

Rosenshein, I.L., Schluter, S.F., Vasta, G.R. and Marchalonis, J.J. 1985. Phylogenetic conservation of heavy chain determinants of vertebrates and protochordates. Dev. Comp. Immunol., 9: 783-795.

Suran, A.A., Tarail, M.H. and Papermaster, B.W. 1967. Immunoglobulins of the leopard shark. I. Isolation and characterization of 17S and 7S immunoglobulins with precipitating activity. J. Immunol. 99: 679-686.

Veterinary Immunology and Immunopathology, 12 (1986) 21–28
Elsevier Science Publishers B.V., Amsterdam — Printed in The Netherlands

PUTATIVE IMMUNOGLOBULIN V_H GENES OF THE GOLDFISH, CARASSIUS AURATUS, DETECTED BY HETEROLOGOUS CROSS-HYBRIDIZATION WITH A MURINE V_H PROBE

MELANIE R. WILSON,[1] DARLENE MIDDLETON,[1] CHARLENE ALFORD,[1] J.T. SULLIVAN,[2] G.W. LITMAN,[3] and G.W. WARR[1,4]

[1]Department of Biochemistry, Medical University of South Carolina, 171 Ashley Avenue, Charleston, SC 29425, USA
[2]Department of Biology, Lamar University, Beaumont, Texas, USA
[3]Showa University Research Institute, St. Petersburg, Florida, USA
[4]To whom reprint requests should be addressed

ABSTRACT

Wilson, M.R., Middleton, D., Alford, C., Sullivan, J.T., Litman, G.W. and Warr, G.W., 1986. Putative immunoglobulin V_H genes of the goldfish, Carassius auratus, detected by heterologous cross-hybridization with a murine V_H probe. Vet. Immunol. Immunopathol., 12: 21-28.

By using a defined cDNA probe for the V_H region of a murine phosphocholine-binding myeloma protein (S107) we have defined a family of distinct cross-hybridizing DNA sequences in genomic DNA of the goldfish. The estimated number of the goldfish putative V_H family detectable by the S107 probe is about 36. By using two putative goldfish V_H probes to analyze, by hybridization, the relationships among seven of the goldfish genomic clones, we have determined that the putative goldfish V_H genes recognized by the S107 probe comprise at least several distinct families that are not closely related.

INTRODUCTION

Nothing is known of the primary structure of the immunoglobulins of the advanced bony fish, nor of the structure, organization and expression of the genes encoding the constituent polypeptide chains of these immunoglobulins.

This paper reports the initial stages of a study to obtain such information for the heavy chain immunoglobulin genes of the goldfish, Carassius auratus, using the approach of heterologous DNA-DNA cross hybridization which has been successfully used in studies of horned shark immunoglobulin genes, (Litman et al., 1985a)

METHODS

DNA Library construction

Goldfish genomic DNA was isolated by the method of Blin and Stafford (1976) as described by Litman et al. (1982). Partial Sau 3A digests of predominant average size of 20 kb were ligated into the Bam H1 site of EMBL-4 λ phage and packaged. (Frischauf et al., 1983) Random screening of phage for inserts, and growth on the selective Escherichia coli strain

*This work was supported by grant PCM 8408484 from the National Science Foundation.

0165-2427/86/$03.50 © 1986 Elsevier Science Publishers B.V.

NM539, indicated that the library comprised approximately $2.5X10^5$ recombinant phage containing the equivalent of 3 haploid genomes; this estimate is based on the figure of $1.4X10^9$ bp/haploid genome for the carp (Cyprinus carpio, Sober, 1968).

Library screening and phage purification

The recombinant phage library was plated on E.coli K802, $hsdR^+$, $hsdM^+$, gal^-, met^-, supE (Wood, 1966), and duplicate plaque lifts on nitrocellulose filter discs were taken and processed for hybridization under reduced stringency conditions as described by Litman et al., (1983). The purified murine S107 V probe (Early et al., 1980) was nick-translated to approximately $1\text{-}2X10^8$ c.p.m./µg. The hybridizing solution included pBR322 at 1µg/mL, polynucleotides (8µg/mL of poly A and poly C), tRNA (0.2 mg/mL), probe (20 ng/mL), and E.coli DNA (10µg/mL); salmon sperm DNA was omitted (Litman et al., 1982). Hybridization was at 65° for 16 hours, and washing was at 52° in 1XSSC (0.15M NaCl, 0.015M Na citrate), 0.1% SDS. Filters were exposed to XAR-5 film for 48 hours at -70° using an intensifying screen.

Plaques yielding positive responses on duplicate filters were cored and purified by successive replatings and screenings. Purified phage suspensions were prepared from 1-6 liter lysates by polyethylene glycol precipitation (Yamamoto et al., 1970) and sedimentation (30 min. at 25000 rpm in a Beckman SW45 rotor) through a two-step glycerol gradient (5% and 40%).

Restriction fragment analysis

DNA from the purified recombinant λ phage was digested with restriction enzymes (Bethesda Research Laboratories, Gaithersburg, MD) in accordance with manufacturers instructions and 1-2 µg were electrophoresed on gels of 1% agarose concentration in 40mM tris-acetate, 20mM sodium acetate, 1mM ethylene diamine tetraacetic acid, pH 8.0. Hind III digests of λ DNA were co-electrophoresed as standards. The gels were stained with ethidium bromide, photographed under UV illumination, depurinated (2 X 15 min washes in 0.25 M HCl) denatured (1 X 30 min wash in 0.6 M NaCl, 0.2 M NaOH) and neutralized (1.5 M NaCl, 1.0 M Tris-HCl, pH 7.5, 1 X 30 min wash) after which the gel was Southern blotted (Southern, 1975) onto nitrocellulose paper, using 10 X SSC, for 16 hours. After drying in a vacuum oven (80°, 2 hours) the nitrocellulose paper was hybridized with the S107 probe and washed as described above. Exposure to XAR-5 film at -70° was for 4-24 hours, using an intensifying screen.

In some experiments the digested, electrophoresed and blotted phage DNA was hybridized with the Pst 1 derived fragments from clones 3 and 5. These fragments, which cross-hybridized with S107 (Fig. 2) and were about 850 and 550 bp in length, respectively, were cloned in pUC 18 and

M13mp18. The isolated purified inserts were nick-translated to specific activities of 1-5 X 10^8 cpm/µg, and hybridized, as described above, to the phage blots. Washing of blots was done either at low stringency (1XSSC at 52° as described above) or at high stringency (65°, 0.1XSSC, 4 washes of 30 minutes to 1 hour each).

RESULTS

Screening of the original, unamplified library yielded 42 recombinant phage that hybridized with the S107 probe. Seven recombinants representing various strengths of hybridization with the S107 probe were studied further. Fig. 1 illustrates the two extremes of intensity of plaque-lift hybridization seen with S107 and two plaque purified clones. The differences in intensity of hybridization between recombinant phages was reproducible in replating of plaques and did not depend upon the size of the phage plaques (which was quite uniform).

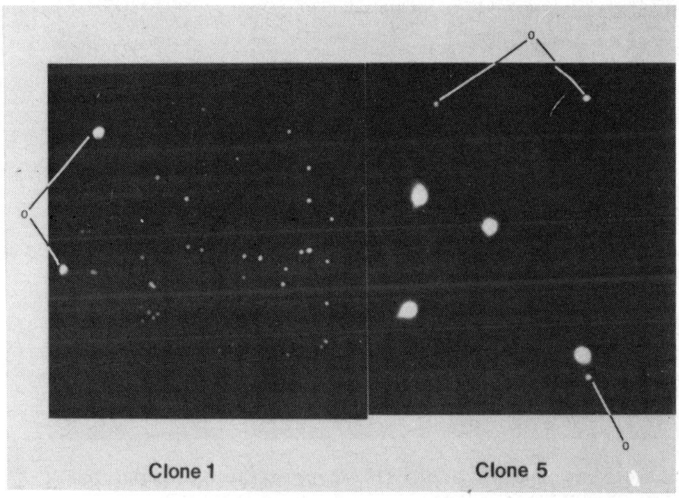

FIGURE 1. Autoradiographs of nitrocellulose filter lifts of plaques produced by lambda clones 1 and 5 hybridized with ^{32}P-labelled S107 DNA. These lifts were taken during plaque purification of the phages, were made at the same time, processed and dried together, hybridized and washed together, and exposed on the same sheet of X-ray film overnight. The S107 probe was labelled to a specific activity of approximately 2 X 10^8 cpm/µg, and the washing conditions were those described for low-stringency conditions by Litman et. al. (1982). The symbol 0 indicates the ink/radioactive orientation marks placed on the filters.

Figure 2 shows the results of the analysis of restriction fragments among cloned DNAs, and their hybridization to the S107 probe. The results of this analysis (Fig. 2) clearly demonstrate that 6 of the recombinant phage studied exhibit unique patterns of restriction fragments under all the restriction digestion conditions utilized. Two clones (6 and 4) appeared to be identical.

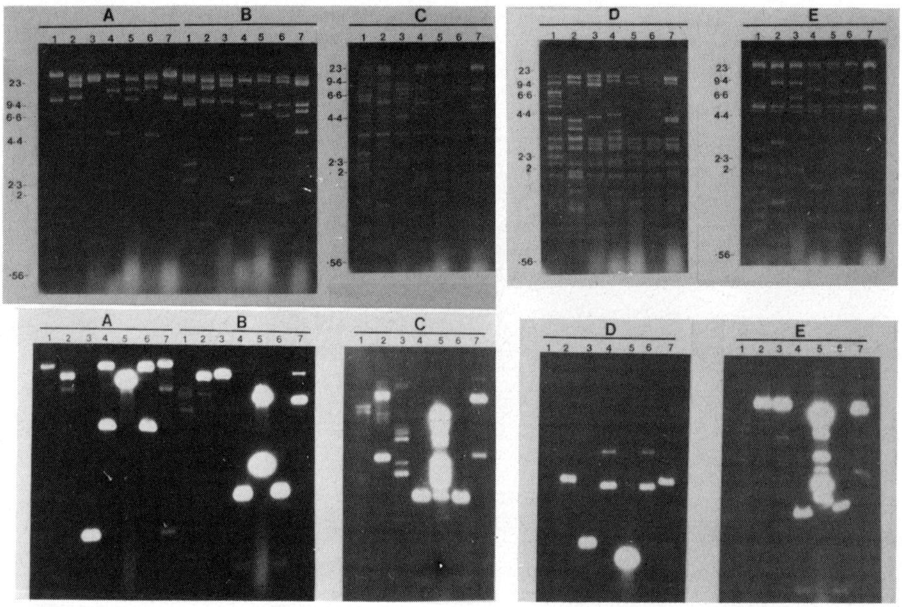

FIGURE 2. Restriction fragment analysis of S107-hybridization using DNA from seven plaque purified recombinant phage.

Upper panels: DNA (∿1μg per lane) from each of seven plaque purified phages (1-7) was digested with a) Bam H1, b) Eco R1 c) Eco R1 plus Sma 1, d) Bam H1 plus Pst 1, and e) Eco R1 plus Hind III. Restriction fragments were electrophoresed on 1% agarose gels and visualized by ethidium bromide staining under UV light. The markers give apparent size in base pairs ($X10^{-3}$)

Lower panels: Hybridization with ^{32}P-labelled S107 of the DNA transferred, from the gels shown in the upper panel, to nitrocellulose sheets. The numbering and lettering of the upper and lower panels correspond exactly.

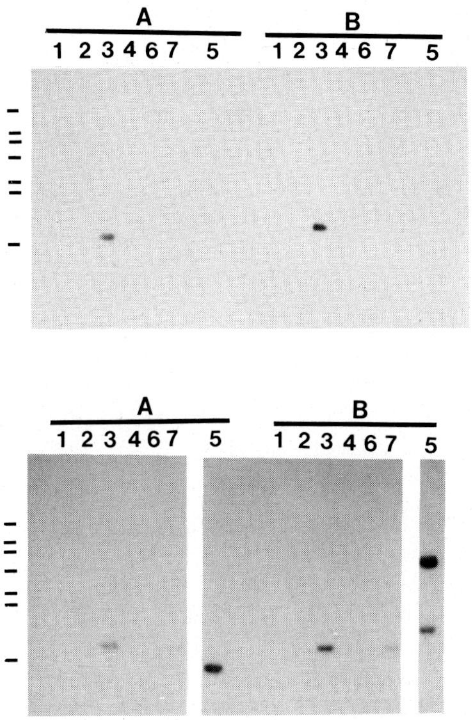

FIGURE 3. Southern blot analysis of DNA from lambda clones 1-7, digested with Bam H1 plus Pst 1 (A) or Bam H1 plus Sst 1 (B) and hybridized with the nick-translated Pst 1 fragment of clone 3. Washing was under high (upper panel) or low (lower panel) stringency conditions. The markers (horizontal lines to the left) are for Kbp values of (from top to bottom) 23,9.4,6.6,4.4,2.3,2 and 0.56.

When the hybridization of the S107 hybridizing Pst 1 fragments of clones 3 and 5 (Fig. 2) with the restriction-digested DNA of the 7 purified clones was examined (Figs. 3, 4) it was observed that under high stringency conditions these probes recognized only the DNA of the clone from which they were derived, thus suggesting that clones 3 and 5 are not closely related in DNA sequence (> 80% identity) either to each other or to the other clones examined. Under low stringency conditions, clone 5 again recognized only its own DNA, whereas clone 3 recognized the DNA of clones 5 and 7 (weakly) in addition to that of clone 3.

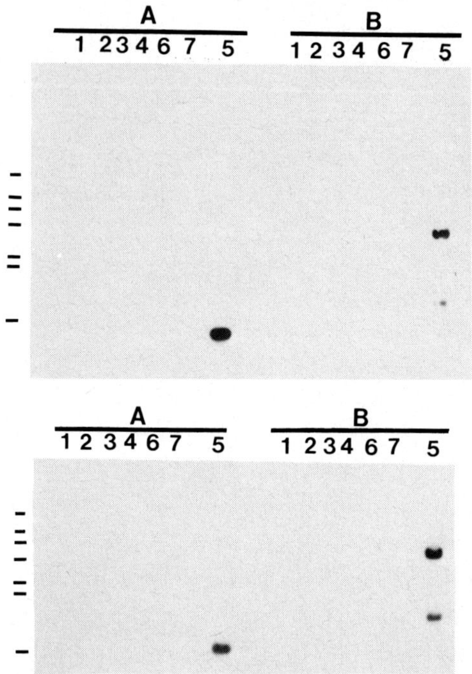

FIGURE 4. Southern blot analysis of DNA from lambda clones 1-7, digested with Bam H1 plus Pst 1 (A) or Bam H1 plus Sst 1 (B) and hybridized with the nick-translated Pst 1 fragment of clone 5. Washing was under high (upper panel) or low (lower panel) stringency conditions. Markers as described in the legend to Fig. 3.

DISCUSSION

The interpretation of the data presented in this report depends upon the validity of using heterologous cross-hybridization of murine S107 cDNA as a means to identify goldfish genomic V_H sequences. Although the S107 probe has been successfully used for such a purpose in the Caiman (Litman et al., 1983, 1985,b) and the horned shark (Litman et al., 1985a), proof of its valid use in the case of the goldfish must await definitive primary structural analysis of the hybridizing sequences. Nevertheless, preliminary partial sequence studies (Warr and Wilson, unpublished) suggest that in two of the phage clones mentioned here, there is sufficient sequence and organizational similarity to S107 DNA to support a conclusion that germline V_H genes (or pseudo-genes) are indeed being detected in this system.

Assuming that the 7 of 42 goldfish S107-hybridizing phage clones chosen by us for more detailed study are representative, a simple calculation suggests that there are in the region of 36 members of the putative goldfish V_H gene family recognized by S107.

Two questions arise: 1) Does the set of genes recognized by S107 represent the total germline putative V_H pool of the goldfish? and 2) Does the cross-hybridization of S107 with goldfish V_H genes have any functional significance relative to our analysis of the immune system of this fish? In considering the first question, we can note that S107 is a member of one of the 7 distinct families of murine V_H genes recognizable by distinct non-overlapping patterns of restriction fragment analysis and hybridization (Brodeur and Riblet, 1984). While it is not possible, at present, to estimate the total size of the putative goldfish germline V_H gene pool, we can conclude that the sequences recognized by S107 do not form a single, closely-related family as defined in the mouse V_H system by Brodeur and Riblet (1984). These authors (Brodeur and Riblet 1984) concluded that under high-stringency conditions sequence identity of > 80% was needed to detect hybridization. Using these criteria, we can tentatively conclude from the data shown in Fig. 3 and 4 that our putative goldfish V_H genes can be considered to represent several families, there being at least three such in the seven clones examined in detail.

The second question, concerning the possible functional significance of S107 hybridization with goldfish genomic sequences arises because S107 is part of the T15 family (Crews et al., 1981) whose encoded proteins express not only common idiotypes (Claflin et al., 1985) but also show binding specificity for the phosphocholine group (Crews et al., 1981). Phosphocholine is an interesting antigen in that it is an expressed and recognized determinant on a wide variety of pathogens and parasites (see, e.g. Pery et al., 1974).

Thus, it would not be surprising if genes related to the T15 family were to be found with a germ-line representation in many vertebrates, since we can assume that selective pressure exerted by the invasion of pathogens and parasites (many of which would be expected to express the phosphocholine determinant) has been quite constant during the evolution of the vertebrates. Although this is an intriguing speculation, it will probably only be possible to provide answers to this question when we can correlate the expression of some of the goldfish V_H genes with functional antibody molecules of known specificity.

Acknowledgements We thank Dr. J.D. Karam for advice, assistance and comments on the manuscript. MRW is in receipt of a studentship from the College of Graduate Studies, Medical University of South Carolina.

REFERENCES

Blin, N. and Stafford, D.W. 1976. A general method for isolation of high molecular weight DNA from eukaryotes. **Nucleic Acids Res. 3, 2303-2308**

Brodeur, P.H. and Riblet, R. 1984. The immunoglobulin heavy chain variable region (Igh-V) locus in the mouse. I. One hundred Igh-V genes comprise seven families of homologous genes. **Eur. J. Immunol. 14,** 922-930

Claflin, J.L., Hudak, S., Maddalena, A. and Bender, T. 1985. Antigen-specific anti-phosphocholine antibodies: binding site studies. **J. Immunol. 134**, 2536-2543

Crews, S., Griffin, J., Huang, H., Calame, K. and Hood, L. 1981. A single V_H gene segment encodes the immune response to phosphorylcholine: somatic mutation is correlated with the class of the antibody. **Cell 25,** 59-66

Early, P., Huang, H., Davis, M., Calame, K. and Hood, L. 1980. An immunoglobulin heavy chain variable region gene is generated from three segments of DNA: V_H, D and J_H. **Cell 19**, 981-992

Frischauf, A.-M., Lehrach, H., Poustka, A. and Murray, N. 1983. Lambda replacement vectors carrying polylinker sequences. **J. Mol. Biol. 170**, 827-842

Litman, G.W., Berger, L. and Jahn, C.L. 1982. Multiple components in restriction enzyme digests of mammalian (insectivore), avian and reptilian genomic DNA hybridize with murine immunoglobulin V_H probes. **Nucleic Acids Res. 10**, 3371-3380

Litman, G.W., Berger, L., Murphy, K., Litman, R., Hinds, K., Jahn, L.L. and Erickson, B.W. 1983. Complete nucleotide sequence of an immunoglobulin V_H gene homologue from Caiman, a phylogenetically ancient reptile. **Nature 303**, 349-352

Litman, G.W., Berger, L., Murphy, K., Litman, R., Hinds, K. and Erickson, B.W. 1985a. Immunoglobulin V_H gene structure and diversity in Heterodontus a phylogenetically primitive shark. **Proc. Natl. Acad. Sci. (USA) 82**, 2082-2086.

Litman, G.W., Murphy, K., Berger, L., Hinds, K. and Erickson, B. 1985b. Complete nucleotide sequence of three V_H genes in Caiman, a phylogenetically ancient reptile: evolutionary diversification in coding segments and variation in the structure and organization of recombination elements. **Proc. Natl. Acad. Sci. (USA) 82**, 844-848

Pery, P., Petit, J., Poulain, J. and Luffan, G. 1974. Phosphorylcholine-bearing components in homogenates of nematodes. **Eur. J. Immunol. 4**, 637-639

Sober, H.A., 1968. (Ed) Handbook of Biochemistry: selected data for molecular biology. Chemical Rubber Company, Cleveland.

Southern, E.M. 1975. Detection of specific sequences among DNA fragments separated by gel electrophoresis. **J. Mol. Biol. 98**, 503-517.

Wood, W.B. 1966. Host specificity of DNA produced by Escherichia coli: Bacterial mutations affecting the restriction and modification of DNA. **J. Mol. Biol. 16,** 118-133

Yamamoto, K.R., Alberts, B.M., Benzinger, R., Lawhorne, L., and Treiber, G. 1970. Rapid bacteriophage sedimentation in the presence of polyethylene glycol and its application to large-scale virus purification. **Virology 40,** 734-744.

Veterinary Immunology and Immunopathology, 12 (1986) 29—38
Elsevier Science Publishers B.V., Amsterdam — Printed in The Netherlands

PRIMARY IN VITRO STIMULATION OF ANTIBODY PRODUCTION BY RAINBOW TROUT LYMPHOCYTES

S. L. KAATTARI, M. J. IRWIN, M. A. YUI, R. A. TRIPP, AND J. S. PARKINS
Microbiology Dept., Oregon State University, Corvallis, OR 97331-3804, USA

ABSTRACT

Kaattari[1], S. L., Irwin, M. J., Yui, M. A., Tripp, R. A., and Parkins, J. S., 1986. Primary *in vitro* stimulation of antibody production by rainbow trout lymphocytes. Vet. Immunol. Immunopathol., 12: 29-38.

Trinitrophenylated (TNP) forms of *E. coli* lipopolysaccharide (LPS) and keyhole limpet hemocyanin (KLH) were used to produce antigen specific plaque-forming cell (PFC) responses with rainbow trout (*Salmo gairdneri*) splenocytes from unprimed fish *in vitro*. The culture system that was developed is described and characterized with respect to the kinetics and dose responses for both the haptenated and unhaptenated forms of the carriers. The induction of the PFC response to TNP-LPS was inhibited with TNP-lysine. Exposure to graded levels of gamma-radiation demonstrated a low dose augmentation of the PFC response with both antigens. Antigen addition experiments reveal that both antigens appear to stimulate the same population of antibody-producing B lymphocytes.

INTRODUCTION

One of the most important advances in the field of cellular immunology has been the development of *in vitro* culture systems that allow for the induction of specific antibody responses. Such a system was originally developed for murine lymphocytes by Mishell and Dutton (1967). Adaptations of this system have been developed most recently for use with the catfish, *Ictalurus punctatus* (Miller and Clem 1984).

In the development of a comparable culture system for salmonid lymphocytes, we chose to use trinitrophenylated (TNP) antigens. A major advantage to the use of such haptenated antigens is that they allow for the examination of the role of various carrier molecules in the production of antibody to a defined antigenic determinant. In the mouse, the use of such defined hapten-carrier conjugates has led to the division of B cells into at least two functionally distinct subpopulations (Lewis and Goodman, 1972; Jennings and Rittenberg, 1976). The use of such conjugates has also greatly aided in the development of our current models of B cell activation and differentiation (Möller, 1975; Coutinho and Möller, 1983).

---

[1]To whom correspondence should be addressed.

0165-2427/86/$03.50 © 1986 Elsevier Science Publishers B.V.

METHODS

Culture media

The tissue culture medium (TCM) consists of RPMI with L-glutamine and bicarbonate, 10% fetal calf serum (hybridoma screened), 100 μg/ml gentamicin, 50 μM 2-mercaptoethanol (MCB, Cincinnati, OH), and the nucleosides; adenosine, uracil, cytosine, and guanosine (10 μg/ml, Sigma, St. Louis, MO). A nutritional cocktail for culture supplementation was also prepared as previously described (Tittle and Rittenberg, 1978) and fed daily to the cultures as described below.

Antigens

A 20 mg/ml stock solution of lipopolysaccharide W (LPS-W) from *E. coli* 055:B5 (Difco, Detroit, MI) was prepared and trinitrophenylated (TNP-LPS) by the method of Jacobs and Morrison (1975) using picrylsulfonic acid (Sigma, St. Louis, MO). Keyhole limpet hemocyanin (generous gift from M. B. Rittenberg) was coupled to TNP by the method of Rittenberg and Amkraut (1966). Sheep red blood cells (SRBC) were trinitrophenylated by the method of Rittenberg and Pratt (1969).

Cell cultures

A single cell suspension was prepared from the spleen of each test animal and washed two times in holding medium (TCM with fetal calf serum and gentamicin only) by centrifugation at 500 x g for 10 minutes at 4°C. The final washed cell pellet was resuspended in the modified Mishell-Dutton tissue culture medium (TCM). Lymphocytes were enumerated by the use of a hemocytometer. Cell viability was determined by trypan blue staining. Triplicate cultures of 4 x 10^6 lymphocytes in 200 μl TCM were added to the wells of a 24-well, flat-bottomed, tissue culture plate (Corning, Corning, NY) containing antigen. The tissue culture plates were then incubated in plastic culture boxes (C.B.S. Scientific, Del Mar, CA) in an atmosphere of 10% CO_2 at 16°C. The cultures were maintained over a nine day period by adding approximately 50 μl of nutritional cocktail daily.

Plaque forming cell assay

Cells were harvested from individual wells and washed once as described above. Cell pellets were resuspended in 0.5 ml holding medium and the lymphocytes enumerated with a Coulter Counter. The Cunningham plaque forming cell assay (Cunningham and Szenberg, 1968) was performed using 100 μl of the lymphocyte suspension, 25 μl of a 10% suspension of SRBC or TNP-SRBC in modified barbital buffer (MBB), and 25 μl of steelhead trout (*Salmo gairdneri*) serum, diluted 1:8 in MBB, as described previously (Kaattari and Irwin, 1985). The Cunningham chambers were incubated for 1-3 h at 16°C. Plaques were enumerated under low power with the aid of a dissecting microscope.

Cell irradiations

Lymphocytes were suspended to 2 x 10^7 cells/ml in holding medium in 5 ml plastic tubes held on ice. The tubes were placed in the low flux region of a Cobalt 60 gamma irradiator at the OSU Radiation Center for the calculated amount of time for each dose. The cells were then rewashed, resuspended in TCM, counted, and plated as described.

RESULTS

In vitro antigen dose responses

Splenic lymphocytes were incubated with various doses of TNP-LPS or TNP-KLH and the number of anti-TNP plaque-forming cells per 10^6 lymphocytes as calculated at the end of a nine day culture period. TNP-LPS induced a response of approximately 800 PFC/10^6 lymphocytes at a peak final concentration of 0.4 μg/ml (Figure 1). TNP-KLH, which usually elicits a lower response than does TNP-LPS, exhibited a response of approximately 150 PFC/10^6 lymphocytes. The LPS carrier demonstrated virtually no stimulation at 0.4 μg/ml (the optimal concentration for the haptenated form of the carrier). However, at a 100-fold increase in LPS (40 μg/ml), the anti-TNP PFC response became significant. It is important to note that at this same concentration of TNP-LPS, the response is declining. In contrast, the free KLH carrier does not stimulate PFC production at any of the tested concentrations.

Hapten-specific inhibition of the PFC response

The plaque-forming response to either TNP-LPS or TNP-KLH can be specifically inhibited by the free hapten, TNP-lysine (Table 1). Comparable concentrations of unhaptenated lysine, and even 10-fold higher molar concentrations were unable to produce any inhibition of plaque formation. These data demonstrate that the antibodies produced by the PFC are specific for TNP. Also, in all assays, the response to unhaptenated sheep red blood cells (SRBC) were insignificant or not present, lending further support for the antigenic specificity of this *in vitro* response.

Hapten-specific inhibition of B cell induction

In an attempt to determine whether the induction of salmonid B cells by TNP-LPS is antigen specific, rather than being due to non-specific carrier

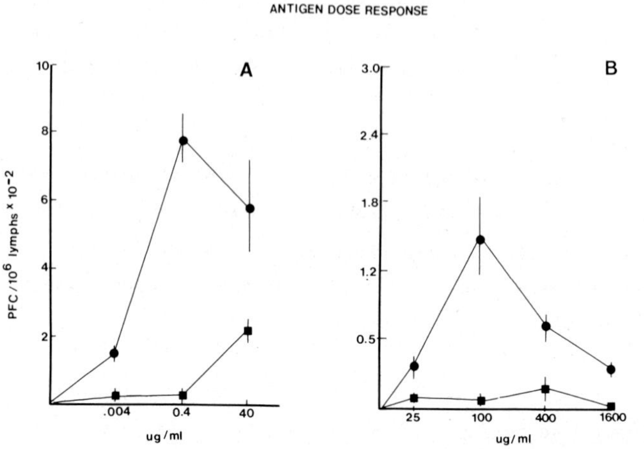

Fig. 1. The plaque forming cell response to TNP-LPS (A) and TNP-KLH (B) was measured on day 9 of culture. Plaque forming values represent the mean values of triplicate cultures. Error bars equal two standard errors about the mean. Responses to the haptenated (●) and unhaptenated (■) carrier are depicted.

stimulation (polyclonal activation), hapten specific inhibition was attempted at the initiation of culture. Concentrations of 40, 8, and 1.6 µg/ml TNP-LPS were incubated with splenocytes in graded amounts of free TNP-lysine. The results show that the highest concentration of TNP-lysine is capable of entirely inhibiting the induction of plaque-forming cells, while a comparable concentration of lysine produces no inhibition (Figure 2). It is of particular importance to note that as the TNP-LPS concentration decreases, less TNP-lysine is required to prevent B cell induction. At TNP-LPS concentrations of 40, 8, and 1.6 µg/ml the concentrations of hapten required to inhibit 50% of the normal response, $[H]_{50}$, is equal to 40, 8, and 1.6 x 10^{-5} M respectively.

Radiation dose response

Since irradiation has been shown to dramatically affect lymphocyte function, the effect of graded doses of radiation was tested to determine if they would have any differential effects on the PFC responses. Figure 3 demonstrates that both TNP-KLH and TNP-LPS responses can be dramatically enhanced by relatively low doses of radiation, with the augmented responses occurring between 100 and 400 rads of gamma irradiation.

TABLE 1

Antigenic specificity of the PFC response

Antigen	PFC			% Inhibition	
	No Inhibition[a]	TNP-lysine (10^{-3}M)	Lysine (10^{-2}M)	TNP-lysine (10^{-3}M)	Lysine (10^{-2}M)
TNP-KLH[b]	68±6	8±2	65±5	88	0
TNP-LPS[c]	130±10	6±2	129±6	95	2

[a]0.25 ml of TCM in a total plaquing mixture of 1.25 ml was used as a control.
[b]TNP-KLH at a concentration of 40 μg/ml was used to induce the PFC response.
[c]TNP-LPS at a concentration of 0.4 μg/ml was used to induce the PFC response.

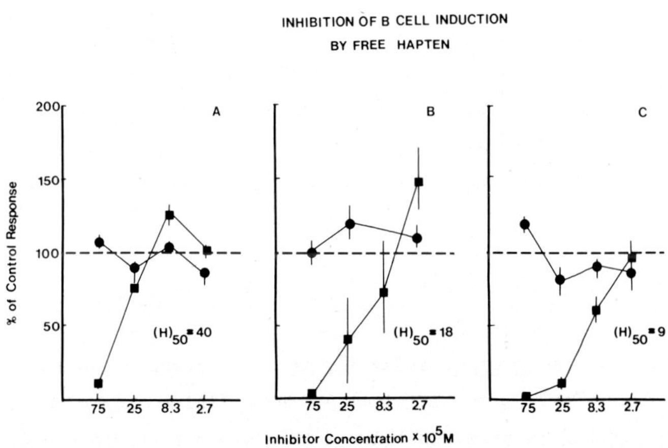

Fig. 2. Hapten inhibition of B cell induction. Cultures of spleen cells wer coincubated with TNP-LPS at 40 (A), 8 (B), and 1.6 (C) μg/ml and decreasing concentrations of TNP-lysine (■) or lysine (●). The broken line represents the PFC control response of TNP-LPS in tissue culture medium alone. Each point represents the mean of triplicate cultures and the error bars represent two standard errors about the mean.

Effects of antigen addition

The population structure of lymphocyte pools were also examined through the use of antigen addition experiments. In these studies the possibility

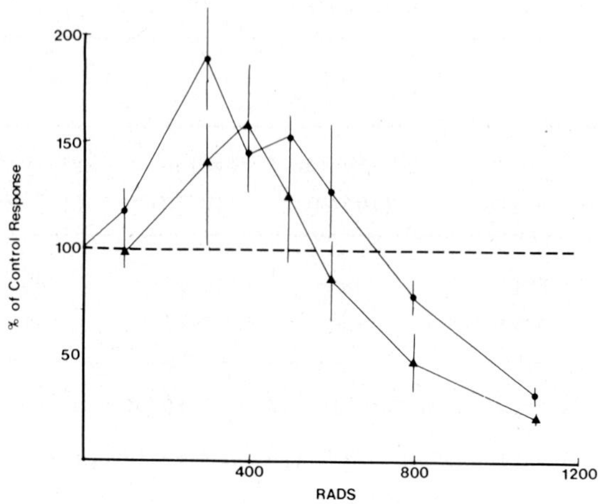

Fig. 3. Radiation dose response. The PFC response of TNP-LPS (●) and TNP-KLH (▲) of spleen cells cultured after exposure to various doses of radiation are depicted. The broken line represents the PFC response of non-irradiated cells. The error bars represent two standard errors about the mean.

that TNP-KLH and TNP-LPS could be stimulating separate subpopulations of anti-TNP B cells was approached by comparing the PFC response from cultures stimulated with optimal doses of TNP-LPS or TNP-KLH alone or in combination. If the antigens stimulate the same population of cells then we should not expect this additive phenomenon. Figure 4 shows that such an addition not only fails to occur, but there is even a lower PFC response than seen with either antigen alone.

DISCUSSION

The importance of an _in vitro_ assay for the production of antibody producing cells lies in the possibilities for the cellular and molecular dissection of the immune response to a level that was not previously available in salmonids. Although these data deal strictly with trinitrophenylated protein and lipopolysaccharide antigens, any antigens can be used as long as the investigators possess a method to detect an antibody response.

An advantage to the use of such defined antigens can be seen in Figure 1. Although we find an optimal dose of TNP-LPS to be 0.4 μg/ml, there is little or no antibody production elicited by the same concentration of LPS

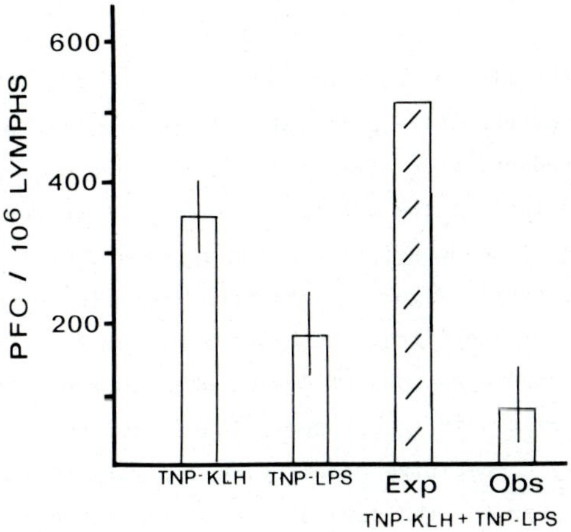

Fig. 4. Antigen addition. The bars for TNP-LPS and TNP-KLH represent the PFC response at 9 days of culture with optimal concentrations of the antigens. The cross-hatched bar depicts the expected PFC value if the responses to TNP-KLH and TNP-LPS were additive (EXP). The observed response to this combination of antigens is shown (OBS). The values shown are the means of triplicate cultures, and the bars represent two standard errors about the mean.

alone. However, a 100-fold increase of the LPS concentration begins to induce an anti-TNP response. This observation seems to corroborate the findings and model proposed by Countinho and Moller (1973). These investigators have theorized that T-independent antigens, such as TNP-LPS, stimulate lymphocytes to antibody production by providing a mitogenic signal. Thus, the TNP epitope simply serves as a targeting agent, which focuses the mitogenic LPS onto the surface of B cells by reaction with anti-TNP receptors. The mitogen then, non-specifically, stimulates the cell to go on to antibody production. One should expect, therefore, that the carrier alone could induce anti-TNP antibodies at high concentrations, since the B cell would no longer require the focusing and concentrating function provided by the haptenic group. In addition, we have found that the concentrations of LPS which induce this possible polyclonal response also induce mitogenesis as determined by the uptake of tritiated thymidine (data not shown).

Figure 1 also reveals the ability of splenocytes from animals not primed to KLH to produce a response to TNP-KLH, which has been determined to be a T-dependent response in mammals. Recent work by Miller et al. (1985) demonstrates that *in vitro* antibody responses to T dependent antigens can be induced with catfish lymphocytes without previous *in vivo* carrier priming, although the responses are considerably lower than those observed with cells from primed animals.

The inhibition of the PFC response demonstrates that the antibodies produced in response to either TNP-KLH or TNP-LPS are specific and not due to non-specific antibody production to SRBC antigens. As can be seen from Table I, 10^{-3} M TNP-lysine can inhibit the entire PFC response, whereas higher concentrations of lysine alone do not affect the response.

We have also demonstrated (Figure 2) that the induction of antibody synthesis to TNP-LPS can be specifically inhibited by the free hapten, TNP-lysine. The comparable concentrations of lysine show no inhibition. As can be seen graphically, or by the $[H]_{50}$ concentrations, the univalent, free hapten acts in a strictly competitive manner with the TNP-LPS (i.e. less antigen requires less hapten for the same degree of inhibition). The most probable explanation for this pattern of inhibition would be simple competition for the antibody receptor on the B cell surface. The decrease in responsiveness cannot be due to any toxic effects due to a high dose of TNP-lysine, since 25×10^{-5} M, does not inhibit antibody production in cells as long as a high dose of antigen is present.

Radiation has been an extremely useful tool in the dissection of the cellular subpopulations of the immune system of mice, due to differential sensitivity of the lymphoid populations (Anderson and Warner, 1975). The work presented here also demonstrates a similar differential sensitivity to radiation doses with salmonid spleen cells. The most striking feature in the data presented (Figure 3) is the presence of an augmented response to both TNP-KLH and TNP-LPS at relatively low doses of radiation (100-600 rads). These data suggest that a relatively radiosensitive cell type may naturally suppress the anti-TNP response. The existence of such a radiosensitive cell type has been seen in the rat (Tada et al., 1971) and appears to be a T suppressor cell. At this point in time, however, although the existence of T cells has been theorized for fish, and even functionally defined with respect to helper function (Miller et al., 1985; Ruben et al., 1977), there is no evidence to suggest that a T suppressor cell population exists in these animals. Experiments are currently underway to ascertain whether a suppressor cell is responsible for this phenomenon.

The addition experiments reveal that when TNP-LPS and TNP-KLH are co-incubated with splenocytes, there was no apparent addition, but rather an observed response that is less than that induced by either antigen alone. This finding would indicate that both antigenic forms affect the same B cell population. A similar observation has been made in the murine system (Lewis and Goodman, 1977). Examination of anti-TNP B cell precursor frequencies revealed no additive effects in the combination of TNP-LPS and TNP-KLH, however, additive responses were observed when TNP-KLH and TNP-ficoll were combined. We are currently characterizing the PFC response to TNP-ficoll to determine whether such a second subpopulation of B cells exists in the rainbow trout.

We feel that the in vitro approaches described here will permit further exploration into the role of carrier molecules, the fine structure and specificity of immunoglobulin receptors on B cells, and the resolution of B lymphocyte subpopulations in salmonids.

ACKNOWLEDGEMENTS

Funding for this study was provided by contract DE-A179-84BP18007 from the Fish and Wildlife program of the Bonneville Power Administration and by fellowships provided by the N. L. Tartar Foundation. Ore. Ag. Exp. Station Tech. Paper No. 7758.

REFERENCES

Anderson, R. E., and Warner, N. L., 1975. Radiosensitivity of T and B lymphocytes III. Effect of radiation on immunoglobulin production by B cells. J. Immunol. 115: 161-167.

Coutinho, A., and Möller, G., 1973. B cell mitogenic properties of thymus-independent antigens. Nature New Biology 245: 12-15.

Cunningham, A. J., and Szenberg, A., 1968. Further improvements in the plaque technique for detecting single antibody-forming cells. Immunology 14: 599.

Jacobs, D. M., and Morrison, D. C., 1975. Stimulation of a T-independent primary anti-hapten response in vitro by TNP-lipopolysaccharide (TNP-LPS). J. Immunol. 144: 360-364.

Jennings, J. J., and Rittenberg, M. B., 1976. Evidence for separate subpopulations of B cells responding to T-independent and T-dependent immunogens. J. Immunol. 117: 1749-1752.

Kaattari, S. L., and Irwin, M. J., 1985. Salmonid spleen and anterior kidney harbor populations of lymphocytes with different B cell repertoires. Dev. Comp. Immunol. 9: 433-444.

Lewis, G. K., and Goodman, J. W., 1977. Carrier-directed anti-hapten responses by B-cell subsets. J. Exp. Med. 146: 1-10.

Miller, N. W., and Clem, L. W., 1984. Microsystem for in vitro primary and secondary immunization of channel catfish (Ictalurus punctatus) leukocytes with hapten-carrier conjugates. J. Immunol. Meth. 72: 1749-1752.

Miller, N. W., Sizemore, R. C., and Clem, L. W., 1985. Phylogeny of lymphocyte heterogeneity: The cellular requirements for in vitro antibody responses of channel catfish leukocytes. J. Immunol. 134: 2884-2888.

Mishell, R. I., and Dutton, R. W., 1967. Immunization of dissociated spleen cell cultures from normal mice. J. Exp. Med. 126: 423-442.

Moller, G. (Editor), 1975. Concepts of B lymphocyte activation. In: Transplantation Reviews, Vol. 23. Munksgaard, Copenhagen.

Rittenberg, M. B., and Amkraut, A. A., 1966. Immunogenicity of trinitrophenyl-hemocyanin: production of primary and secondary anti-hapten precipitans. J. Immunol. 87:421-430.

Rittenberg, M. B., and Pratt, K., 1969. Anti-trinitrophenyl (TNP) plaque assay. Primary response of BALB/c mice to soluble and particulate immunogen. Proc. Soc. Exp. Biol. Med. 132: 575-581.

Ruben, L. N., Warr, G. W., Decker, J. M., and Marchalonis, J. J., 1977. Phylogenetic origins of immune recognition: Lymphoid heterogeneity and the hapten/carrier effect in the goldfish, Carassius auratus. Cell. Immunol. 31: 266-283.

Tada, T., Taniguchi, M., and Okumura, J. M., 1971. Regulation of homocytotropic antibody formation in the rat II. Effect of X-irradiation. J. Immunol. 106: 1012-1018.

Tittle, T. V., and Rittenberg, M. B., 1978. Expression of IgG memory response in vitro to thymus-dependent and thymus-independent antigens. Cell. Immunol. 35: 180-190.

Veterinary Immunology and Immunopathology, 12 (1986) 39—45
Elsevier Science Publishers B.V., Amsterdam — Printed in The Netherlands

SALMONID B LYMPHOCYTES DEMONSTRATE ORGAN DEPENDENT FUNCTIONAL HETEROGENEITY

MICHAEL J. IRWIN AND STEPHEN L. KAATTARI[1]
Oregon State University, Corvallis, Oregon 97331-3804, USA

ABSTRACT

Irwin, M. J. and Kaattari, S. L., 1986. Salmonid B lymphocytes demonstrate organ dependent functional heterogeneity. Vet. Immunol. Immunopathol., 12: 39-45.

The passive hemolytic plaque assay was used to examine the functional heterogeneity of antibody producing cells in salmonid immune organs. In this study, the antibody response to Vibrio anguillarum antigens was induced by the injection of a somatic antigen extract. This antigen was also coated onto sheep red blood cells (SRBC) for plaque forming cell (PFC) determination. Previous studies have demonstrated that this response is antibody dependent and antigen specific (Kaattari and Irwin, 1985). The present study was focused upon the heterogeneity of antibody producing cells that arise in the spleen, anterior and posterior kidney of immunized coho salmon (Oncorhynchus kisutch). The functional heterogeneity of lymphocytes was assessed by histogram analysis of the antigen inhibition profiles of the plaque forming responses. These analyses have revealed that the anterior kidney lymphocytes possess a much more restricted profile of antibody specificities than do lymphocytes from the posterior kidney or spleen. These data suggest that B cell repetoires differ among the immune organs of salmonids.

INTRODUCTION

Studies on the ontogeny of the immune response in fish have been limited to the physical characterization of cell types and the structure of immune organs at different times during fish maturation (Zapata, 1979; Grace and Manning, 1980). Information from these studies have indicated that the anterior kidney is the lymphopoietic organ of teleosts, analogous to the bone marrow of mammals (Zapata, 1979). Functional characterization of the lymphocytes residing in the lymphoid organs of teleosts could demonstrate where the maturation of immune cells occurs. In the murine system, such characterizations were accomplished by employing the use of differential antigen inhibition of antibody producing cells (APC). Claflin and Merchant (1973), Goidl and Siskind (1974), and Marshall-Clarke and Playfair (1978)

[1] To whom correspondence should be addressed

0165-2427/86/$03.50 © 1986 Elsevier Science Publishers B.V.

have used antigen inhibition analyses to study ontogeny of the immune response in mice. This technique is useful in that the plaque forming cell (PFC) assay allows one to visualize the individual PFC and characterize these cells by inhibition with graded doses of antigen.

Previous work in our laboratory has shown PFC responses can be generated in coho salmon (*Oncorhynchus kisutch*) to an O-antigen extract of *Vibrio anguillarum* (Kaattari and Irwin, 1985). PFC from the spleen, anterior kidney and the thymus were detected by means of a passive hemolytic plaque assay. In this study we again examine inhibition profiles of PFC from the spleen and anterior kidney and extend this analysis to lymphocytes from the posterior kidney. Inhibition histograms indicate that the anterior kidney contains a homogeneous PFC population responsive to *Vibrio* antigens in both yearling and two to three year old coho salmon. In contrast, splenic and posterior kidney derived lymphocytes demonstrate a more heterogeneous APC population from the same animals.

METHODS

Materials and methods used are the same as previously described (Kaattari and Irwin, 1985). Briefly, O-antigen extracts used in immunizations, coating SRBC, and antigen inhibitor were prepared from *Vibrio anguillarum* (LS-174). Fish were immunized intraperitoneally with 10 μg of powdered antigen in 0.1 ml phosphate buffered saline (PBS). Spleens, anterior kidneys and posterior kidneys were removed one to three weeks post immunization, at which time they were tested for PFC using a modified Cunningham plaque assay (Cunningham and Szenberg, 1968). Free antigen inhibition of PFC was assessed using serial dilutions of soluble Vibrio antigen incorporated into the plaquing mixture. Histogram plots depict the resulting inhibition profiles and the variance from the mean of the log transformed data was calculated.

RESULTS

The heterogeneity or antigen specificity of antibody producing cells from coho salmon was investigated by the use of free antigen inhibition of plaque formation. Inhibition histograms were generated for PFC from splenic, anterior kidney and posterior kidney lymphocytes. Previous work (Kaattari and Irwin, 1985) has demonstrated that a more restricted population of PFC resides in the anterior kidney as opposed to the spleen. Application of the technique described above to PFC derived from the posterior portion of the kidney has produced unexpected results. Figure 1 shows inhibition histograms generated from splenic, anterior and posterior kidney derived lymphocytes.

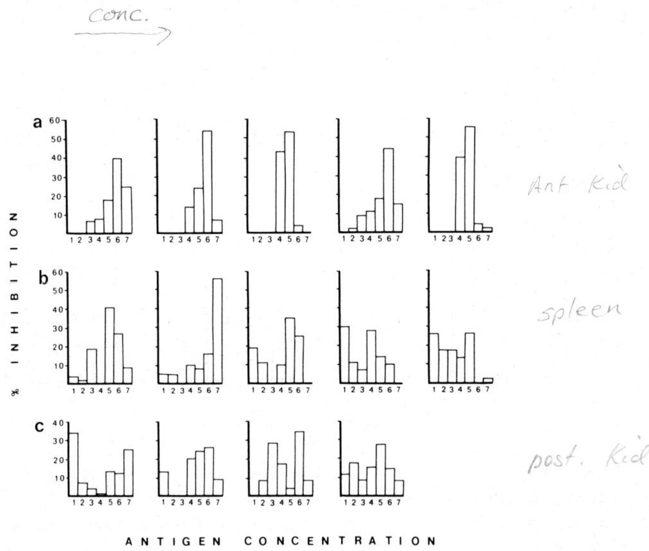

Figure 1. Histograms showing inhibition profiles of PFC from the anterior kidney (a), spleen (b), and posterior kidney (c). Each frame represents inhibition profiles generated from 2-3 fish pools of the designated lymphocyte source. The numbers on the abscissa represent three fold serial dilutions of the free antigen inhibitor concentrations used: 1) 0.09 μg/ml, 2) 0.26, 3) 0.8, 4) 2.4, 5) 7, 6) 21, and 7) 64 μg/ml. Histogram bars represent the increase in percent plaque forming cell inhibition with respect to the increase in free antigen inhibitor concentration.

PFC from the posterior kidney can be seen to have a very heterogeneous inhibition profile as compared to that seen in the anterior kidney. In fact, the heterogeneity profiles of the posterior kidney more closely resemble those of the spleen, rather than those of the anterior kidney. The variance from the mean of the log transformed data (data obtained from histogram analyses) was used to describe the degree of heterogeneity of PFC obtained from these lymphoid tissues (Zar, 1984). Figure 2 shows compiled data obtained from an average of five histograms from the anterior kidney, and the spleen and four experiments from the posterior kidney. Each experiment used organs from two to three fish pools.

The average variance calculated for the anterior kidney was 0.22, while the spleen and posterior kidney gave variances of 0.90 and 0.84 respectively. The posterior kidney is therefore shown, statistically, to house PFC of essentially the same heterogeneity as splenic PFC in response to Vibrio antigens, while both are more heterogeneous than responding PFC from the anterior kidney.

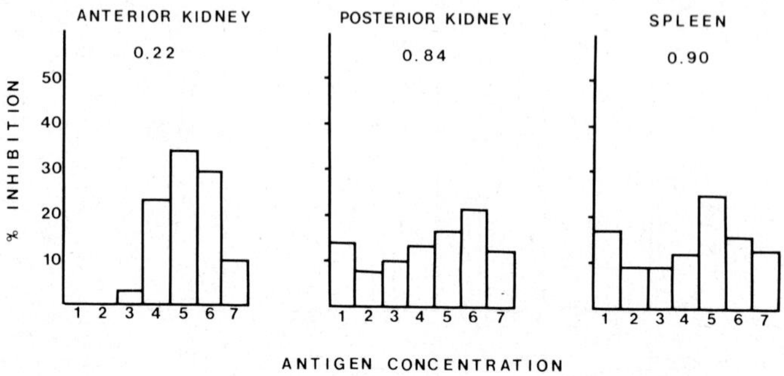

Figure 2. Compiled data of the inhibition profiles obtained in Figure 1 from, anterior kidney, posterior kidney, and splenic derived lymphocytes. Values shown at the top of each plot represent the variance from the mean of log transformed data.

CONCLUSION

Immunologists working with the murine system have used the technique of free antigen inhibition of antibody responses with graded doses of antigen to characterize PFC populations as to their affinity and heterogeneity (Claflin and Merchant, 1973; Goidl and Siskind, 1974; Marshall-Clarke and Playfair, 1978). Free antigen inhibition studies on PFC generated to Vibrio antigens in yearling and 2-3 year coho salmon have yielded unexpected results. Histograms generated by inhibition analyses have shown the spleen and posterior kidney to contain a more heterogeneous responding PFC population than the anterior kidney. Mathematical analysis, using variance from the mean of log transformed data, describes the relative heterogeneity. We prefer to describe our data in this manner because we feel it more accurately describes relative heterogeneity than does the Shannon heterogeneity index, the method of choice in some murine studies (Kaattari and Irwin, 1985).

It is of interest that lymphocytes obtained from different sections of a continuous organ, such as the kidney, would house PFC with vastly different specificities or affinities. Histological evidence exists that supports the contention that the anterior kidney of teleosts is the hematopoietic center of teleosts (Zapata, 1979). Zapata (1979) also discusses the dichotomy of function in the anterior and posterior kidneys of teleosts, and refers to the anterior kidney of the teleost as being equivalent to mammalian bone marrow.

Our data lends evidence to these arguments by demonstrating more restricted or homogeneous PFC in the anterior kidney.

An alternate hypothesis that could explain these differences found between the immune organs could be that only lower concentrations of antigen are able to reach the anterior kidney. The ability of immune organs of rainbow trout to take up and sequester bacterial antigens was approached by Secombes and Manning (1980) and by Nelson et al. (1985). Both of these groups found that the antigens under investigation could be detected in the spleen and anterior kidney of fish at the earliest assay time. Nelson (1985) used a Vibrio anguillarum bacterin and immunofluorescence to study the localization of the bacterin in rainbow trout tissues. Vibrio bacterin was shown to have disseminated to all tissues of the fish by one minute post intraperitoneal injection. Moreover, the antigen was cleared from the tissues and localized in the spleen and throughout the kidney by day 14 post immunization. Thus, on the basis of these studies there appears to be no difference in the distribution of antigen. Furthermore, we feel that this alternate hypothesis is not likely, since we would expect that the limiting amounts of antigen would preferentially bind high affinity receptor bearing lymphocytes (Andersson, 1970). Thus, if there were a relatively low concentration of antigen in the anterior kidney, we should expect to see a restricted response in the high affinity (i.e. low free antigen) end of the inhibition plot, not in the low affinity end, which was the case in this study.

An alternate model can be developed from concepts about the circulation of lymphocytes through lymphoid tissues. As lymphocytes mature in the anterior kidney, they may be immediately dispatched to the circulation, then localize in either the posterior kidney or the spleen. This phenomenon might occur in much the same way that lymphocytes mature in the bone marrow of mammals, enter the circulation and finally localize in secondary immune organs (Brahim and Osmond, 1970). However, in mammals recirculation occurs through the bone marrow, thereby causing lymphocyte populations to take on a more mature appearance later in fetal life (Goidl and Siskind, 1974). In contrast, we observed a restricted, and possibly immature PFC population in the anterior kidney in both yearling and 2-3 year coho salmon. Therefore, our model of maturation and migration from the pronephros may also explain the observed absence of mature PFC in the anterior kidney, or alternatively, why the population of mature lymphocytes are seemingly depleted from this region.

Thymocytes have long been known to exert dramatic effects on antibody responses in higher vertebrates. Although, in fish immune systems, a strictly defined T cell has not yet been demonstrated, T-like functions have been shown to play an integral role in certain fish immune responses (Ruben et al., 1977; Miller et al., 1985). Work by Doenhoff et al. (1979) has demonstrated that in order to produce a mature, heterogeneous antibody response in mice, T cells are required. Tatner (1985) has shown a preferential migration of thymocytes to the spleen and to a much lesser extent to the anterior kidney. We might expect that the observed heterogeneous PFC response in the spleen might be due to a cell-cell interaction that cannot occur in the anterior kidney because either a particular thymocyte is absent, or does not migrate in large enough numbers to this region. If this alternative is true then a crucial experiment would be to measure the relative level of thymocyte migration to both the anterior and posterior kidney regions.

ACKNOWLEDGEMENTS

Funding for this study was provided by the N. L. Tartar Foundation. Ore. Ag. Exp. Station Tech. Paper No. 7757.

REFERENCES

Andersson, B., 1970. Studies on the regulation of avidity at the level of the single antibody-forming cell. The effect of antigen dose and time after immunization. J. Exp. Med. 132: 77-88.

Brahim, F. and Osmond, D. G., 1980. Migration of bone marrow lymphocytes demonstrated by selective bone marrow labelling with thymidine-H^3. Anat. Rec. 168: 139-151.

Claflin, L. and Merchant, B., 1973. Antibody binding characteristics at the cellular level. II. Presence of cells secreting high affinity antibody at the onset of the immune response. J. Immunol. 110: 252-261.

Cunningham, A. J. and Szenberg, A., 1968. Further improvements ini the plaque technique for detecting single and body-forming cells. Immunology 14:599.

Doenhoff, M. J., Musallam, R., Keeler, K. D., and Dresser, D. W., 1979. Restricted heterogeneity of antibody synthesized by T-cell deprived mice. Immunology 38: 57-62.

Goidl, E. A. and Siskind, G. W., 1974. Ontogeny of B lymphocyte function. I. Restricted heterogeneity of the antibody response of B lymphocytes from neonatal and fetal mice. J. Exp. Med. 140: 1285.

Grace, M. F. and Manning, M. J., 1980. Histogenesis of the lymphoid organs in rainbow trout, *Salmo gairdneri*. Dev. and Comp. Immunol. 4: 255-64.

Kaattari, S. L. and Irwin, M. J., 1985. Salmonid spleen and kidney harbor populations of lymphocytes with different B-cell repertoires. Dev. and Comp. Immunol. 9: 433-444.

Marshall-Clarke, S. and Playfair, J. H. L., 1978. Ontogeny of murine B-lymphocytes. Avidity of antigen binding cells in neonatal and adult mice. Immunology 34: 1089.

Miller, N. W., Sizemore, R. C., and Clem, L. W., 1985. Phylogeny of lymphocyte heterogeneity: The cellular requirements for *in vitro* antibody responses of channel catfish leukocytes. J. Immunol. 134: 2884-2888.

Nelson, J. S., Rohovec, J. S., and Fryer, J. L., 1985. Tissue location of *Vibrio* bacterin delivered by intraperitoneal injection, immersion and oral routes to *Salmo gairdneri*. Fish Pathol. 19: 263-269.

Ruben, L. N., Warr G. W., Decker, J. M., and Marchalonis, J. J., 1977. Phylogenetic origins of immune recognition: Lymphoid heterogeneity and the hapten/carrier effect in the goldfish, *Carassius auratus*. Cell. Immunol. 31: 266-83.

Secombes, C. J. and Manning, M. J., 1980. Comparative studies on the immune system of fishes and amphibians: Antigen localization in the carp, *Cyprinus carpio* L. J. Fish Dis. 3: 399-412.

Tatner, M. F. 1985. Themigration of labelled thymocytes to the peripheral lymphoid organs in the rainbow trout, *Salmo gairdneri* Richardson. Dev. and Comp. Immunol. 9: 85-91.

Zapata, A. 1979. Ultrastructural study of the teleost fish kidney. Dev. and Comp. Immunol. 3: 55-65.

Zar, J. H. 1984. Measures of dispersion and variability. Indices of diversity. In: Biostatistical Analysis. Second edition. Prentice-Hall, Englewood Cliffs, New Jersey.

Veterinary Immunology and Immunopathology, 12 (1986) 47—58
Elsevier Science Publishers B.V., Amsterdam — Printed in The Netherlands

PHYLOGENETIC STUDIES ON LYMPHOKINES. FISH LYMPHOCYTES RESPOND TO HUMAN IL-1 AND EPITHELIAL CELLS PRODUCE AN IL-1 LIKE FACTOR

M.M. SIGEL, B.A. HAMBY and E.M. HUGGINS, Jr.,

Department of Microbiology and Immunology, USC School of Medicine, Columbia, South Carolina 29208, USA

ABSTRACT

Sigel, M.M., Hamby, B.A. and Huggins, E.M., Jr., 1986. Phylogenetic studies on lymphokines. Fish lymphocytes respond to human IL-1 and epithelial cells produce an IL-1 like factor. Vet. Immunol. Immunopathol., 12: 47-58.

The results obtained indicate, that catfish peripheral blood lymphocytes recognize and respond to human IL-1. The second part of this report is dealing with a substance produced by carp epidermal cells with functional similarities to mammalian IL-1.

INTRODUCTION

Interleukin-1 (IL-1), a cytokine that acts as an initiator of a number of physiological reactions, is known to cross species barriers as evidenced by IL-1 from one mammalian species interacting with cells of other mammalian species. Since fish are capable of mounting immune responses through lymphocytes and macrophages, it is reasonable to assume that cellular interactions in these species are mediated by cytokines similar to those described for phylogenetically higher vertebrates. In fact, previous studies have demonstrated the existence of regulatory cytokines in fish. For example, production of interferon by the grunt was reported by Beasley and Sigel (1967). More recently, the presence of a proliferation promoting factor for carp T-like cells was shown by Caspi and Avtalion (1984). This factor has functional similarities to Interleukin 2 (IL-2).

IL-1 serves as a starting point for a number of physiological events in mammals which form cascades of interdependent reactions. These involve a variety of cells, molecular products and signals. For example, IL-1 acts on T cells, increasing the expression of their receptors for IL-2 which leads to proliferation (Kaye et al., 1984). Activated T cells release lymphokines, some of which can act on macrophages/monocytes, stimulating these in turn to produce IL-1 (Chao et al., 1977; Bernheim et al., 1980; Dinarello, 1981). Another kind of cascade encompasses the augmentation of production of prostaglandins (For review see Dinarello 1984).

The initial part of our studies was focused on the effect of human IL-1 on catfish peripheral blood lymphocytes (PBL) as measured by the proliferative response in the presence and absence of T cell mitogens. The

0165-2427/86/$03.50 © 1986 Elsevier Science Publishers B.V.

results obtained indicate that fish lymphocytes recognize and respond to human IL-1 thus providing evidence for the early phylogenetic emergence of a mechanism (receptor?) for the recognition of IL-1.

Next we proceeded to determine whether fish cells were capable of producing IL-1. The second part of this report will present preliminary findings on a substance produced by carp epidermal cells with functional similarities to mammalian IL-1 as judged by: 1-its mitogenic effect on fish PBL and its co-mitogenic effect on murine thymocytes; 2-the ability to stimulate production of thromboxane; and 3-the ability to induce IL-2.

MATERIALS & METHODS

Fish: Channel catfish (*Ictalurus punctatus*) were obtained from local catfish farmers and acclimated in 30 gallon aquaria for 2 weeks at 24°C before use. Catfish were fed every other day with fresh beef liver to satiation. Carp (*Cyprinus carpio*) were obtained from a local aquaculturist, acclimated for 2 weeks at 24° prior to use and fed commercial fish pellets every other day.

Mice: Male Balb/c mice, aged 4-8 weeks, were obtained from Harlan Sprague Dawley, (Indianapolis, Ind.).

IL-1: Two different preparations of human IL-1 were utilized in these studies. The first, a gift from Dr. L. B. Lachman at M.D. Anderson Cancer Center, was obtained from monocytes isolated from patients with acute myelomonocytic lymphoma (Lachman, 1983). The second IL-1 preparation was generously provided by Dr. Charles A. Dinarello at Tufts University Medical School and was isolated from normal peripheral blood monocytes (Dinarello, 1981). Dr. Dinarello also kindly furnished anti-human IL-1 rabbit antibody.

EPC fish cell line: The EPC (*Epithelioma Papulosum Cyprini*) cell line was derived from hypertrophic skin lesions of carp. This epithelial cell line, first described by Fijan, et al., (1983), has now been maintained in culture for over 100 passages and has demonstrated signs of transformation such as change in chromosome number and the acquisition of ability to grow in soft agar. This line was obtained through the courtesy of Dr. B. Lindgerding at National Fish Health Research Laboratory, Kearneysville, W.Va., and was maintained in Eagle's Minimal Essential Medium (MEM) with 10% FBS and 50μg/ml gentamicin at 24°C. Cultures were fed weekly and supernatants were collected and frozen at -70°C.

Catfish PBL Proliferation Assay: The method of Faulmann et al., (1983) was used. Catfish were anesthetized by immersion into water containing Tricaine (Sigma) and bled from the caudal sinus into 1ml of catfish RPMI 1640 (9 parts RPMI and 1 part distilled H_2O) containing sodium heparin (100U/ml of blood). The blood was layered over Lymphoprep (Nyegaard and Co.) in a ratio of 4 parts blood to 3 parts Lymphoprep and centrifuged for 20 minutes at 400g at room temperature. The resulting interface band, predominantly WBC, was recovered and washed three times in catfish RPMI-1640. Viable WBC were enumerated by trypan blue dye exclusion and adjusted to $5X10^6$/ml in complete catfish blastogenic medium (RPMI-1640 with 10% heat inactivated human serum, 5% heat inactivated catfish serum, 2mM glutamine, and 1X penicillin-streptomycin). WBC were added to individual wells of 96 well flat bottomed tissue culture plates (Linbro) in a volume of 0.1ml. 0.1ml of IL-1 or EPC supernatants at various dilutions was then added, as was 0.05ml of Concanavalin-A (ConA) at the appropriate concentrations. Antibody neutralization of the comitogenic effects of IL-1 was performed by preincubating various dilutions of IL-1 with IL-1 Ab at a 1:50 dilution for 1 hr. prior to addition to the wells. The plates were then incubated for 72 hrs. at 27° in 5% CO_2 before pulsing with 0.5μCi/well of ^{3}H-Thymidine (ICN). Eighteen hrs. after pulsing, the individual wells were harvested onto glass filtermats with a Skatron Automated Cell Harvester (Skatron, Inc.). The filtermats were dried and the contents from individual wells were placed into Omni-vials (Wheaton) containing 2ml of scintillation fluid and counted in a Beckman LS 8100 liquid scintillation counter. Results are expressed as mean counts per min. (CPM) per group of four wells ± one standard deviation (SD).

Carp PBL Proliferation Assay: The same procedure for catfish PBL was followed except the medium used was Dulbecco's MEM with 5% heat inactivated carp serum, 1X pencillin - streptomycin, 2mM glutamine, fungisone, and 2-mercaptoethanol ($5X10^{-5}$M).

Murine thymocyte assay: Thymocytes were separated with a glass tissue grinder and washed in RPMI-1640 with 10% FBS. RBC were lysed by osmotic shock with Tris-ammonium chloride lysing solution, followed by 3 washes in medium. Viable WBC were adjusted to $10X10^6$/ml in RPMI-1640 with 10% FBS,

2mM glutamine, 1X pencillin-streptomycin, and $2.5X10^{-5}$M 2-mercaptoethanol. Wells were loaded as above and incubated for 72 hrs. at 37°C in 5% CO_2 before pulsing with 0.5μCi of ^{3}H-Thymidine.

Corneal epithelial cell line (SIRC) and Chicken chondrocytes:

The rabbit corneal epithelial cell line was obtained from ATCC, Rockville, MD. Chicken chondrocytes were from a primary culture. Cells were grown at 37°C in 5% CO_2. The medium was RPMI 1640 supplemented with 1X penicillin-streptomycin, 2mM glutamine, non-essential amino acids, pyruvate, and 10% FBS. For induction of thromboxane (Tx), cells were grown in either 24 well tissue culture plates seeded with $3\text{-}5X10^4$ cells/well or in $25cm^2$ tissue culture flasks seeded with $8X10^5\text{-}1X10^6$ cells/flask.

RIA for TxB_2

96 hr. old cultures of SIRC or chicken chondrocytes were washed and fed with serum free culture medium. Wells received either human IL-1 (from Dr. Lachman), EPC supernatants or cell extracts, or serum free growth medium. Plates/flasks were incubated for 16-18 hrs. at 37°C in 5% CO_2. Supernatants were harvested and subjected to RIA for TxB_2. The protocol for the competitive RIA was a modification of the procedure of Burch et al., (1979). The concentration of TxB_2 in each sample is expressed in pg/100μl.

RESULTS:

Effects of human IL-1 on Catfish PBL

Earlier experiments had established that a final concentration of 4μg/ml of ConA was a suboptimal dose for catfish PBL in our system. Therefore, this concentration was used for costimulation of the mitogenic response by human IL-1. As shown in Table 1, both preparations of IL-1 were effective at causing costimulation of the catfish PBL response to the mitogenic effect of suboptimal doses of ConA. The costimulatory effect was evident at high dilutions of IL-1. These dilutions were considerably higher than those obtained in mouse thymocyte assays (data not shown).

To ensure that the costimulatory effect on catfish PBL was due to human IL-1, a set of experiments using anti-human IL-1 antibodies to attempt to neutralize IL-1 was performed. A representative experiment is illustrated in Table 2. Preincubation of various dilutions of IL-1 with anti-human IL-1 antibody resulted in diminution of the costimulatory effect of the IL-1 on catfish PBL that were exposed to suboptimal concentrations of ConA. Thus, the increased mitogenic response of catfish PBL in the presence of low doses of ConA was due to human IL. These findings were confirmed in other tests.

TABLE 1

COMITOGENIC EFFECT OF HUMAN IL-1 ON CATFISH PBL

	no ConA	+ ConA 4 μg/ml[a]
PBL	338 ± 106[b]	9932 ± 1784
PBL + D[c] 1:5120	407 ± 91	30840 ± 4474
PBL + D 1:20480	577 ± 239	35098 ± 2931
PBL + D 1:81920	318 ± 58	29972 ± 6548
PBL + L[d] 1:800	391 ± 130	42371 ± 3056
PBL + L 1:3200	587 ± 117	40001 ± 9486
PBL + L 1:12800	392 ± 117	42879 ± 5802

[a] Suboptiomal dose
[b] Mean of 4 wells ± 1SD
[c] Dinarello IL-1
[d] Lachman IL-1

TABLE 2

INHIBITION OF BLASTOGENIC EFFECT OF IL-1 ON CATFISH PBL BY ANTI-HUMAN ANTIBODY

	no ConA	ConA 4 μg/ml[a]
	732 ± 245[b]	3757 ± 1623
L[c] 1:800	9642 ± 1986	21997 ± 1524
L 1:800 + Ab[d]	2348 ± 879	8227 ± 2204
L 1:3200	2807 ± 400	19844 ± 1642
L 1:3200 + Ab	1792 ± 336	6186 ± 1717
L 1:12800	8157 ± 2979	21418 ± 4499
L 1:12800 + Ab	1240 ± 132	5011 ± 962

[a] Supoptimal dose
[b] Mean of 4 wells ± 1 SD
[c] Lachman IL-1
[d] Anti-human-IL-1 Ab (1:100 final dilution; incubated 1 hour with IL-1 before adding to wells)

In a few experiments we obtained an indication of lymphocyte stimulation by IL-1 without the addition of lectin. The experiment depicted in Table 2 is one such experiment in which human IL-1 caused stimulation and proliferation of catfish PBL even in the absence of ConA.

Effect of EPCF on blastogenic responses

The response of catfish PBL to human IL-1 prompted us to search for a similar substance produced by fish cells. Since mammalian epithelial cells have been shown to produce an IL-1 like substance, the EPC cell line was used in our search for fish IL-1. The EPC cell line is derived from carp, therefore, the initial experiments looking for a growth factor were performed using carp PBL. As shown in Table 3, both supernatant (conditioned medium) from confluent EPC cells as well as extracts from disrupted cells increased the proliferation of carp PBL in the absence of mitogen. The cell extract was much more effective at stimulating proliferation of carp PBL than was the supernatant, although both enhanced the uptake of ^{3}H-thymidine at least four-fold.

TABLE 3

EFFECT OF EPC SUPERNATANT AND CELL EXTRACT ON CARP PBL

PBL	182 ± 35[a]
PBL + EPC sup. 1:2[b]	773 ± 70
PBL + EPC sup. 1:4	894 ± 199
PBL + EPC sup. 1:8	933 ± 25
PBL + EPC cell extract 1:2[c]	1674 ± 94
PBL + EPC cell extract 1:4	1367 ± 202
PBL + EPC cell extract 1:8	1315 ± 304

[a]Mean of 4 wells ± 1 SD
[b]Supernatant from 16 day old EPC culture
[c]Cells from 16 day old EPC culture disrupted by freeze-thaw method in acetone and dry ice

Further experiments were performed utilizing catfish PBL as the target for EPCF. The factor greatly increased the proliferation of catfish PBL as shown in Table 4. Once again, more growth-promoting activity was observed in samples from disrupted cells than from supernatant.

Since human and murine IL-1 have been shown to retain activity across species barriers, we hypothesized that if the factor produced by the EPC cell line was related to IL-1, it should also be recognized by mammalian cells. Consequently, the supernatant from the EPC line was tested for proliferation promoting activity on murine thymocytes. Table 5 shows that while there was little or no direct effect of EPCF on thymocytes in the absence of suboptimal doses of mitogen, a costimulatory effect was observed in the presence of ConA and, more visibly, PHA.

TABLE 4

EFFECT OF EPC SUPERNATANT AND CELL EXTRACT ON CATFISH PBL

PBL	82 ± 19[a]
PBL + EPC sup. 1:2[b]	1912 - 205
PBL + EPC sup. 1:8	1584 ± 345
PBL + EPC cell extract 1:2[c]	7398 ± 1290
PBL + EPC cell extract 1:8	3199 ± 405

[a]Mean of 4 wells ± 1 SD
[b]Supernatant from 16 day old EPC culture
[c]Cells from 16 day old EPC culture disrupted by freeze-thaw method in acetone and dry ice

TABLE 5

EFFECT OF EPC SUPERNATANT ON MOUSE THYMOCYTES

	no ConA or PHA	+ ConA 1μg/ml[a]	+ PHA 1μg/ml[b]
THYMOCYTES	91 ± 40[c]	9131 ± 2016	730 ± 135
THYMO + EPC sup 1:2[d]	284 ± 77	13870 ± 1545	2005 ± 595
THYMO + EPC sup. 1:4	202 ± 83	1506 ± 2515	1707 ± 209
THYMO + EPC sup. 1:8	186 ± 44	16618 ± 4008	1838 ± 720

[a]Suboptimal dose
[b]Suboptimal dose
[c]Mean of 4 wells ± 1 SD
[d]Supernatant from 16 day old EPC culture

Effects of EPCF on TxB_2 production by SIRC and chicken chondrocytes

IL-1 has previously been shown to activate the cyclooxygenase pathway leading to the production of PGs and Tx from arachidonic acid. The enhanced production of TxB_2 by IL-1 in both the corneal epithelial cells and chicken chondrocyte systems can be seen in Tables 6 and 7. IL-1 (at a 1:100 dilution) increased TxB_2 production up to 5X that of the control level in chicken chondrocytes and 13X in the corneal epithelial cells (Table 6). The IL-1 effect on TxB_2 production in corneal epithelial cells was found to be dose dependent as shown in Table 7. EPC cell extract was tested for its ability to induce an increased release of TxB_2 in these cell systems. In Table 6, it can be seen that the cell extract increased TxB_2 release at least 3 fold in chondrocytes and approximately 4 fold in corneal epithelial cells. In another experiment (Table 7), both cell extract and supernatant enhanced TxB_2 release in corneal epithelial cells. The response appears to be dose dependent, but further determinations are necessary.

TABLE 6

RIA FOR THROMBOXANE B_2

CELLS	SUPERNATANT TESTED	Pg TxB_2/100μl	
		EXP. 1	EXP. 2
Chicken chondrocytes	Control	52	78
	Human IL-1 (1:100)[a]	288	330
	EPC cell extract (1:4)[b]	168	190
Rabbit corneal epithelial cells	Control	36	45
	Human IL-1 (1:50)	475	608
	EPC cell extract (1:4)	163	213

[a]Lachman IL-1
[b]Cells from 16 day old EPC cultures disrupted by freeze-thaw method in acetone and dry ice

DISCUSSION:

One of the accepted principles of phylogeny and ontogeny is that inherent to the evolution or development of a system of cellular immunity are the abilities to recognize foreign antigens, to respond in an appropriate manner to such insult, and to be able to regulate said response as situations dictate. It is therefore not surprising to find that in lower vertebrates as well as in invertebrates one can encounter cellular products capable of mediating or modifying a number of biochemical and physiological activities which in higher species are frequently regulated by lymphokines. Interferon is one such substance and its presence had previously been documented by the studies of Gravell and Malsberger (1965), Beasley, et al., (1966), and Beasley and Sigel (1967).

TABLE 7

RIA FOR THROMBOXANE B_2

Cells	Supernatants Tested	Pg TxB_2/100µl
Rabbit corneal epithelial cells	Control	43
	Human IL-1 (1:50)[a]	618
	Human IL-1 (1:100)	365
	Human IL-1 (1:200)	190
	Human IL-1 (1:400)	131
	Human IL-1 (1:800)	85
	Human IL-1 (1:1600)	84
	EPC cell extract 1:2[b]	149
	EPC cell extract 1:8	62
	EPC sup 1:2[c]	180
	EPC sup 1:8	101

[a]Lachman IL-1
[b]Cells from 16 day old EPC culture fractured by freeze-thaw method with acetone and dry ice
[c]Supernatant from 16 day EPC culture

This paper reports on the ability of fish lymphocytes to recognize and to respond to mammalian IL-1. The studies also present preliminary evidence that a fish epithelial cell line is capable of producing an IL-1 like substance (EPCF). Thus the characterization of EPCF being IL-1 like is based on the following considerations: 1 - it causes proliferation of fish PBL; 2 - it augments the proliferative response of mouse thymocytes to suboptiomal doses of ConA and PHA; 3 - it causes an increase in production of thromboxane as measured by RIA; and 4 - it induces production of IL-2 as determined in the EL-4/CTLL-20 assay system (Simon, 1984; tests performed as a courtesy by Dr. John C. Lee).

IL-1 causes many effects including induction of fever, (Dinarello and Wolff, 1982) induction of release of acute phase reactants from liver, (Dinarello, 1984) induction of neutrophilia (Kampschmidt et al., 1972), alteration of levels of divalent cations in plasma (Kampschmidt and Upchurch, 1969), and immunoregulatory effects on T & B cells (Dinarello, 1984). Some effects are elicited by mediators released by cells stimulated by IL-1. Some of these are products from the breakdown of arachidonic acid including prostaglandins, thromboxane, and prostacyclins. They exert a number of effects on the vasculature, on smooth muscle, on cell growth, and on immune responses.

In the context of effects on the immune responses, we should add another family of products derived from arachidonic acid, the leukotrienes, which are generated via the lipoxygenase pathway. It is of special interest that some of these substances can interact in a protagonistic or antagonistic manner. For example, PMN and eosinophil chemotaxis, which is promoted by leukotriene LTB_4, can be enhanced by PGs of the E series and inhibited by other leukotrienes. Chemotaxis can also be modulated by thromboxane which increases leukocyte adherence (Payan et al., 1984). Prostaglandin may cause immunosuppression partly by inhibiting the expression of Ia glycoprotein on macrophages. Thromboxane antagonizes this effect (Snyder et al., 1982).

Of special interest is the sea star factor (SSF) which was first described by Prendergast and Suzuki (1970). This factor has a number of biological effects similar to lymphokines (Liu et al., 1983). In a recent report, Donnelly et al., (1985) refer to the SSF as being a primitive IL-1 like monokine. This reference was based on their finding that SSF leads to the inhibition of expression of Ia on macrophages. This inhibition has been associated with the action of PGs of the E series. The inhibition of Ia expression by SSF could be blocked by addition of indomethecin.

Another phylogenetically early sign of recognition of IL-1 was described for the desert iguana (Bernheim and Kluger, 1977). The body temperature of this animal was significantly increased after injection with rabbit endogenous pyrogen (IL-1).

Our present work provides evidence for the early evolutionary origin and conservation of the gene coding for IL-1. A molecule such as IL-1 in fish probably plays a number of important roles in initiation and/or regulation of physiologic functions. These may include regulation of immune responses either directly through action on lymphocytes or indirectly by way of activation of the various sequences of reactions which lead to the production of other important mediators such as IL-2, thromboxanes, and prostaglandins.

REFERENCES

Beasley, A. R. and Sigel, M. M., 1967. Interferon production in cold-blooded vertebrates. In Vitro, 3:154-165.

Beasley, A. R., Sigel, M. M. and Clem, L. W., 1966. Latent infection in marine fish cell tissue cultures. Proc. Soc. Exp. Biol. Med., 121: 1169-1174.

Bernheim, H. A. and Kluger, M. J., 1977. Endogenous pyrogen-like substance produced by reptiles. J. Physiol., 267:659-666.

Bernheim, H. A., Block, L. H., Francis, L. and Atkins, E., 1980. Release of endogenous pyrogen-activating factor from Concanavalin-A-stimulated human lymphocytes. J. Exp. Med., 152:1811-1816.

Burch, R. M., Knapp, D. R. and Halushka, P. V., 1979. Vasopressin stimulates thromboxane synthesis in the toad urinary bladder: Effects of imidazole. J. Pharmacol. and Exp. Ther., 210:344-348.

Caspi, R. R. and Avtalion, R. R., 1984. Evidence for the existence of an IL-2 like lymphocyte growth promoting factor in a bony fish, *Cyprinus carpio*. Dev. and Comp. Immunol., 8:51-60.

Chao, P., Francis, L. and Atkins, E., 1977. The release of an endogenous pyrogen from guinea pig leukocytes in vitro. J. Exp. Med., 145:1288-1298.

Dinarello, C. A., 1981. Demonstration of a human pyrogen-inducing factor during mixed leukocyte reactions. J. Exp. Med., 153:1215-1224.

Dinarello, C. A. and Wolff, S. M., 1982. Molecular basis of fever in humans. Am. J. Med., 72:799-819.

Dinarello, C. A., 1984. Interleukin-1. Rev. Infect. Dis., 6:51-95.

Donnelly, J. J., Vogel, S. N. and Prendergast, R. A., 1985. Down-regulation of Ia expression on macrophages by sea star factor. Cell. Immunol., 90:408-415.

Faulmann, E., Cuchens, M. A., Lobb, C. J., Miller, N. W. and Clem, L. W., 1983. An effective culture system for studying *in vitro* mitogenic responses of channel catfish lymphocytes. Trans. Am. Fish. Soc., 112:673-679.

Fijan, W., Sulimanovic, D., Bearzotti, M., Muzinic, D., Zwillenberg, L. O., Chilmonczyk, S., Vautherot, J. F. and deKinkelin, P., 1983. Some properties of the *Epithelioma Papulosum Cyprini* (EPC) cell line from carp *Cyprinus carpio*. Ann. Virol. (Inst. Pasteur), 134E:207-220.

Gravell, M. and Malsberger, R. G., 1965. A permanent cell line from the fathead minnow (Pimephalis promelas). Ann. N.Y. Acad. Sci., 126: 555-565.

Kampschmidt, R. F., Long, R. D., and Upchurch, H. F., 1972. Neutrophil releasing activity in rats injected with endogenous pyrogen. Proc. Soc. Exp. Biol. Med., 139:1224-1226.

Kampschmidt, R. F. and Upchurch, H., 1969. Lowering of plasma iron concentration in the rat with leukocytic extracts. Am. J. Physiol., 216:1287-1291.

Kaye, J., Gillis, S., Mizel, S. B., Shevach, E. M., Malek, T. R., Dinarello, C. A., Lachman, L. B. and Janeway, C. A., Jr., 1984. Growth of a cloned helper T cell line induced by a monoclonal antibody specific for the antigen receptor: Interleukin 1 is required for the expression of receptors for interleukin 2. J. Immunol., 133:1339-1345.

Lachman, L. B., 1983. Human interleukin 1: Purification and properties. Fed. Proc., 42:2639-2645.

Liu, S. H., McChesney, M. D. and Prendergast, R. A. 1983. Kinetics of tumor cell cytostasis by sea star factor - activated macrophages. Dev. and Comp. Immunol., 7:545-554.

Payan, D. G., Goldman, D. W. and Goetzl, E. J., 1984. Biochemical and cellular characteristics of regulation of human leukocyte function by lipoxygenase products of arachidonic acid. In: L. W. Chakrin and D. M. Bailey (Editors), The Leukotrienes: Chemistry and Biology. Academic Press, Orlando, pp. 231-245.

Prendergast, R. A. and Suzuki, M., 1970. Invertebrate protein simulating mediators of delayed hypersensitivity. Nature (London), 227:277-279.

Simon, P. L., 1984. Calcium mediates one of the signals required for interleukin 1 and 2 production by murine cell lines. Cell. Immunol., 87:720-726.

Snyder, D. S., Beller, D. I. and Unanue, E. R., 1982. Prostaglandins modulate macrophage Ia expression. Nature, 299:163-165.

Veterinary Immunology and Immunopathology, 12 (1986) 59—67
Elsevier Science Publishers B.V., Amsterdam — Printed in The Netherlands

MODULATION OF NONSPECIFIC HOST DEFENSES IN FISH

T. C. FLETCHER
N.E.R.C. Institute of Marine Biochemistry, St. Fittick's Road,
Aberdeen, AB1 3RA (U.K.)

ABSTRACT

Fletcher, T.C., 1986. Modulation of nonspecific host defenses in fish. Vet. Immunol. Immunopathol., 12: 59-67.

Seasonal, nutritional and hormonal effects on fish nonspecific protective mechanisms have been reviewed, together with the influence of some environmental pollutants. In the plaice (*Pleuronectes platessa* L.), the serum concentration of lysozyme and the acute phase reactant, C-reactive protein (CRP) and in vitro neutrophil migration have been used as indicators of the ability of test substances to modulate nonspecific defense mechanisms. Cortisol and adrenalin appear to be implicated in the production of CRP, and cortisol, at concentrations found in naturally stressed plaice, significantly reduces the migration of peritoneal neutrophils. Exposure to sub-lethal concentrations of inorganic mercury reduce circulating levels of lysozyme. The results provide further support for an association between environmental stressors and the disease susceptibility of fish populations. Phagocytic cell function, as measured by chemiluminescence, migration or phagocytic index, emerges as a useful test system.

INTRODUCTION

An awareness of the importance of nonspecific mechanisms of protection in fish is apparent in the work of Olivier et al. (1985), where macrophages appear to contribute to the protection elicited against *Aeromonas salmonicida* in coho salmon injected with adjuvant alone. The topic of phagocytic macrophages and neutrophils in fish has been reviewed by MacArthur and Fletcher (1985) and non-antibody humoral factors with a putative protective role, listed by Fletcher (1982). With few exceptions, experimentation has not been directed towards elucidating the mechanisms which modulate the production and functioning of these factors in fish. There can be little doubt however, that they will be influenced by the genetic constitution, age, sex, nutritional status and hormonal balance of the fish with the additional impact of environmental variables, both natural and man-induced (Sindermann, 1984). An example of the environmental modulation, of what must be recognised as a protective protein in fish, is provided by metallothionein. Not only is the synthesis of this protein induced by metals but fish from polluted areas have been found to be more resistant to heavy metals, suggesting adaptation to environmental contamination (Klaverkamp et al., 1984).

Most of the experiments described from our own work concern the responses of the plaice (*Pleuronectes platessa*). This demersal, marine flatfish is

0165-2427/86/$03.50 © 1986 Elsevier Science Publishers B.V.

readily available throughout the year from Scottish inshore waters and amenable to injection and blood sampling.

SEASON

The occurrence of disease in fish is often seasonal and can be due to influences not only on the host but also on the life cycle of the disease organism. Temperature is usually implicated in the seasonal incidence of disease because of its known effects on antibody production. In the summer flounder (*Paralichthys dentatus*), infected throughout the winter with *Trypanoplasma bullocki*, an increased trypanoplasmacidal lytic activity of the plasma was observed with elevated water temperature. This was responsible for the annual spring decline in the prevalence and eventual elimination of the hemoflagellate infection (Sypek and Burreson, 1983). In the plaice, circulating levels of lysozyme (Fletcher and White, 1976) and C-reactive protein (CRP: White et al., 1983) are at their highest in late summer, coincidental with the highest water temperatures and also with the peak condition of the plaice, following their active feeding period from March to October (White and Fletcher, 1985a). The total protein concentration of the serum is also highest in late summer (White et al., 1983) and the concentration of circulating antibody to metacercariae of a digenean parasite of the plaice has been observed to peak in October (Cottrell, 1977).

The seasonal pattern of CRP production in relation to cortisol levels in the plaice is shown in Fig. 1. Their cortisol levels reach a maximum during the peak spawning period (Wingfield and Grimm, 1977) but as cortisol can affect the immune response of fish (Anderson et al., 1982), then the importance of studying seasonal hormonal patterns is apparent.

Studies on the seasonal variation of the packed cell volume of plaice blood have been reported by Preston (1960) but no comparable examination of their leucocyte numbers or activities appears in the literature. As an indicator of phagocytic efficiency and of reticuloendothelial activity, the kinetics of particle clearance from the circulation provides a useful measure. Russell et al. (1976) reported that circulating bacteriophage was more rapidly cleared from nurse sharks in the summer than in the winter period. This was mainly due to the enhancing effect of the antibody produced at the higher temperatures because MacArthur et al. (1983) found no significant difference in the rate at which abiotic particles were cleared from plaice acclimated at 5°, 12° and 19°C. This would suggest that phagocytosis is relatively temperature insensitive and can function at periods when antibody production is slow. Sypek and Burreson (1983) observed active phagocytosis

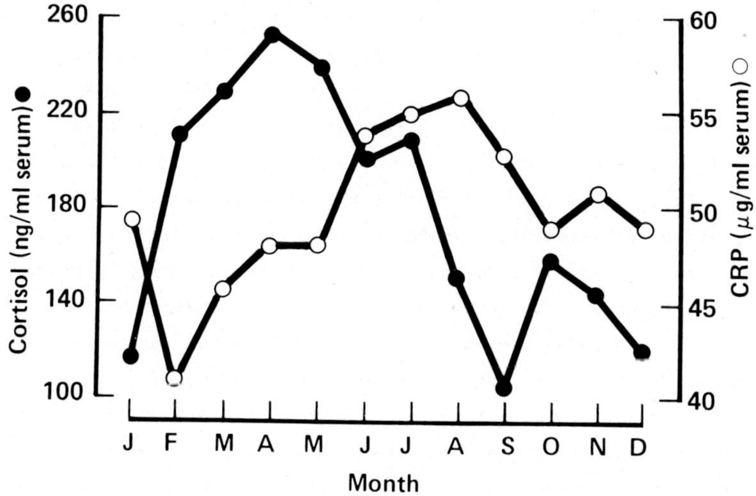

Fig. 1. Seasonal serum levels of C-reactive protein and cortisol in plaice between January (J) and December (D). Values plotted from White et al. (1983) and White and Fletcher (1984).

of Trypanoplasma in summer flounders at 5°C that did not display lytic activity in their plasma at this temperature.

NUTRITION

The late summer condition peak and elevated serum protein levels described above, reflect the nutritional status of wild plaice. It appears axiomatic that a well fed fish is a healthy fish and for cultured animals this means the formulation of nutritionally balanced diets, if protective factors are to be synthesized and cell function maintained. Cho (1983) has summarized the recommended nutrient levels for salmonid diets, together with a list of 68, mainly histopathological, nutritional deficiency signs in finfish. Few studies however, have examined dietary influences on immunity and nonspecific protective factors in fish.

Ascorbic acid and α-tocopherol appear to be the only dietary constituents so far examined for their role in immunity in fish. Durve and Lovell (1982) found that levels of ascorbic acid higher than the minimum dietary requirement for normal growth provided increased resistance in channel catfish fingerlings to the pathogenic bacterium Edwardsiella tarda, especially at low temperatures. Li and Lovell (1985) extended these studies, demonstrating the important role that dietary vitamin C can have on nonspecific defense mechanisms. The sera of channel catfish fed an ascorbic acid-deficient diet had significantly lower levels of complement hemolytic activity than those of fish fed diets supplemented with 30-300 mg ascorbic acid/Kg, with megadoses (3000 mg/Kg) almost doubling the rate of activity found at 30-300 mg. Ascorbic acid deficiency also significantly reduced the number of bacteria engulfed by blood phagocytes although supplementation at 30-3000 mg/Kg gave similar enhancement. Ascorbic acid deficiency did not however affect the intracellular bactericidal activity of the phagocytes. Blazer and Wolke (1984) working with rainbow trout, showed that resident peritoneal macrophages from fish fed a diet deficient in α-tocopherol for 16 weeks, exhibited significantly decreased phagocytosis of latex beads.

There has been increasing interest in the role of dietary lipids in the mammalian immune response (Johnston and Marshall, 1984). This interest does not yet seem to have extended to fish, although experimentation could give further support for the concept that nutrition influences immunity in fish. Deficiencies in dietary polyunsaturated fatty acids have marked effects on the mortality and pathology of turbot (Bell et al., 1985). A study of the functioning of defense mechanisms in fish fed diets of various fatty acid composition would provide a useful adjunct to the elucidation of immunity in ectotherms and a possible means of manipulating their protective systems.

HORMONES

The homeostatic systems of fish are continuously challenged by the demands of the aquatic environment and the primary response to stressors involves the release of catecholamines and corticosteroids (Wedemeyer et al., 1984). Cortisol is the major corticosteroid in the plaice (White and Fletcher, 1984) and we have studied its effects on CRP production and phagocytic function.

The lipopolysaccharide endotoxins extractable from the cell wall of gram-negative bacteria, cause an increase in the concentration of both circulating CRP (White et al., 1981) and cortisol (White et al., 1984) in the plaice, within 24h of an i.p. injection. Cortisol also stimulates CRP production directly (White and Fletcher, 1982) and the possibility therefore exists that CRP levels are controlled by cortisol. We have not however, been able to confirm this attractive hypothesis (White and Fletcher, 1985b). There does not appear to be any dose response of CRP to injected cortisol or correlation between circulating cortisol and CRP levels. Also, ACTH which caused significant elevation of cortisol, did not stimulate CRP. If cortisol is involved in CRP control, then it is probably as part of a chain of reactions that could involve interleukins (White and Fletcher, 1985b) and prostaglandins (White et al., 1984). Adrenalin also causes a significant elevation of CRP and cortisol levels (White and Fletcher, 1985b) so that hormonal factors are convincingly implicated at some stage of acute phase protein production in fish.

TABLE I
Effect of cortisol on in vitro migration of plaice peritoneal inflammatory neutrophils

Preincubation concentration of cortisol (ng/ml)	No. of cells moving through filter†	
	Randomly	10^{-6}M FMLP gradient
0	1029 ± 36	1269 ± 53
200	684 ± 135	757 ± 124
400	450 ± 12*	508 ± 20*
600	727 ± 27*	815 ± 73*

† mean cell numbers per 10 high power fields ± s.e.m. (3 experiments: each in triplicate)
* $p < 0.001$ compared with controls

The effects of cortisol on leucocyte function in the plaice are more clearcut. MacArthur et al. (1984) found that cortisol injection and environmentally-induced stress, caused a significant reduction ($p < 0.01$) in the total leucocyte numbers present in the peritoneal cavity of plaice, 3 days after the induction of an inflammatory response with glycogen. We therefore investigated the effect of cortisol on leucocyte migration in vitro. In collaboration with K. A. Nash and using the system described by Nash, Fletcher and Thomson (this volume), glycogen-induced inflammatory neutrophils, harvested from the peritoneal cavity of plaice, were incubated with 0, 200, 400 or 600 ng cortisol/ml for 1.5h at 12°C. The cells were then washed, resuspended in Gey's solution and assayed in a microchamber against Gey's solution or 10^{-6}M N-formylmethionyl-leucyl-phenylalanine (FMLP). Table I shows that incubation with 400 and 600 ng cortisol/ml caused significant ($p < 0.001$) reduction in both random and peptide-induced migration, compared with controls. Cortisol at 400 ng/ml was also significantly more inhibitory than 600 ng. These results provide a possible explanation for the reduced inflammatory response found in stressed fish by MacArthur et al. (1984).

Another aspect of the role of cortisol in modulating nonspecific defense mechanisms of fish, is shown by the work of Stave and Roberson (1985) with phagocytic leucocytes from the pronephros of the striped bass (*Morone saxatilis*). Chemiluminescence of phagocytes can be used as a sensitive indicator of microbicidal activity. Stave and Roberson (1985) found that preincubation of the cells with cortisol at 280 μg/ml led to 80% suppression of the chemiluminescent response of phagocytes stimulated with *Aeromonas hydrophila*. Despite the use of non-physiological amounts of cortisol, their results give some indication that cortisol-induced suppression of microbicidal activity could contribute to the susceptibility of fish to disease following exposure to stressors. The concentration of 400 ng of cortisol found to be effective in our migration studies is comparable to levels found in stressed plaice (MacArthur et al., 1984).

POLLUTANTS

There is an extensive literature on the induction of pathological lesions in fish by experimental exposure to chemical contaminants but it is difficult to quantify the extent to which environmental stressors are responsible for the transformation of an infection into a disease. However, any reports of the impairment of the immune function of fish by pollutants adds to the growing evidence of the association between disease and environmental contamination (Sindermann, 1983). Examination of fish from naturally polluted areas and sublethal exposure in the laboratory yield the most relevant results because pollutants rarely cause an obvious fish kill and their action is usually much more insidious.

Weeks and Warinner (1984) have isolated kidney macrophages from the hogchoker (*Trinectes maculatus*) and the spot (*Leiostomus xanthurus*) taken from clean and polluted rivers. They found a significant reduction ($p < 0.05$) in the phagocytosis of killed bacteria by macrophages from fish taken from the polluted areas. Robohm and Nitkowski (1974) reported that cadmium at 12 ppm increased the rate of bacterial uptake by phagocytes in the liver and spleen of the cunner (*Tautogolabrum adspersus*) but significantly decreased the rates of bacterial killing.

Plaice have been exposed to mercury at 0.3 ppm as $HgCl_2$ and the effect on circulating lysozyme examined (Fletcher and White, unpublished observations). There was a steady decline in serum lysozyme over 7 days exposure and a concomitant lysozymuria. There was also a significant increase in spleen index by day 6 of exposure. Mercuric chloride has been reported as mitogenic on human lymphocytes (Caron et al., 1970) and as mercury is concentrated in the plaice spleen (Pentreath, 1976) the possibility exists that

$HgCl_2$ could stimulate proliferation of plaice splenic lymphoid tissue. Although we did not examine the phagocytes from our Hg-exposed plaice, a relevant report may be that of Malamud et al. (1985). They found that low levels of Hg (10-100 ng/ml) inhibit the respiratory burst of human neutrophils and suggest that this cation may compromise the normal protective functions of neutrophils.

CONCLUSIONS

A fact that has emerged from an examination of the literature, is the growing attention being directed towards phagocytic cells of fish. Phagocytosis is an important element in host defenses against invading micro-organisms and, as illustrated, phagocytic cell functions provide a useful experimental model for assessing the effects of pollutants and hormones on the nonspecific protective mechanisms of fish. Perhaps, because the protective role of many of the humoral factors is only putative, less attention appears to have been directed to understanding the mechanisms involved in their control. An awareness of the seasonal influences on the protective mechanisms of fish is becoming more apparent and should be recognised in the interpretation of results from fish collected at different times of the year.

REFERENCES

Anderson, D.P., Roberson, B.S. and Dixon, O.W., 1982. Immunosuppression induced by a corticosteroid or an alkylating agent in rainbow trout (Salmo gairdneri) administered a Yersinia ruckeri bacterin. Dev. Comp. Immunol., Suppl. 2: 197-204.

Bell, M.V., Henderson, R.J., Pirie, B.J.S. and Sargent, J.R., 1985 Effects of dietary polyunsaturated fatty acid deficiencies on mortality, growth and gill structure in the turbot, Scophthalmus maximus. J. Fish Biol., 26: 181-191.

Blazer, V.S. and Wolke, R.E., 1984. The effects of α-tocopherol on the immune response and non-specific resistance factors of rainbow trout (Salmo gairdneri Richardson). Aquaculture, 39: 1-9.

Caron, G.A., Poutala, S. and Provost, T.T., 1970. Lymphocyte transformation induced by inorganic and organic mercury. Int. Arch. Allergy Appl. Immunol., 37: 76-87.

Cho, C.Y., 1983. Nutrition and fish health. In: F.P. Meyer, J.W. Warren and T.G. Carey (Editors), Health Management in the Great Lakes Basin. Great Lakes Fishery Commission, Ann Arbor, Michigan, pp. 63-73.

Cottrell, B., 1977. The immune response of plaice (Pleuronectes platessa L.) to the metacercariae of Cryptocotyle lingua and Rhipidocotyle johnstonei. Parasitology, 74: 93-107.

Durve, V.S. and Lovell, R.T., 1982. Vitamin C and disease resistance in channel catfish (Ictalurus punctatus). Can. J. Fish. Aquat. Sci., 39: 948-951.

Fletcher, T.C., 1982. Non-specific defence mechanisms of fish. Dev. Comp. Immunol., Suppl. 2: 123-132.

Fletcher, T.C. and White, A., 1976. The lysozyme of the plaice *Pleuronectes platessa* L. Comp. Biochem. Physiol., 55B: 207-210.

Johnston, D.V. and Marshall, L.A., 1984. Dietary fat, prostaglandins and the immune response. Prog. Food Nutr. Sci., 8: 3-25.

Klaverkamp, J.F., Macdonald, W.A., Duncan, D.A. and Wagemann, R., 1984. Metallothionein and acclimation to heavy metals in fish: a review. In: V.W. Cairns, P.V. Hodson and J.O. Nriagu (Editors), Contaminant effects on fisheries. John Wiley and Sons, Chichester/New York, pp. 99-113.

Li, Y. and Lovell, R.T., 1985. Elevated levels of dietary ascorbic acid increase immune responses in channel catfish. J. Nutr., 115: 123-131.

MacArthur, J.I. and Fletcher, T.C., 1985. Phagocytosis in fish. In: M.J. Manning and M.F. Tatner (Editors), Fish Immunology. Academic Press, New York/London, pp. 29-46.

MacArthur, J.I., Fletcher, T.C., Pirie, B.J.S., Davidson, R.J.L. and Thomson, A.W., 1984. Peritoneal inflammatory cells in plaice, *Pleuronectes platessa* L.: effects of stress and endotoxin. J. Fish Biol., 25: 69-81.

MacArthur, J.I., Fletcher, T.C. and Thomson A.W., 1983. Distribution of radiolabeled erythrocytes and the effect of temperature on clearance in the plaice (*Pleuronectes platessa* L.). J. Reticuloendothel. Soc., 34: 13-21.

Malamud, D., Dietrich, S.A. and Shapiro, I.M., 1985. Low levels of mercury inhibit the respiratory burst in human polymorphonuclear leukocytes. Biochem. Biophys. Res. Commun., 128: 1145-1151.

Olivier, G., Evelyn, T.P.T. and Lallier, R., 1985. Immunity to *Aeromonas salmonicida* in coho salmon (*Oncorhynchus kisutch*) induced by modified Freund's complete adjuvant: its non-specific nature and the probable role of macrophages in the phenomenon. Dev. Comp. Immunol., 9: 419-432.

Pentreath, R.J., 1976. The accumulation of inorganic mercury from sea water by the plaice, *Pleuronectes platessa* L. J. exp. mar. Biol. Ecol., 24: 103-119.

Preston, A., 1960. Red blood values in the plaice (*Pleuronectes platessa* L.). J. mar. biol. Ass. U.K., 39: 681-687.

Robohm, R.A. and Nitkowski, M.F., 1974. Physiological responses of the cunner, *Tautogolabrus adspersus*, to cadmium. IV. Effects on the immune system. U.S. Dept. Commer., NOAA Tech. Rep. NFMS SSRF-681: 15-20.

Russell, W.J., Taylor, S.A. and Sigel, M.M., 1976. Clearance of bacteriophage in poikilothermic vertebrates and the effect of temperature. J. Reticuloendothel. Soc., 19: 91-96.

Sindermann, C.J., 1983. An examination of some relationships between pollution and disease. Rapp. P.-v. Réun. Cons. int. Explor. Mer., 182: 37-43.

Sindermann, C.J., 1984. Fish and environmental impacts. Arch. Fischereiwiss, 35: 125-160.

Stave, J.W. and Roberson, B.S., 1985. Hydrocortisone suppresses the chemiluminescent response of striped bass phagocytes. Dev. Comp. Immunol., 9: 77-84.

Sypek, J.P. and Burreson, E.M., 1983. Influence of temperature on the immune response of juvenile summer flounder, *Paralichthys dentatus*, and its role in the elimination of *Trypanoplasma bullocki* infections. Dev. Comp. Immunol., 7: 277-286.

Wedemeyer, G.A., McLeay, D.J. and Goodyear, C.P., 1984. Assessing the tolerance of fish and fish populations to environmental stress: the problems and methods of monitoring. In: V.W.Cairns, P.V.Hodson and J.O. Nriagu (Editors), Contaminant effects on Fisheries. John Wiley and Sons, Chichester/New York, pp. 163-195.

Weeks, B.A. and Warinner, J.E., 1984. Effects of toxic chemicals on macrophage phagocytosis in two estuarine fishes. Mar. Environ. Res., 14: 327-335.

White, A. and Fletcher, T.C., 1982. The effects of adrenal hormones, endotoxin and turpentine on serum components of the plaice (Pleuronectes platessa L.). Comp. Biochem. Physiol., 73C: 195-200.

White, A. and Fletcher, T.C., 1984. Radioimmunoassay of serum cortisol in the plaice. (Pleuronectes platessa L.). Gen. Comp. Endocrinol., 53: 410-417.

White, A. and Fletcher, T.C., 1985a. Seasonal changes in serum glucose and condition of the plaice, Pleuronectes platessa L. J. Fish Biol., 26: 755-764.

White, A. and Fletcher, T.C., 1985b. The influence of hormones and inflammatory agents on C-reactive protein, cortisol and alanine aminotransferase in the plaice (Pleuronectes platessa L.). Comp. Biochem. Physiol., 80C: 99-104.

White, A., Fletcher, T.C. and Pepys, M.B., 1983. Serum concentrations of C-reactive protein and serum amyloid P component in plaice (Pleuronectes platessa L.) in relation to season and injected lipopoly-saccharide. Comp. Biochem. Physiol., 74B: 453-458.

White, A., Fletcher, T.C., Pepys, M.B. and Baldo, B.A., 1981. The effect of inflammatory agents on C-reactive protein and serum amyloid P-component levels in plaice (Pleuronectes platessa L.) serum. Comp. Biochem. Physiol., 69C: 325-329.

White, A., MacArthur, J.I. and Fletcher, T.C., 1984. Distribution of endotoxin and its effect on serum concentrations of C-reactive protein and cortisol in the plaice (Pleuronectes platessa L.). Comp. Biochem. Physiol., 79C: 97-101.

Wingfield, J.C. and Grimm, A.S., 1977. Seasonal changes in plasma cortisol, testosterone and oestradiol-17β in the plaice, Pleuronectes platessa L. Gen. Comp. Endocrinol., 31: 1-11.

Veterinary Immunology and Immunopathology, 12 (1986) 69—74
Elsevier Science Publishers B.V., Amsterdam — Printed in The Netherlands

FURTHER STUDIES ON THE ALPHA-PRECIPITINS OF THE ATLANTIC SALMON (SALMO SALAR)

J.B. ALEXANDER and N. AL-SHAKARCHI

Department of Biological Sciences, University of Salford, Salford, M5 4WT, UK

ABSTRACT

ALEXANDER, J.B. and AL-SHAKARCHI, N., 1986. Further studies on the alpha-precipitins of the Atlantic salmon (*Salmo salar*). Vet. Immunol. Immunopathol., 12: 69-74.

The alpha-precipitins of the Atlantic salmon have been isolated by a combination of chromatography and gel filtration. A monospecific antiserum has been raised and this has been used to measure the concentration of the antigen in 925 fish sera by CELISA. The results were analysed for the effects of sex and disease state of the animal, time of year and year of collection, and the part of the UK from which they were collected. Significant differences were found in all cases.

The components of alpha-precipitin were investigated by the isoelectric focusing of pure alpha-precipitin, whole serum and serum heated for 18 h at 95 ^{o}C. Multiple banding occurred in the acid region of the gels; the number, relative strength and position of the bands depended upon the animal from which the serum was isolated.

INTRODUCTION

The serum of the Atlantic salmon (*Salmo salar*) contains a number of precipitins, with alpha- and beta-globulin mobilities, which react with extracts of fungi, bacteria, amylopectin and amylose (Alexander, 1976). The precipitins exist in serum as both monomer and polymer. The dominant protein in the alpha-region, alpha-precipitin, has a monomeric molecular weight of 170000 D and exists as a number of apparently antigenically identical forms (Alexander, 1982). The total concentration of those components which react with the constituents of soluble starch have been shown to vary according to the sex and state of health of the animal, the year and season of collection, and the location of the collection point (Alexander, 1976; 1980). These proteins are not unique to the Atlantic salmon and similar precipitins have been found in all species of vertebartes examined, although not necessarily in all members of the same species.

With the isolation of alpha-precipitin and the production of a monospecific antiserum in rabbits, it was decided to investigate further the concentration of

0165-2427/86/$03.50 © 1986 Elsevier Science Publishers B.V.

that protein in the serum of the Atlantic salmon.

MATERIALS & METHODS

Sera

The isolation of sera from the Atlantic salmon, the locations of the collection points and the techniques of immunoelectrophoresis, gel diffusion, and antiserum production in rabbits have been described elsewhere (Alexander, 1976; 1980; 1982).

Alpha-precipitin isolation

Alpha-precipitin was isolated by a combination of DEAE-cellulose chromatography and gel filtration. The pooled sera were dialysed against 20 mM phosphate buffer, pH 8, and applied to the top of a DE52-cellulose column (Whatman Chromedia) equilibrated in the same buffer. Components were eluted at 40 mlh^{-1} and 10 ml fractions were collected. Those fractions positive by gel diffusion for alpha-precipitin (47 to 66) were pooled, concentrated and dialysed against 100 mM sodium acetate buffer, pH 8. The pool was applied to the top of a Sephacryl S300 column (Pharmacia Fine Chemicals), 900 mm long by 15 mm diameter, and eluted at 10 mlh^{-1} with the same buffer. Those fractions which eluted between 100 and 150 ml were pooled, concentrated, and fractionated through the same column. The first few fractions, which contained protein, were found to be pure alpha-precipitin by immunoelectrophoresis.

Alpha-precipitin analysis

The concentration of alpha-precipitin was measured by the method of competition enzyme-linked immunosorbent assay (CELISA) developed by Yorde *et al.* (1976). The plates were coated with 50 ul, 5 $ugml^{-1}$ alpha-precipitin. The salmon sera were diluted either 1:4000 or 1:10000 and 100 ul were added to 100 ul of a 1:100 dilution of monospecific anti-alpha-precipitin.

After incubation for 2 h at room temperature the amount of unreacted anti-alpha-precipitin was measured by the ELISA test.

Isoelectric focusing

Isoelectric focusing was performed on whole sera, heated sera and isolated alpha-precipitin by the method of Gorg *et al.* (1980). The gel contained a mixture of ampholytes (Ampholine, Pharmacia Fine Chemicals) made as follows: pH 4 to 6, 0.02 ml; pH 5 to 7, 0.02 ml; pH 9 to 11, 0.04 ml; pH 3.5 to 11, 0.28 ml. Electrophoresis was carried out initially at 500 volts for 30 min, then at 1000 volts for 1 h and finally at 1500 volts for 30 min. The gels were maintained at 4 ^{o}C. They were stained with Coomassie brilliant blue R250 (BDH Ltd).

RESULTS

The concentration of alpha-precipitin was determined in the serum of some 925 fish collected from the rivers and estuaries of Lancashire, South-west England, Northern Ireland and Wales in the years 1967 to 1975, and from the sea off the North-west coast of Northern Ireland. A large number of these fish were infected with the disease ulcerative dermal necrosis (UDN) and/or *Saprolegnia*. The numbers, means and standard errors of the means are given in Table I. In all cases significant differences were obtained between the various subsets.

TABLE I
The mean concentration (mgml^{-1}), standard error of the mean (SE) and numbers of fish examined, analysed for sex and state of health, year and season of collection, and source.

Condition	Female animals			Male animals		
	n	mean	SE	n	mean	SE
Diseased	219	4.75	0.46	356	11.99	0.59
Year						
1968	39	1.39	0.30	19	2.47	0.75
1969	72	2.01	0.30	47	6.95	0.65
1970	38	12.66	1.04	31	18.76	3.13
1971	30	0.64	0.22	12	3.21	1.61
1972	34	8.46	1.77	65	18.60	2.20
1973	5	5.76	1.24	87	12.99	0.64
1974	5	7.33	1.21	96	10.05	0.38
Season						
Spring	6	0.54	0.36			
Summer	5	2.58	1.71	1	12.0	
Autumn	214	4.84	0.47	357	11.97	0.59
Location						
Lancashire	193	5.11	0.51	334	11.73	0.54
NI (Freshwater)	12	2.10	0.62	3	8.24	4.18
SW England	13	2.08	1.13	12	22.02	8.47
Wales	7	2.06	1.49	9	8.79	2.21
NI (Marine)*	102	55.33	4.86			

* the sex of these animals is not known

The isolated alpha-precipitin gave a number of bands in the acid region of the gels (Figure 1a) and these were not affected by heating at 95 ^{0}C for 18 h. When serum and heated serum were examined in similar gels it was found that the apparent changes in banding observed could be attributed to the denaturation of unrelated proteins. It can be seen in Figure 1b that the number of bands in heated sera and the relative strengths of the bands varied from animal to animal.

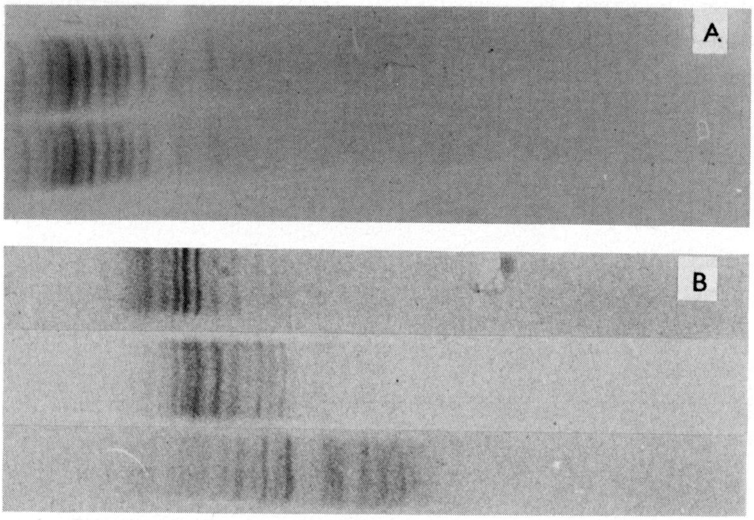

Fig. 1. Isolectric focusing results for (A) isolated alpha-precipitin and (B) heated serum from the Atlantic salmon to demonstrate the variations in the number and concentration of the different components.
The acidic end of the gel is to the left.

DISCUSSION

Alexander (1980) observed that the concentration of alpha-precipitin in serum varies significantly between the two sexes. The differences he found were smaller than those reported here. However, the amylopectin used by Alexander to measure the concentration does not react with all alpha-precipitin molecules. Therefore, the concentration measured will be lower than if a technique was used that measured the total concentration. The CELISA method used in the present study is such a technique. As the fish sera used in the two studies were subsets of the same population, it would appear that there are larger differences between the concentrations of the non-amylopectin-reacting components of alpha-precipitin than of those which do react with amylopectin.

Because of the differences between the sexes, it was necessary to analyse for the effects of other parameters in male and female fish separately. When this was done, the results were still very significant for the other parameters and so confirm the observations reported by Alexander (1980).

The dominant proteins in the sera of Atlantic salmon which react mainly with carbohydrate-containing antigens are alpha-precipitins. There is more than one alpha-precipitin and more than one component in this region which reacts with these antigens, because it has been found that sera which react with amylopectin do not react with fungal extracts and vice versa (Alexander, 1980). Also upon heating one of the two arcs produced in this region upon immunoelectrophoresis against the components of soluble starch disappears, although it has been demonstrated that alpha-precipitin is not affected by this treatment. Alexander (1982) showed that crude extracts of alpha-precipitin contained at least 7 components when subjected to isoelectric focusing. This has been confirmed by the results presented here using pure alpha-precipitin which have shown that alpha-precipitin contains at least 14 components.

The number of components present in individual fish varies from animal to animal. Also the relative concentration of the different components similarly varies. In fish infected with UDN and/or *Saprolegnia*, the number and concentration of the bands are much reduced. However, it is not possible at the moment to state whether this reduction is due to absorption by the antigens of the disease-causing agent or because the overall concentration is reduced resulting in weaker bands not being detected by the stain.

At the present it is not possible to say whether the variations between the relative strengths of the different components detected by isoelectric focusing and the differences in concentration found by CELISA are due to genetic variation between the individual fish or due to antigenic stimulation. However, work is in hand in an attempt to resolve this question.

The authors would like to acknowledge the ELISA facilities provided by Dr C. Smith of the North Wales Institute of Science and Technology.

REFERENCES

Alexander, J.B., 1976. The serum proteins of the Atlantic salmon (*Salmo salar*) with special reference to precipitins. PhD. thesis, University of Salford.

Alexander, J.B., 1980. Precipitins in the serum of the Atlantic salmon. Dev. Comp. Immunol., 4: 641 - 651.

Alexander, J.B., 1982. The antibody-mimetic precipitins of fish. Dev. Comp. Immunol., Suppl., 2: 133 - 138.

Gorg, A, Postel, W. and Westermeier, R., 1980. Ultrathin-layer protein mapping combining horizontal isoelectric focusing and horizontal electrophoresis in ultrathin-layer polyacrylamide gels on foils. Sci. Tools, 27: 14 - 18.

Yorde, D.E., Sasse, E.A., Wang, T.Y., Hussa, R.O. and Garancis, J.C., 1976. Competitive enzyme-linked immunoassay with the use of soluble enzyme/antibody complexes for labeling. I. Measurement of human choriogonadotropin. Clin. Chem., 22: 1372 - 1377.

Veterinary Immunology and Immunopathology, 12 (1986) 75—82
Elsevier Science Publishers B.V., Amsterdam — Printed in The Netherlands

PRELIMINARY STUDIES ON THE CHEMOTACTIC POTENTIAL OF DOGFISH (SCYLIORHINUS CANICULA) LEUCOCYTES USING THE BIPOLAR SHAPE FORMATION ASSAY

T.C. Hunt & A.F. Rowley

Biomedical & Physiological Research Group, School of Biological Sciences, University College of Swansea, Singleton Park, Swansea, SA2 8PP, U.K.

ABSTRACT

Hunt, T. and Rowley, A.F., 1986. Preliminary studies on the chemotactic potential of dogfish (*Scyliorhinus canicula*) leucocytes using the bipolar shape formation assay. Vet. Immunol. Immunopathol., 12: 75-82.

The bipolar shape formation assay, previously used to determine the chemotactic potential of various factors for mammalian leucocytes, was tested in the present study with granulocytes of the lesser spotted dogfish, *Scyliorhinus canicula*. Bipolar shape formation was found to be a temperature dependent process with maximal formation observed at 30°C. Addition of the formyl peptide, *N*-formyl-methionyl-phenylalanine failed to induce any bipolar forms at all temperatures and concentrations tested.

INTRODUCTION

For a cell to respond chemotactically, it must be capable of motility and thus be able to mobilize its locomotor machinery in response to a chemoattractant. Such a mobilization is often manifested by a change in cell shape. For example, cells usually elongate and align themselves in a chemical gradient with a broad lamellipodium anteriorly, and a narrower, often tapering uropod, posteriorly (Zigmond, 1977). Mammalian neutrophils when exposed to a chemoattractant are capable of exhibiting such changes in suspension (Jadwin et al., 1981). It has been shown, for example, that both human and dog neutrophils in suspension will assume a bipolar shape, in contrast to their normal spherical form, when exposed to known chemotactic factors (Jadwin et al., 1981; Stickle et al., 1985). Induction of bipolar shape formation (BSF) in cells by a particular factor may well be a reliable indicator of whether

0165-2427/86/$03.50 © 1986 Elsevier Science Publishers B.V.

that factor is chemotactic to those cells. Results obtained for human neutrophils using the BSF assay have corresponded to those from traditional chemotaxis assays such as the Boyden chamber. A positive result in the BSF assay for a particular factor usually correlates with a positive display of chemotaxis against the same factor and the converse is also true (Jadwin et al., 1981; Stickle et al., 1985). Thus, the BSF assay may be a rapid and simple method for evaluating the chemotactic potential of a putative chemoattractant and of assessing chemotactic function/dysfunction of a particular cell type.

Factors of bacterial origin are known to induce chemotaxis of mammalian leucocytes (Wilkinson, 1982) and these are probably one of the most fundamental stimuli such cells are likely to encounter. It has been demonstrated that certain chemotactic constituents of bacterial culture filtrates are structurally similar to synthetic formyl-methionyl peptides (Marasco and Becker, 1982) which are also potent chemoattractants for neutrophils of certain mammals (e.g. Schiffman et al., 1975).

Little is known about the effect of synthetic formyl-methionyl peptides upon fish leucocytes. Nash et al. (1986) described enhanced chemokinesis of plaice neutrophils upon exposure to *N*-formyl-methionyl-leucyl-phenylalanine, while Hunt and Rowley (in prep.) failed to demonstrate chemotaxis or chemokinesis of dogfish leucocytes to a range of concentrations of *N*-formyl-methionyl-phenylalanine (f-Met-Phe) using the migration under agarose assay of Nelson et al. (1975). Furthermore, Obenauf and Hyder Smith (1985) failed to observe chemotaxis of nurse shark leucocytes to bacterial culture filtrates.

The present study, using blood from the lesser spotted dogfish, *Scyliorhinus canicula*, was designed to investigate the potential of the BSF assay in determining the response of fish granulocytes to the synthetic peptide f-Met-Phe. This, in turn, will hopefully provide information on the chemotactic potential of the synthetic peptide for these cells.

METHODS

Test Chemotactic Factor

F-Met-Phe (Sigma Chemical Co. Ltd.) was used at a final concentration of either 2 x 10^{-7} M or 4 x 10^{-7} M respectively.

Blood Collection

Collection of dogfish was as described previously (Mainwaring and Rowley, 1985). The fish were subsequently maintained in large circular tanks containing continuously recirculating sea water at 15 ± 3°C and fed twice weekly on chopped plaice. Blood (0.9 ml) was taken from the caudal sinus using a 1 ml syringe containing 1.5 mg EDTA in 0.1 ml ice-cold Ca^{2+}/Mg^{2+} free elasmobranch saline (Mainwaring and Rowley, 1985). The syringe was then inverted several times to ensure thorough mixing of blood and anticoagulant, and the sample dispensed into a vial containing the f-Met-Phe. The blood was swirled to facilitate dissolution of the peptide and then incubated at either 15, 20, 25 or 30°C. Controls were run in an identical manner, but without the putative chemotactic factor. Following 10, 30 or 60 min incubation, blood smears were prepared, rapidly air-dried, fixed for 2-3 min in 95% methanol and stained with Wright's stain.

Granulocyte Shape Evaluation

Following incubation, the granulocytes were categorised as either spherical, amorphous or bipolar (see Jadwin et al., 1981), and the percentage frequency of each shape determined. A minimum of 100 G1 and G3 granulocytes (as classified by Morrow and Pulsford, 1980; Mainwaring and Rowley, 1985) were counted per smear. A Students t-test was used to determine the significance of paired means.

BSF Formation With Human Granulocytes

As a positive control, whole human blood collected from healthy volunteers, was tested against 2 x 10^{-7} M f-Met-Phe at 22°C.

RESULTS

Of the dogfish leucocytes, the two granulocytes designated G1 and G3 were regarded as the most likely contenders to respond in the BSF assay. This is because *in vitro* both cell types are adherent and are capable of locomotion (Mainwaring and Rowley, 1985). Consequently, these two cell types were examined in this assay.

It was found that in a normal blood smear 60.5 ± 5.1% (mean value ± SE, n=4) of G1 granulocytes are spherical, with a regular cell surface and no cytoplasmic blebs or protrusions. Such cells are therefore classified as spherical. The nucleus is eccentric and the cytoplasm is homogeneously filled with spherical

TABLE 1

Bipolar shape formation of dogfish G3 granulocytes incubated with 2×10^{-7} M f-Met-Phe at 30°C

Time (min)	Cell morphology (mean % frequency ± SE)					
	Spherical		Amorphous		Bipolar	
	F-Met-Phe	Control	F-Met-Phe	Control	F-Met-Phe	Control
0	53.0 ± 13.6[a]	49.6 ± 13.9	46.4 ± 13.8	49.1 ± 12.4	0.6 ± 0.1[b]	1.3 ± 0.1
10	17.6 ± 3.6	21.1 ± 2.9	65.4 ± 17.5	57.4 ± 11.9	17.0 ± 1.8[b]	21.5 ± 3.0
30	26.9 ± 3.1	20.4 ± 2.2	32.3 ± 3.7	37.5 ± 3.4	40.8 ± 3.2[b]	42.1 ± 5.2
60	36.0 ± 6.2	39.2 ± 3.9	48.5 ± 3.4	45.8 ± 4.3	15.5 ± 4.3[b]	15.0 ± 4.4

[a]n = 4 in all cases [b]No significant difference compared to control

eosinophilic granules. Bipolar shaped G1 granulocytes (Fig. 1) are only rarely seen in normal blood smears (<1%). These forms are elongated, constricted and polarized. At one pole is a lamellipodium, which usually contains the nucleus, and at the other end a long, often tapering uropod, sometimes with a light blue agranular cytoplasmic tip. Except for the tip of the uropod and a thin peripheral rim of ectoplasm the cytoplasm of the bipolar G1 contains granules. The G1 classified as amorphous, falls into

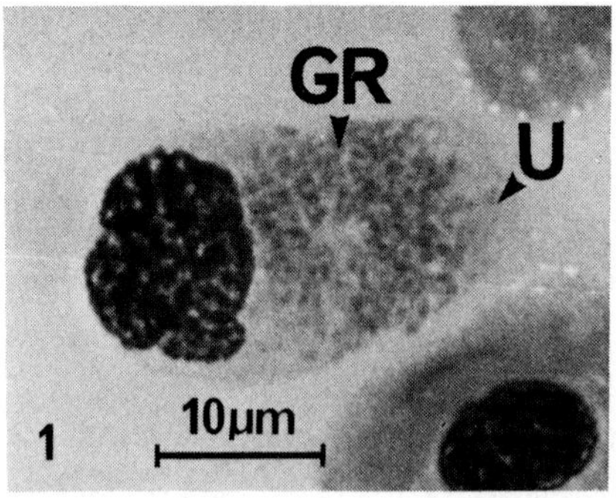

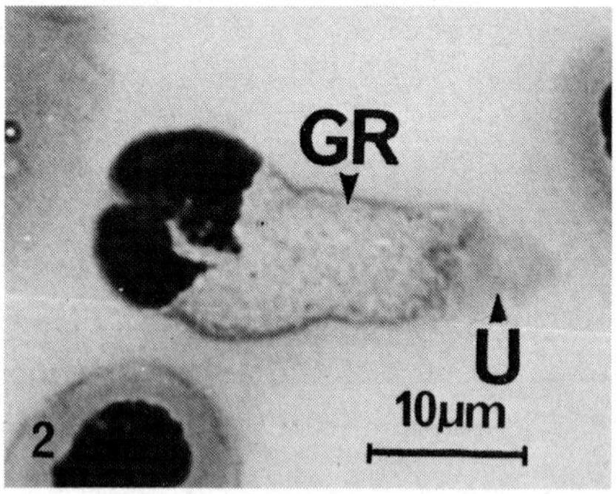

Fig. 1. Bipolar G1 granulocyte after 30 min incubation with f-Met-Phe. Note granules in cytoplasm (GR) and agranular uropod(U).

Fig. 2. Bipolar G3 granulocyte after 30 min incubation with f-Met-Phe. Granule mass(GR) and uropod(U).

neither of the two aforementioned categories and is usually an intermediary form. Often, amorphous G1s have prominent pseudopodia or cytoplasmic blebs and are markedly asymmetrical or distended in shape.

The spherical G3 granulocyte comprises ca. 53% of the normal G3s in smears (Table 1). The nucleus of these cells is polymorphic with up to five lobes and is peripherally situated in the cells. The cytoplasm is replete with elongate, eosinophilic granules. Bipolar forms (Fig. 2) are constricted and elongate and comprises ca. 1% of the normal G3 population in smears (Table 1). The nucleus is usually within the anterior lamellipodium and there is a long, frequently tapering uropod often with a protracted agranular cytoplasmic tip. The amorphous G3 granulocyte is distorted in shape compared to the spherical form and may possess cytoplasmic blebs and pseudopodia.

When blood was incubated with both concentrations of f-Met-Phe at 15, 20, 25 and 30°C, the numbers of G1 and G3 granulocytes assuming the bipolar shape was maximal at the highest temperature (Table 1 & 2). More significantly, there was no difference between the number of bipolar forms of either G1 or G3 granulocytes in the experimental and control smears at any of these temperatures (Table 2)

When blood was incubated with 2 x 10^{-7}M f-Met-Phe at 30°C there was an increase in the percentage frequency of G3 bipolar forms with time (Table 1). However, this increase was mirrored in the control smears and there was no significant difference between the two sets of results. Similar results (original data not presented here) were obtained using f-Met-Phe at a concentration of 4 x 10^{-7}M. Counts for BSF formation by G1 granulocytes at 30°C with both concentrations of f-Met-Phe revealed comparable trends (results not shown here). The only notable differences in the assumption of a bipolar shape by the G1 and G3 granulocytes was that the peak number of G3 bipolar forms was seen at 30 min followed by a decline, whereas maximal G1 bipolar forms were seen at 60 min. There was also a greater percentage frequency of bipolar G3s than of bipolar G1s at higher temperatures (Table 2). Finally, in control experiments human neutrophilic granulocytes tested alongside the dogfish cells showed elevated BSF in the presence of f-Met-Phe.

TABLE 2

Effect of temperature on bipolar shape formation of dogfish G1 and G3 granulocytes incubated with 2×10^{-7} M f-Met-Phe for 30 min

Temp (°C)	Cell morphology (mean % frequency ± SE)											
	G1 Granulocytes						G3 Granulocytes					
	Spherical		Amorphous		Bipolar		Spherical		Amorphous		Bipolar	
	f-Met-Phe	Control	f-Met-Phe	Control	f-Met-Phe	Control	f-Met-Phe	Control	f-Met-Phe	Control	f-Met-Phe	Control
15	58.0 ± 11.6[a]	53.1 ± 8.2	33.2 ± 9.7	39.5 ± 7.0	8.8 ± 7.0	7.4 ± 5.3	45.6 ± 12.4	48.8 ± 6.8	54.0 ± 3.1	49.8 ± 4.3	0.4 ± 0.6	1.4 ± 0.4
20	40.0 ± 12.4	37.6 ± 6.6	49.1 ± 15.6	47.8 ± 9.6	10.9 ± 3.2	14.6 ± 6.9	44.5 ± 11.7	43.0 ± 13.8	40.1 ± 13.4	38.1 ± 10.3	15.4 ± 4.8	18.9 ± 2.1
25	36.6 ± 7.3	38.6 ± 6.7	50.8 ± 8.7	48.0 ± 6.9	12.6 ± 5.4	13.4 ± 7.6	38.7 ± 4.4	34.6 ± 6.6	38.2 ± 7.0	45.1 ± 6.6	23.1 ± 8.1	20.3 ± 6.3
30	31.4 ± 8.7	35.1 ± 10.4	51.6 ± 4.1	48.7 ± 6.6	17.0 ± 5.1	16.2 ± 3.9	26.9 ± 3.1	20.4 ± 2.2	32.3 ± 3.7	37.5 ± 3.4	40.8 ± 3.2	42.1 ± 5.2

[a] n = 4 in all cases

DISCUSSION

The results show that both G1 and G3 granulocytes are capable of assuming a bipolar shape *in vitro*. This shape was most readily assumed however, at 30°C, a temperature outside the normal extremes likely to be encountered by dogfish. Bipolar shape formation does not appear to have been induced by the synthetic formyl peptide used, as the percentage of bipolar forms in the control groups was not significantly different. This was also the case when the assay was performed at lower temperatures i.e. 15, 20 and 25°C. Thus it seems that for dogfish granulocytes BSF is purely a temperature induced process. Experiments with dogfish monocytes gave similar results (Hunt and Rowley, unpub. observations) showing an apparent lack of reactivity to f-Met-Phe.

Neutrophils in human blood incubated at 22°C with 5 x 10^{-6}M f-Met-Phe showed a peak of 43.8% bipolar forms at 60 min after which their percentage frequency declined (Jadwin et al., 1981). This compares with the peak of 40.8% bipolar G3 granulocytes seen at 30 min in our assay, after which their percentage frequency also begins to decline. Such comparisons however, are somewhat misleading as in the study of Jadwin et al. (1981), very few (<2%) bipolar forms were seen in the controls.

Human neutrophils are known to possess receptors for *N*-formyl peptides (Williams et al., 1977) and can respond chemotactically to them (Schiffman et al., 1975) so their responsiveness in the BSF assay is a reflection of this. The lack of response to f-Met-Phe by the dogfish granulocytes is in agreement with our inability to demonstrate their chemotaxis to this same peptide by the migration under agarose assay (Hunt and Rowley, in prep.). This may be indicative of an absence of receptors for f-Met-Phe, which is not surprising, as even in mammals there are interspecies differences in the capacity to respond to various synthetic formyl peptides (Aswanikumar et al., 1977; Chenoweth et al., 1980; Stickle et al., 1985).

We are presently using the BSF assay to evaluate the potential chemotactic ability of a range of other factors. Initial results, however, have failed to demonstrate BSF following incubation with microbially-activated dogfish immune serum and plasma and this reflects similar findings using the chemotaxis under agarose method of Nelson et al. (1975). Further experiments are planned with other synthetic peptides and leukotriene B4.

Acknowledgements

We are grateful to the British Society for Immunology, the Royal Society and the organising committee for FISH for financial support.

REFERENCES

Aswanikumar, S., Corcoran, B., Schiffman, E., Day, A.R., Freer, R.J., Showell, H.J., Becker, E.L. and Pert, C.B., 1977. Demonstration of a receptor on rabbit neutrophils for chemotactic peptides. Biochem. Biophys. Res. Commun., 74: 810-817.

Chenoweth, D.E., Lane, T.A., Rowe, J.G., and Hugli, T.E., 1980. Quantitative comparisons of neutrophil chemotaxis in four animal species. Clin. Immunol. Immunopathol., 15: 525-535.

Jadwin, D.F., Smith, C.W. and Meadows, T.R., 1981. Neutrophil bipolar shape formation in whole blood. A simple and rapid method for the assessment of neutrophil leucocyte responsiveness. Am. J. Comp. Pathol., 76: 395-402.

Mainwaring, G. and Rowley, A.F., 1985. Separation of leucocytes in the dogfish (Scyliorhinus canicula) using density gradient centrifugation and differential adhesion to glass coverslips. Cell Tissue Res., 241: 283-290.

Marasco, W.A. and Becker, E.L., 1982. Anti-idiotype as antibody against the formyl peptide chemotaxis receptor of the neutrophil. J. Immunol., 128: 963-968.

Morrow, W.J.W. and Pulsford, A., 1980. Identification of peripheral blood leucocytes of the dogfish (Scyliorhinus canicula) by electron microscopy. J. Fish Biol., 17: 461-475.

Nash, K.A., Fletcher, T.C. and Thomson, A.W., 1986. Migration of fish leucocytes in vitro. Vet. Immunol. Immunopath. (this volume).

Nelson, R.D., Quie, P.G. and Simmons, R.L., 1975. A new and simple method for measuring chemotaxis and spontaneous migration of human polymorphonuclear leucocytes. J. Immunol., 115: 1650-1656.

Obenauf, S.D. and Hyder Smith, S., 1985. Chemotaxis of nurse shark leucocytes. Dev. Comp. Immunol., 9: 221-230.

Schiffman, E., Corcoran, B.A. and Wahl, S.M., 1975. N-Formyl-methionyl peptides are chemotactic for leucocytes. Proc. Natl. Acad. Sci. U.S.A., 72: 1059-1062.

Stickle, J.E., Kwan, D.K. and Smith, C.W., 1985. Neutrophil function in the dog: shape change and response to a synthetic tripeptide. Am. J. Vet. Res., 46: 225-228.

Wilkinson, P.C., 1982. Chemotaxis and Inflammation. Churchill Livingstone, 2nd edn., Edinburgh/London/Melbourne/New York, 249pp.

Williams, L.T., Snyderman, R., Pike, M.C. and Lefkowitz, R.J., 1977. Specific receptor sites for chemotactic peptides on human polymorphonuclear leucocytes. Proc. Natl. Acad. Sci. U.S.A., 74: 1204-1208.

Zigmond, S.H., 1977. Ability of polymorphonuclear leucocytes to orient in gradients of chemotactic factors. J. Cell Biol., 75: 606-616.

Veterinary Immunology and Immunopathology, 12 (1986) 83—92
Elsevier Science Publishers B.V., Amsterdam — Printed in The Netherlands

MIGRATION OF FISH LEUCOCYTES IN VITRO: THE EFFECT OF FACTORS WHICH MAY BE INVOLVED IN MEDIATING INFLAMMATION

K.A.NASH[a], T.C.FLETCHER[a], and A.W.THOMSON[b]
[a]N.E.R.C., Institute of Marine Biochemistry, Aberdeen AB1 3RA.
[b]Department of Pathology, University of Aberdeen, Aberdeen, AB9 2ZD, U.K.

ABSTRACT

Nash, K.A., Fletcher,T.C. and Thomson, A.W., 1986. Migration of fish leucocytes in vitro: the effect of factors which may be involved in mediating inflammation. Vet. Immunol. Immunopathol., 12: 83-92.

Plaice (Pleuronectes platessa L.) neutrophils were isolated from the kidney on a discontinuous Percoll gradient and from the peritoneal cavity at the peak of a glycogen-elicited inflammatory response. The migratory ability of neutrophils was assessed using a 48-well microchemotaxis chamber, with an incubation of 1.5 h at 12°C.

The two neutrophil populations showed different responses to N-formylmethionyl-leucyl-phenylalanine (FMLP). Whereas kidney neutrophils only showed a significant enhancement of migration at 10^{-7} M, inflammatory neutrophils exhibited a bimodal response, with one peak of migratory activity at 10^{-9} M and a second at $>10^{-6}$ M.

Kidney neutrophils showed a consistent response with various concentrations of a 24 h culture supernatant of Vibrio alginolyticus. In every case increased migration was observed with 5-, 10- and 100-fold dilutions, with the latter two conditions producing a significant enhancement ($p<0.01$ and $p<0.05$ respectively). The undiluted and 2-fold diluted supernatant caused a decreased cell migration compared with control values.

The supernatant from kidney neutrophils cultured with serum-opsonized, heat-killed V. alginolyticus produced greater migratory activity than neutrophils or the treated bacteria incubated alone (the controls). In each case, the enhanced activity of the supernatant was detectable by 1 h of incubation. By 4 h, the activity of the neutrophil/bacteria supernatant was significantly higher than that of the controls ($p<0.01$), but by 24 h had fallen to control levels.

There was no evidence for a chemotactic response with FMLP, the bacterial supernatant or the neutrophil-derived factor and the responses were therefore assumed to be chemokinetic.

INTRODUCTION

Migration of leucocytes from the blood or surrounding tissue to a site of

0165-2427/86/$03.50 © 1986 Elsevier Science Publishers B.V.

infection or tissue damage is a crucial step in inflammation since it is these cells that provide the effector role in the response. A study of the conditions that affect leucocyte migration can therefore contribute to the understanding of inflammation as a whole.

Leucocyte migration can be assessed both in vivo (reviewed by Issekutz, 1983) and in vitro (for review: Wilkinson, 1982; Gee, 1984), although, assessing migration in vitro can give greater control over the assay conditions and thus, be potentially more informative. However, it is only since Boyden (1962) first described a simple, reproducible assay that the study of leucocyte migration in vitro has become wide-spread. There is now a vast amount of published work in this field (Wilkinson, 1982), although, understandably, most of this has been devoted to mammalian systems.

To our knowledge, there are only three independent reports on the chemotactic/kinetic migration of fish leucocytes in vitro. Obenauf and Hyder Smith (1985) found that blood granulocytes from the nurse shark (Ginglymostoma cirratum) responded with enhanced migration to endotoxin-activated (E-A) rat serum, E-A nurse shark serum and a partially purified nurse shark complement pool. However, whereas the response appeared to be chemotactic to the E-A rat serum, the response to E-A shark serum was only chemokinetic. In the rainbow trout (Salmo gairdneri) blood neutrophils appeared to show enhanced, chemotactic migration to heat-treated immune serum containing Aeromonas salmonicida with fresh serum as a complement source (Griffin, 1984) . MacArthur et al. (1985) found that peritoneal neutrophils and splenic macrophages from the plaice (Pleuronectes platessa) showed enhanced migration to E-A plaice serum and peritoneal exudate fluid, although no evidence of a chemotactic response was found. These data show that fish leucocytes can respond to an activatable serum component, possibly part of the complement cascade. There appears to be little evidence, however, to suggest that fish leucocytes can respond to other substances possibly important in mediating inflammation. Thus, the aim of this study was to investigate the migration of plaice neutrophils in the presence of N-formylmethionyl-leucyl-phenylalanine (FMLP : a synthetic compound based on bacterial peptide products), Vibrio alginolyticus culture supernatant and a neutrophil product; factors that are likely to be involved in the regulation of the inflammatory response.

MATERIALS AND METHODS

Experimental animals

Plaice were caught off the east coast of Scotland and maintained in an aquarium in recirculating seawater at 12°C.

Cell preparation

Tissue leucocytes were obtained by gently disrupting the whole kidney over a nylon mesh and the resulting suspension allowed to stand for 5 min on ice to remove large cell clumps and tissue debris. The remaining suspension was then layered over a one step discontinuous Percoll gradient (1.060 and 1.075 g/ml) and spun for 40 min at 400g (4°C). The interface cells were washed and resuspended in plaice Ringer (containing penicillin G 40 U/ml and streptomycin 7.35 U/ml). Peritoneal exudate cells (PEC) were harvested three days after an ip injection of 3 ml 10% w/v oyster glycogen (BDH Chemicals Ltd., Poole, U.K.) using the method of MacArthur et al. (1984) with the following modifications. The peritoneal cavity was lavaged with 4 ml of 5 U/ml heparin (preservative-free) in plaice Ringer, the fish being bled by caudal venipuncture before aspirating the peritoneal fluid. These procedures were found to minimise haemorrhagic contamination and clot formation of the peritoneal fluid. Both the kidney cells and the PEC comprised 70 - 90% neutrophils, as defined by PAS and Giemsa staining.

N-formylmethionyl-leucyl-phenylalanine (FMLP)

A stock solution was prepared by adding dimethyl sulphoxide (DMSO) to give an FMLP (Sigma chemicals Co. Ltd., Poole, U.K.) concentration of 10^{-2} M. This was further diluted with saline to a concentration of 10^{-4} M before storing at -20°C.

Bacterial culture supernatant

Vibrio alginolyticus was seeded into 10 ml of plaice Ringer (antibiotic free) to an initial density of about 10^{8} cfu/ml and left for 24 h at 12°C. The bacteria were then pelleted and the supernatant stored at -70°C until use. The control supernatant was obtained by pelleting the bacteria immediately afer inoculation.

Endogenous neutrophil factor production

Kidney neutrophils, at a final concentration of $5x10^{6}$ cells/ml, were incubated for 1, 2, 3, 4 and 24 h at $12^{o}C$ either with or without plaice serum-opsonized (60 min at $12^{o}C$), heat-inactivated (30 min at $60^{o}C$) *V. alginolyticus* (HO *Vibrio*) at a cell:bacteria ratio of 1:50. To ascertain the role of the inactivated bacteria, an incubation of the serum opsonized bacteria alone was also run. Lactate dehydrogenase (LDH) was determined as described in Sigma Technical Bulletin no. 500 (Sigma Chemical Co.).

Migration assay

A 48-well microchemotaxis chamber (Neuro Probe, Inc., Maryland, U.S.A.) was used to assess the migratory activity of the neutrophils. The lower wells of the apparatus were filled with 26 µl of test substance and then covered with a polyvinylpyrrolidone-free, nitrocellulose filter (3 µm pore size). The upper wells were placed in position and 45 µl of cell suspension ($4x10^{6}$ cells/ml for the kidney cells and $2x10^{6}$ cells/ml for the inflammatory cells) added. The apparatus was incubated for 90 min at $12^{o}C$ (conditions which appeared to give an optimal response). After incubation, the apparatus was dismantled and the non-migrated cells on the upper surface of the filter removed. The filter was then air-dried, fixed for 60 min in methanol and stained with 10% Giemsa (BDH Chemicals, Poole, U.K.). The number of cells attached to the lower surface (i.e. the migrated cells) was assessed for each individual well by counting the number of neutrophils in 10 high power fields (HPF) at x400 magnification. The cells obtained from individual fish were tested separately and assayed in triplicate in as many of the test conditions as possible. Each condition was tested using the cells from 5 different fish, and a mean and standard error calculated.

Chemotaxis/kinesis assay

Whether the cells were responding tactically was assessed by observing the ability of the cells to detect the direction of a gradient of test substance by the way they orientated in the gradient. This was done using an orientation slide (Zigmond, 1977), incubated for 60 min at $12^{o}C$ (conditions found to give optimal results). The response was quantified by comparing the number of cells orientating in the 180° sector towards the test source, with the number of cells showing orientation in any direction (excluding those at right angles to the test gradient).

RESULTS

Migration to FMLP

Fig. 1 shows that the responses of the two cell populations differ, with kidney neutrophils showing a single peak of activity and inflammatory neutrophils revealing a more complex, bimodal response. Unfortunately, the responses to FMLP concentrations greater than 10^{-6} M could not be reliably ascertained due to the interference of the DMSO, used to dissolve the FMLP.

Using the orientation slide, the percentage number of cells orientating towards the FMLP source for the kidney neutrophils was 51% $\pm$ 2 (n=5) and for the inflammatory neutrophils was 56% $\pm$ 2 (n=5). These values were for a gradient of 0 - 10^{-6} M FMLP and were the highest for any of the conditions used. These results show no significant difference from that which would be expected if the cells were orientating randomly in the gradient (i.e. 50%). Thus, no evidence was found for a chemotactic response to FMLP for either of the cell populations.

V. alginolyticus culture supernatant

Fig. 2 shows that significant enhancement of migration occurs with the supernatant at low concentrations. With undiluted and 2-fold dilutions (i.e. concentrations of 50 - 100%) the response was always lower than that for the control supernatant.

No significant deviation from random orientation was found with the supernatant using the orientation slide. Thus, again providing no evidence of chemotaxis.

Endogenous neutrophil attractants

The supernatant produced by kidney neutrophils cultured with HO Vibrio produced an enhanced migration of neutrophils, compared with cells cultured alone. That the active factor(s) in the supernatant were not due solely to the HO Vibrio was shown by incubating the bacteria alone (data not shown). The active factor(s) in the supernatant were unlikely to have been released from damaged or dead cells since the cytosol marker, (LDH), remained constant throughout the period of the incubations.

Despite the lack of a significant difference, there was in every case detectable activity in the supernatant by 1 h of incubation, which had reduced to control levels by 24 h.

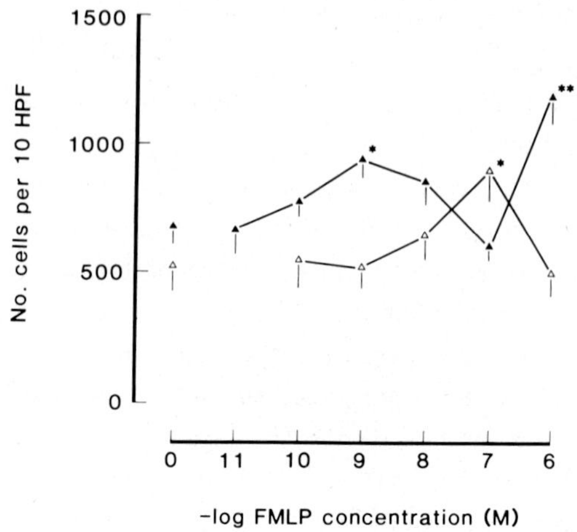

Fig. 1. The effect of various concentrations of FMLP on the migratory activity of inflammatory neutrophils used at 2×10^6 cells/ml (▲——▲), and kidney neutrophils used at 4×10^6 cells/ml (△——△). Each point represents the mean ± S.E.M. of 5 fish. *$p<0.05$; **$p<0.01$, compared with media alone.

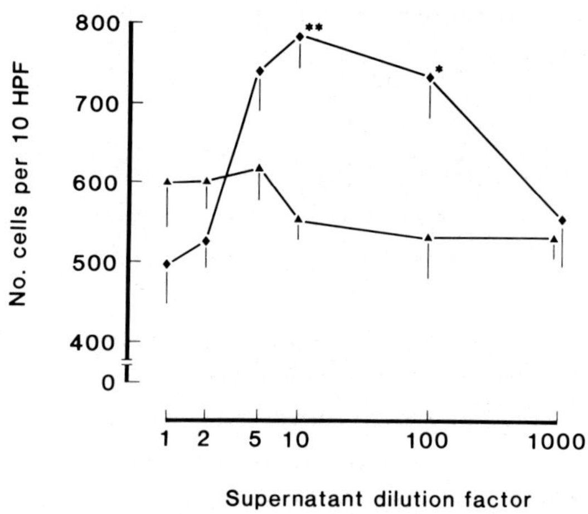

Fig. 2. The effect on the migration of kidney neutrophils of the 24 h *V. alginolyticus* culture supernatant (◆——◆) and the control supernatant (▲——▲). *$p<0.05$; **$p<0.01$.

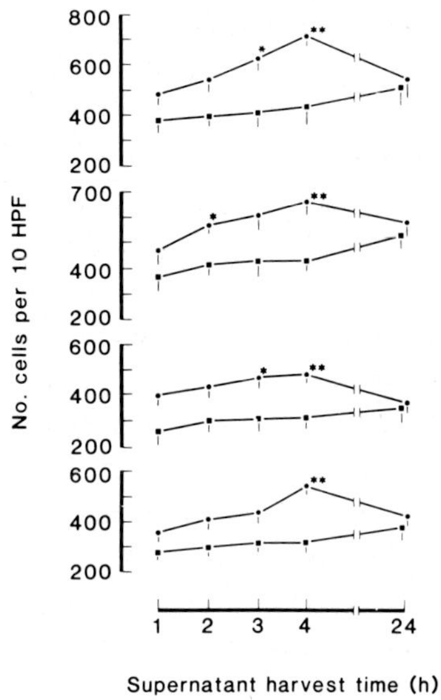

Fig. 3. The effect on kidney neutrophil migration of supernatants harvested at various time from the kidney neutrophil - HO *Vibrio* culture (●——●) and from the neutrophils cultured alone (■——■). The 4 graphs represent supernatant produced by the cells of 4 different fish. Each point represents the mean no. of cells migrating ± S.E.M. from 5 fish. *$p<0.05$; **$p<0.01$.

As with the other attractants tested, no significant difference from random orientation was observed.

DISCUSSION

The underlying mechanisms mediating the infiltration to and the eventual emigration from the site of invasion during inflammation can be divided into two broad catagories: those where microbe-derived factors directly cause leucocyte accumulation at the focus, and those that are dependent on host-derived factors. Although this division is artificial in that both catagories will be, to some extent, interdependent on each other, it does help in the understanding of this complex response.

One substance that has attracted interest, since its first description as a potent modulator of leucocyte function, is FMLP (Showell et al., 1976). This substance was originally used as an analogue of bacterial peptide products, but it has recently been shown to be present in bacterial secretions (Marasco et al., 1984). The potency of this substance in mammalian systems can be illustrated by the fact that it produced an increase in migration of human blood PMN at concentrations as low as 10^{-9} M (Harvath et al. 1980). Our results, using the same assay system, show that 10^{-9} M FMLP can cause a significant enhancement of migration with plaice inflammatory neutrophils. With kidney neutrophils, the lowest active concentration of FMLP appears to be 100 times higher. This difference in response between the two neutrophil populations is not unique to the plaice. Mammalian inflammatory neutrophils showed a greater response than "unstimulated", blood-borne neutrophils at FMLP concentrations of 10^{-10} and 10^{-9} M (Keller and Cottier, 1984). For the mammalian cells, this difference seems to be due to a 6- to 7-fold increase in the binding of FMLP to inflammatory neutrophils compared with blood-borne neutrophils. Whether plaice cells have an FMLP receptor is unknown, but the difference in response of the two cell populations suggests that they do.

Since factors released by V. alginolyticus can cause enhanced migration of plaice neutrophils, one can expect such substances to be involved in mediating the infiltration of cells to the site of a bacterial invasion. However, at higher concentrations, the bacterial exudates cause a reduction in the apparent migration of the neutrophils. Whether this is due to inhibition of locomotion is not known, but it does suggest that different substances become predominant at higher concentrations (i.e. nearer the bacteria focus). Perhaps we see the effect of a cytotoxin such as that produced by Pseudomonas aeruginosa, which has been shown to cause several destructive effects on leucocyte function, including a reduction in migratory activity of the cells (Baltch et al., 1985). However, the interpretation of our results in terms of inflammation is unclear, although such a reduction in migration would provide a mechanism for trapping leucocytes at a bacterial focus.

There is now evidence that the host cells can also release chemicals in response to the invasion, capable of modulating leucocyte function, including migration. Mammalian PMN can be stimulated to release such factors (either of protein or leukotriene nature) by the presence of FMLP (Clancy et al. 1983), opsonized zymosan (Kurihara et al. 1984; Ishibashi and Yamashita, 1985), and the fungus Paracoccidiodes brasiliensis (Calich et al. 1985). This function appears to be present in fish, although, as yet the chemical nature of the factor(s) involved is unknown and requires further investigation.

Fig. 3 shows that although the supernatant appears to be active by 1 h of incubation, by 24 h the activity has decreased to control levels. This decrease cannot be explained in terms of stimulus removal, since phagocytosis by the kidney cells is not fast enough to remove a great many of the bacteria from the suspension. A possible explanation may be that the relevant factor(s) have a short half life and that by 24 h the constant invagination of the cell membrane during phagocytosis reaches a rate high enough to prevent any further release of the factor(s) into the medium. Alternatively, the rate of production of the factor(s) in the supernatant may remain constant, but as the concentration increases so the activity of the supernatant decreases, as with FMLP and the live bacteria culture supernatant. This therefore seems to be evidence for a negative feedback mechanism. There is evidence for a prostaglandin based negative feedback mechanism for several leucocyte functions in mammalian systems (Kunkel and Chensue, 1984). The effect of such a mechanism may well directly control migration as well as chemoattractant production. In the context of the inflammatory response, such mechanisms may be vital in the modulation of the underlying processes.

With the knowledge we now have on the mechanisms of acute inflammation in the plaice, we can begin to build a model for the infiltration of leucocytes. The initial inoculation of bacteria invading the tissue will produce chemoattractants which will draw neutrophils to the infection site. Perhaps simultaneously, neutrophils already present in the tissue will be stimulated to release their own factors. The output of chemoattractants will increase further as more neutrophils are attracted to the site, producing an avalanche effect, characteristic of many immune processes. Once the invasion has been contained, the response will be gradually shut down by some form of negative feedback mechanism, thus preventing unnecessary damage to the hosts own tissue by a prolonged inflammatory response.

This highly simplified and incomplete model draws attention to several questions. For example, how long after the initial microbial invasion are the attractants first active in the tissue and are they bacteria or host derived? How do the different substances produced by the host leucocytes and the invaders integrate within the response with time? When does the shut down of the host response begin, and does the microbe and its products have a role in it? These and other questions are not just relevant immunologically, but also to the understanding of the evolution of host-parasite relationships.

ACKNOWLEDGEMENTS

We thank Mr. J.W.Adron for making the orientation slides, and also the Natural Environment Research Council for their grant to K.A.N.

REFERENCES

Baltch, A.L., Hammer, M.C., Smith, R.P., Obrig, T.G., Conroy, J.V., Bishop, M.B., Egy, M.A. and Lutz, F., 1985. Effects of Pseudomonas aeruginosa cytotoxin on human serum and granulocytes and their microbicidal, phagocytic, and chemotactic functions. Infection and Immunity, 48: 498-506.

Boyden, S.V., 1962. The chemotactic effect of mixtures of antibody and antigen on polymorphonuclear leucocytes. J. exp. Med., 115:453-466.

Calich, V.L.G., Vaz, C.A.C. and Burger, E., 1985. PMN chemotactic factor produced by glass-adherent cells in the acute inflammation caused by Paracoccidioides brasiliensis. Br. J. exp. Path., 66: 57-65.

Clancy, R.M., Dahinden, C.A. and Hugli, T.E., 1983. Arachidonate metabolism by human polymorphonuclear leukocytes stimulated by N-formyl-met-leu-phe or complement component C5a is independent of phospholipase activation. Proc. Natl. Acad. Sci. USA., 80: 7200-7204.

Gee, A.P., 1984. Advantages and limitations of methods for measuring cellular chemotaxis and chemokinesis. Molecular and Cellular Biochemistry, 62: 5-11.

Griffin, B.R., 1984. Random and directed migration of trout (Salmo gairdneri) leukocytes: activation by antibody, complement, and normal serum components. Dev. Comp. Immunol., 8: 589-598.

Harvath, L., Falk, W. and Leonard, E.J., 1980. Rapid quantitation of neutrophil chemotaxis: use of a polyvinylpyrrolidone-free polycarbonate membrane in a multiwell assembly. J. Immunol. Methods., 37: 39-45.

Ishibashi, Y. and Yamashita, T., 1985. Purification and characterization of a phagocytosis-stimulating factor from phagocytosing polymorphonuclear neutrophils: comparison with granule basic proteins. Infection and Immunity, 48: 799-805.

Issekutz, A.C., 1983. Quantitation of acute inflammation in the skin: recent methodological advances and their application to the study of inflammatory reactions. Surv. Synth. Path. Res., 1: 89-110.

Keller, H.U. and Cottier, H., 1984. Comparison of locomotion, chemotaxis and adhesiveness of rabbit neutrophils from blood and peritoneal exudates. Blood Cells, 10: 45-57.

Kunkel, S.L. and Chensue, S.W., 1984. Prostaglandins and the regulation of immune responses. In: I. Otterness, R. Capetola and S. Wong (editors), Advances in inflammation Research, Vol 7, Raven Press, New York, pp. 93-108.

Kurihara, A., Ojima, F. and Tsurufuji, S., 1984. Chemotactic factor production by rat polymorphonuclear leukocytes: stimulation with opsonized zymosan particles and inhibition by dexamethazone. Biochem. Biophys. Res. Comm., 119: 720-725.

MacArthur, J.I., Fletcher, T.C., Pirie, B.J.S., Davidson, R.J.L. and Thomson, A.W., 1984. Peritoneal inflammatory cells in plaice Pleuronectes platessa L; effects pf stress and endotoxin. J. Fish. Biol., 25: 69-81.

MacArthur, J,I., Thomson, A.W. and Fletcher, T.C., 1985. Aspects of leucocyte migration in the plaice, Pleuronectes platessa L. J. Fish. Biol., in press.

Marasco, W.A., Phan, S.H., Krutzsch, H. Showell, H.J., Feltner, D.E., Nairn, R., Becker, E.L. and Ward, P.A., 1984. Purification and identification of formyl-methionyl-leucyl-phenylalanine as the major peptide neutrophil chemotactic factor produced by Escherichia coli. J. Biol. Chem., 259:5430-5439.

Obenauf, S.D. and Hyder Smith, S., 1985. Chemotaxis of nurse shark leukocytes. Dev. Comp. Immunol., 9: 221-230.

Showell, H.J., Freer, R.J., Zigmond, S.H., Schiffmann, E., Aswanikumar, S., Corcoran, B. and Becker, E.L., 1976. The structure-activity relations of synthetic peptides as chemotactic factors and inducers of lysosomal enzyme secretion for neutrophils. J. exp. Med., 143: 1154-1169.

Wilkinson, P.C., 1982. Chemotaxis and Inflammation, 2nd edition. Chirchill Livingstone, Edinburgh/London/Melbourne/New York, 249pp.

Zigmond, S.H., 1977. Ability of polymorphonuclear leukocytes to orient in gradients of chemotactic factors. J. Cell Biol., 75: 606-616.

Veterinary Immunology and Immunopathology, 12 (1986) 93—105
Elsevier Science Publishers B.V., Amsterdam — Printed in The Netherlands

THE ONTOGENY OF HUMORAL IMMUNITY IN RAINBOW TROUT, SALMO GAIRDNERI

MARY F. TATNER

Institute of Aquaculture, University of Stirling, Stirling FK9 4LA, Scotland.

ABSTRACT

Tatner, M.F., 1986. The ontogeny of humoral immunity in rainbow trout, *Salmo gairdneri*. Vet. Immunol. Immunopathol., 12: 93-105.

The ontogeny of the humoral immune response to a 'thymus dependent' and a 'thymus independent' antigen, human gamma globulin (HGG) and *Aeromonas salmonicida* (AS) respectively, was investigated in the fry of rainbow trout, *Salmo gairdneri*, by direct immersion vaccination in the antigens (dose 5mg/L HGG; 10^8 cells/ml AS; 30 minutes) at known ages/weights from 7 days post hatch, and at 1, 2, 3, and 4 months post hatch. Half the fry in each group were tested for antibodies 4 weeks after vaccination, the remainder were reimmunised and tested again after a further 4 weeks. Appropriate controls to test for tolerance induction and memory responses were included. The results indicate that fry are capable of mounting a humoral immune response very early in ontogeny. There is a period of 'unresponsiveness' which persists for longer against HGG, than against AS, though it was not thought to be tolerance as such. Memory could be detected to HGG in fry given a first immunisation at 2 months. The results are compared with preliminary experiments in which fry were first thymectomised 4 weeks before the first immunisation. In fry thymectomised at 1 month post hatch, and tested for primary and secondary responses at 2 and 3 months, the primary response to HGG is unaltered, but the secondary response is reduced. Both the primary and secondary response to AS is unaltered. When thymectomy is performed later, the effect on the secondary response to HGG is no longer apparent, but the primary response to AS is slightly reduced.

INTRODUCTION

Several studies have been performed which indicate that fish, at an early stage in their development, can mount a humoral immune response to various antigens (Dorson, 1974; Paterson and Fryer, 1974; Khalifa and Post, 1976). In some cases, tolerance induction has been reported against antigens which are

0165-2427/86/$03.50 © 1986 Elsevier Science Publishers B.V.

thymus dependent in mammals. The soluble antigen, human gamma globulin (HGG) has been shown to be tolerogenic in rainbow trout fry (Secombes, 1981), although the period in which tolerance can be induced is of short duration (Mughal and Manning, 1985), and in carp, tolerance can be induced to sheep red blood cells (Van Loon et al., 1981). The ability to respond to different antigens develops sequentially, as Etlinger et al. (1979) have shown that the ability to respond to thymus independent antigens precedes that to thymus dependent antigens in trout.

The previous studies have involved injecting antigens. However, young fry are hatched into a hostile environment with an immature immune system, and it is of interest to see how they cope with antigens as they would naturally encounter them i.e. in the water. In order to study the natural development of the immune system, it was also felt to be important to conduct experiments at the rising water temperatures the fish would naturally encounter in their first few months of life. Two test antigens were chosen in the present study, human gamma globulin (HGG), a thumus dependent antigen, and *Aeromonas salmonicida* (AS), a thymus independent antigen, which were presented to fry of various ages and known weights by direct immersion immunisation. The primary and secondary responses were then monitored. The priming and challenge routes were both by direct immersion, as Lamers and de Haas (1985) have suggested that for memory to be established the routes must be the same. Also, tolerance might be induced by one route which might not be tested for if the challenge was by a different route. Appropriate controls were set up to test that any tolerance observed was specific. Since the immune response matures with age, any heightened response after secondary vaccination could simply be a reflection of this maturation and not a true memory effect. Therefore, at each reimmunisation, appropriate controls with fish of the same age and at the same temperature were included for comparison.

The effect of thymectomy on the ontogeny of immune responses in fish has received little attention, mostly due to the difficulty in thymectomising very young fry. Salendri (1973) thymectomised two month old *Tilapia mossambica* of 0.7g. After a further 2 months they were immunised with sheep red blood cells, and the plaque forming cell response was found to be totally abolished. In the present study, preliminary experiments were performed in which groups of rainbow trout fry were thymectomised by microcautery at 1, 2 and 3 months old, left for one month, and then their primary and secondary responses to HGG and AS were determined. The fry could be compared with intact fry receiving the immunisation schedule at the same age.

MATERIALS AND METHODS

Fish

Eyed ova of rainbow trout, *Salmo gairdneri*, were purchased from Clone Hatcheries, Auchterarder, Scotland, and hatched in the aquarium on stainless steel grids in flowing, aerated water. Fry from the same batch were then purchased at 1, 2, 3 and 4 months for use in later experiments, and maintained in small tanks with a flow through of water. The water temperature was monitored daily and rose from 4°C to 14°C by the end of the experiments.

Experimental Design

Starting with sac fry at 7 days post hatch, groups of 100 fish were immunised for 30 minutes in either HGG at a dose of 5mg/L (GpA); in formalin killed AS, strain 838, at a dose of 10^8 cells/ml (GpB) (the bacteria having been grown for 24h in brain heart infusion broth at 20°C); or 2 groups in bovine serum albumin at a dose of 5mg/L (GpC and GpD). The fry were maintained for one month, then half of GpA and half of GpB were sampled. The remaining fry of GpA, GpC fry, plus a further control group of fry of the same age/weight, GpE, were immunised with HGG as before. The remaining fry in GpB, GpD fry, plus a further control, GpF, were immunised with AS as before. All groups were maintained for a further 4 weeks, and then sampled. Hence, Gps A and B received two immunisations of HGG or AS respectively to test their primary and secondary responses. Gps C and D, initially immunised with BSA and then with HGG or AS acted as controls to test that any tolerance observed was specific. Gps E and F acted as controls to test that any heightened responses in Gps A and B following the second immunisation was a true memory effect and not simply a reflection of the increasing maturity of the response as the fish aged. At each immunisation, the average weight of the fish was recorded. The experimental design is illustrated in Fig. 1. The experiment was repeated 4 times, commencing with fry of 1, 2, 3 and 4 months post hatch.

First Immunisation at time x	Response at x + 4 weeks	Immunised at x + 4 weeks	Response at x + 8 weeks
Gp A (HGG)	1/2 Gp A	1/2 Gp A (HGG)	1/2 Gp A (HGG)
Gp B (AS)	1/2 Gp B	1/2 Gp B (AS)	1/2 Gp B (AS)
Gp C (BSA)		Gp C (HGG)	Gp C (AS)
Gp D (BSA)		Gp D (AS)	Gp D (AS)
		Gp E (HGG)	Gp E (HGG)
		Gp F (AS)	Gp F (AS)

Fig. 1. The Ontogeny of Humoral Immunity in Rainbow Trout

Sampling procedure and tests for antibody production

Since the fry were too small to bleed, samples were obtained by macerating whole fry (after emptying the gut contents) in 0.1ml 0.85% saline, and then pooling the macerates in groups of three. The samples were centrifuged, the supernatants decanted, and frozen until tested. Although this method of sampling introduces a dilution factor to any titre obtained, titres between groups could be compared as the dilution factor remained constant throughout the experiments. It has the advantage that not only serum antibody is included, but the spleen, kidney, gut and skin are also tested for any antibodies resulting from the direct immersion immunisation. The samples were serially diluted in microtitre plates and tested against HGG or AS as appropriate, using the passive haemagglutination and bacterial agglutination tests respectively. Titres were expressed as - Log 2. The number of positive samples within each group was noted.

Thymectomy experiments

Fry were thymectomised by microcautery at 1, 2 and 3 months post hatch, and maintained in tanks to which antibiotics had been added for 24h before being put on a flow through system. Mortalities were high; the % survival following thymectomy was 10% at 1 month, 43% at 2 months and 48% at 3 months. Thymectomised fish were weighed on immunisation one month later. There was no significant difference in weight between the thymectomised fish and control fish of the same age. Following immunisation, the fish were tested for their primary and secondary responses to HGG and AS, after a further 4 and 8 weeks. The experimental design is illustrated in Fig. 2.

Thymectomised	First Immunisation at time x	Response at x + 4 weeks	Immunised at x + 4 weeks	Response at x + 8 weeks
x - 4 wks	Gp 1 (HGG)	1/2 Gp 1	1/2 Gp 1 (HGG	1/2 Gp 1 (HGG)
	Gp 2 (AS)	1/2 Gp 2	1/2 Gp 2 (AS)	1/2 Gp 2 (AS)

Fig. 2. The Effect of Thymectomy on the Ontogeny of Humoral Immunity in Trout

Analysis of results

Significant differences in titre between groups were tested, where possible, using the students 't' test for nonpaired data.

RESULTS

Experiment 1 (Table 1)

Sac fry of 1 week post hatch which had been immunised with either HGG (GpA) or AS (GpB) had no detectable antibodies to HGG when tested at 1 month old though a slight response to AS was noted (3 out of 5 samples). After reimmunisation, the remaining fry were tested after a further month when they were 2 months old. No response to HGG was detected, neither was there a response in the GpC fry which had received BSA initially and then HGG. In the control 2 month old fry (GpE), a very slight response was noted (1 in 10 samples). The A. salmonicida GpB fish demonstrated a positive response on secondary immunisation, with GpD and GpF fish also showing positive titres, but there was no significant differences between the titres of GpB, GpD and GpF.

TABLE 1 Response of rainbow trout immunised at 1 week post hatch. Numbers in parentheses indicate number of positive samples

First immunisation 1 week post hatch Sac fry	Response at 1 month Mean titre		2nd Immunisation 1 month	Response at 2 months Mean titre	
HGG (GpA)	0	(0/5)	HGG	0	(0/15)
AS (GpB)	0	(3/5 neat)	AS	0.23 ± 0.83	(3/13)
BSA (GpC)			HGG	0	(0/4)
BSA (GpD)			AS	0.80 ± 0.30	(4/5)
			HGG(GpE)	0.20 ± 0.63	(1/10)
			AS (GpF)	1.71 ± 1.70	(5/7)

Experiment 2 (Table 2)

In fry immunised with HGG at 1 month old, no response was detected one month later at 2 months; following reimmunisation, a response was seen at 3 months. This did not differ from the control fish response of Gps C and E at 3 months. Against A. salmonicida, a primary immune response was seen at 2 months, but no heightened response at 3 months occurred after boosting, there being no difference in titres between the GpB fish at 3 months, and Gps D and F.

TABLE 2 Response of rainbow trout immunised at 1 month post hatch

First Immunisation 1 month post hatch Wgt. 0.13±0.02g	Response at 2 months Mean titre		2nd Immunisation 2 months	Response at 3 months Mean titre	
HGG (GpA)	0	(0/10)	HGG	2.16±0.75	(6/6)
AS (GpB)	0.30±0.94	(4/10)	AS	1.60±1.83	(8/10)
BSA (GpC)			HGG	2.00±0.0	(4/4)
BSA (GpD)			AS	1.66±1.50	(4/6)
			HGG(GpE)	1.25±1.03	(8/8)
			AS (GpF)	1.62±1.99	(5/8)

Experiment 3 (Table 3)

Fry immunised with HGG at 2 months post hatch gave a positive primary response when tested at 3 months, and a heightened response after boosting at 4 months. This appeared to be a true memory effect as it was significantly different from the control four month response of GpE fish ($P<0.05$). The fish initially immunised with BSA and then with HGG failed to respond at 4 months however. Against A. salmonicida, a primary response was detected at 3 months, and a heightened secondary response at 4 months. Again, this appeared to be a true memory effect as the response was significantly different both from the fish receiving BSA initially and then AS, GpD, ($P<0.05$), and from the control four month response of GpF ($P<0.01$).

TABLE 3 Response of rainbow trout immunised at 2 months post hatch

First Immunisation 2 months post hatch Wgt. 0.26±0.04g	Response at 3 months Mean titre		2nd Immunisation 3 months	Response at 4 months Mean titre	
HGG (GpA)	1.92±1.03	(13/13)	HGG	4.60±2.60	(12/12)
AS (GpB)	2.72±2.10	(10/11)	AS	2.18±1.40	(9/11)
BSA (GpC)			HGG	0	(0/7)
BSA (GpD)			AS	0.85±1.21	(3/7)
			HGG(GpE)	2.45±1.75	(11/11)
			AS (GpF)	0.63±1.12	(3/11)

Experiment 4 (Table 4)

Fish immunised against HGG at 3 months failed to show a positive titre at 4 months (though three of the six samples were positive when tested undiluted). After boosting, a response was seen at 5 months, but no statistically significant memory effect could be demonstrated on this occasion. Positive responses were detected against A. salmonicida at 4 and 5 months, but there was no significant difference between the primary and secondary response.

TABLE 4 Response of rainbow trout immunised at 3 months post hatch

First Immunisation 3 months post hatch Wgt. 0.47±0.11g	Response at 4 months Mean titre		2nd Immunisation 4 months	Response at 5 months Mean titre	
HGG (GpA)	0	(3/6)neat	HGG	1.75±0.95	(4/4)
AS (GpB)	2.4±1.26	(9/10)	AS	1.50±1.64	(3/6)
BSA (GpC)			HGG	3.00±1.51	(7/8)
BSA (GpD)			AS	1.20±1.22	(6/10)
			HGG(GpE)	3.33±1.60	(6/6)
			AS (GpF)	0.80±1.31	(4/11)

Experiment 5 (Table 5)

Some of the groups were lost midway through this experiment due to a white spot infection, so no results could be obtained concerning the response to HGG in fish given primary and secondary doses at 4 and 5 months. Fish receiving a first dose at 5 months (Gps C and E) responded well to this antigen. Against A. salmonicida, a primary response was obtained at 5 months, although still at a fairly low level, but no significant memory was demonstrated at 6 months in this instance.

TABLE 5 Response of rainbow trout immunised at 4 months post hatch

First Immunisation 4 months post hatch Wgt. 1.05±0.22g	Response at 5 months Mean titre		2nd Immunisation 5 months	Response at 6 months Mean titre	
HGG (GpA)	Lost		HGG	Lost	
AS (GpB)	1.14±0.69	(6/7)	AS	0.63±0.92	(5/12)
BSA (GpC)			HGG	3.75±1.75	(7/8)
BSA (GpD)			AS	1.13±1.13	(5/8)
			HGG(GpE)	3.30±0.50	(3/3)
			AS (GpF)	3.00±0	

Thymectomy experiments

The results from these experiments are summarised in Table 6. In experiment A, fish were thymectomised at 1 month post hatch, immunised at 2 months, and tested for primary and secondary responses at 3 and 4 months. Against HGG, there was no difference in primary response between thymectomised and control fish, although following reimmunisation, the secondary response was significantly reduced in the thymectomised fish. There was no difference in the response of thymectomised and control fish to A. salmonicida. In experiment B, the fry were thymectomised at 2 months post hatch, and immunised at 3 months. Again, there was no secondary response to HGG in the thymectomised fry (though this may be simply an effect of the small sample size). In this instance, a suppression of the primary response to *A. salmonicida* in the thymectomised fry was noted. In fry thymectomised at 3 months, and immunised at 4 months (Exp.C), the thymectomised fry did respond to HGG after both a first and second immunisation, although unfortunately the corresponding controls of intact fish were lost. Against *A. salmonicida*, there was no primary response detected in the thymectomised fish, compared to the controls. After secondary immunisation, the response of thymectomised and control fry was not significantly different.

TABLE 6 Effect of thymectomy on the humoral immune response to HGG and *A. salmonicida* in rainbow trout

Exp. A Thymectomised 1 month post hatch

Immunised at 2 months		Response at 3 months Mean titre		Response at 4 months Mean titre	
HGG	Tx	1.0 ± 1.4	(1/2)	0.33 ± 0.57	(1/2)
HGG	Controls	1.92 ± 1.03	(13/13)	4.67 ± 2.61	(12/13)
AS	Tx	1.0 ± 1.4	(1/2)	1.00 ± 1.73	(1/3)
AS	Controls	2.73 ± 2.1	(10/11)	2.18 ± 1.40	(9/11)

Exp. B Thymectomised 2 months post hatch

Immunised at 3 months		Response at 4 months Mean titre		Response at 5 months Mean titre	
HGG	Tx	1.6 ± 1.14	(5/5)	0	(0/4)
HGG	Controls	0	(3/6neat)	1.75 ± 0.95	(4/4)
AS	Tx	0.6 ± 0.54	(3/5)	0.50 ± 1.22	(1/5
AS	Controls	2.4 ± 1.26	(9/10)	1.50 ± 1.64	(3/6)

Exp. C Thymectomised 3 months post hatch

Immunised at 4 months		Response at 5 months Mean titre		Response at 6 months Mean titre	
HGG	Tx	1.75 ± 1.5	(4/4)	5.30 ± 1.1	(3/3)
HGG	Controls	Lost		Lost	
AS	Tx	0	(6/6)	0.14 ± 0.37	(1/7)
AS	Controls	1.14 ± 0.69	(6/7)	0.58 ± 0.90	(5/12)

DISCUSSION

The results presented here confirm previous reports that young fish can mount a humoral immune response at an early stage in their development, and that the ability to respond to different antigens develops sequentially (Etlinger et al., 1979; Secombes, 1981; Mughal and Manning, 1985). The response to the soluble antigen, human gamma globulin, regarded as a thymus dependent antigen develops later than that to the particulate antigen Aeromonas salmonicida, a thymus independent antigen. A positive response was detected to AS by 2 months of age, and to HGG at 3 months of age at the naturally rising water temperatures used in the experiments. Tolerance to HGG has been demonstrated in some studies (Secombes, 1981; Mughal and Manning, 1985) but in these instances, the fry were presented with the antigen by intraperitoneal injection. When presented by direct immersion in a manner similar to which fry would naturally encounter antigens in their environment, no 'tolerance' effect was seen to either HGG or AS. There was a period of 'unresponsiveness' which was longer for HGG than for AS, but it does not appear to be the same as tolerance in the strict mammalian sense of the word. It would appear to be more a refractory state during which antigen is simply not taken up, because the immune system is immature and not able to cope with it. Some evidence for this has been provided by immersing rainbow trout fry in a radiolabelled bacterial vaccine and measuring antigen uptake directly (Tatner and Horne, 1984), and it has been suggested that the mechanism whereby the antigen is excluded is the phagocytic ability that was noted in the gills of young, but not adult, trout (Tatner and Manning, 1985). Mughal and Manning (1985) have also shown that young carp are refractory to HGG uptake from direct immersion vaccination for the first four weeks of life, although immersion in A. salmonicida at the same age yields positive immunity (Manning and Mughal, 1985). It is therefore important to know at exactly what stage it is possible to vaccinate fry by direct immersion for it to be effective. Following the refractory period, which appears to be different for different antigens - possibly depending on their physical state - positive immunity was obtained against both the antigens used in the present study, with no sign of tolerance induction.

From 2 months onwards, a response was obtained against A. salmonicida, which did not seem to mature as the fish aged to any extent, but remained at the fairly low levels of antibody titre usually reported for bacterial antigens given by direct immersion. The response to HGG, commencing at 3 months, was fairly vigorous and appeared to increase gradually as the fish matured. However, at some stages, negative results would be obtained, such as the four month response to HGG. On examination of the number of samples which gave a positive result at each sampling period, the large individual variation within groups of fish becomes apparent. At all stages, some samples were 'non responders'. Without very large sample sizes, it is difficult to demonstrate conclusively exactly what is occurring at each stage. Although each group of fish was as similar as possible and of the same age, a range of weights was apparent within each age group. There is some evidence to show that, in fact, it is not the age of the fish which determines its immunological maturity, but its body weight (Johnson et al., 1982; Tatner and Horne, 1983). The latter authors suggested that the onset of different immune capabilities was a function of the attainment of a certain critical number of immunocompetent cells. The number of cells in the developing rainbow trout fry shows a closer correlation to body weight than to age (Tatner and Manning, 1983).

The existence of memory in fish has been called into question following the results of Dunier (1985), who using the appropriate controls, could detect no memory effect in adult trout injected intraperitoneally with DNP-KLH or DNP-Ficoll in saline or adjuvant. In the present study, a positive memory effect was seen towards HGG at 4 months. There was also a suggestion of memory against A. salmonicida at 4 months. In the later experiments where the sample sizes were smaller, it was not possible again to demonstrate a significant memory effect.

The development of the various responses in young trout is illustrated in Figure 3. Whether it is the age of the fish, its weight, or simply the rising water temperature that correlates with its state of immunological maturity remains to be determined. Of interest however, the period just prior to the first antibody detection (marked with a star in Fig. 3) corresponds to a body weight of approximately 0.24g. It was at around this weight that, in a previous study on the growth of the lymphoid organs, that the weight of the thymus reaches its maximum percentage body weight, and the number of cells in the thymus reaches a peak (Tatner and Manning, 1983).

The thymectomy experiments reported here are preliminary, and still in progress. Due to the high mortalities following the operation, it is even more difficult to maintain a sufficiently large sample size throughout an experiment, to draw a definite conclusion. However, the following effects were noted and warrant further investigation. Thymectomy at 1 month of age had no effect on the primary response to HGG, but the secondary response at 4 months (when memory was first detected in intact controls) was reduced. There was no effect at all on the response to A. salmonicida. Thymectomy at 2 months again resulted in no secondary response to HGG at 5 months, and the primary response to AS was slightly depressed. After thymectomy at three months, the slight reduction in primary response to AS was again apparent. Unfortunately, the controls for the HGG thymectomised fry were lost. However, the secondary response to HGG in the thymectomised fry was higher than the primary response in the thymectomised fry, which might suggest that the effect of thymectomy on the secondary response had

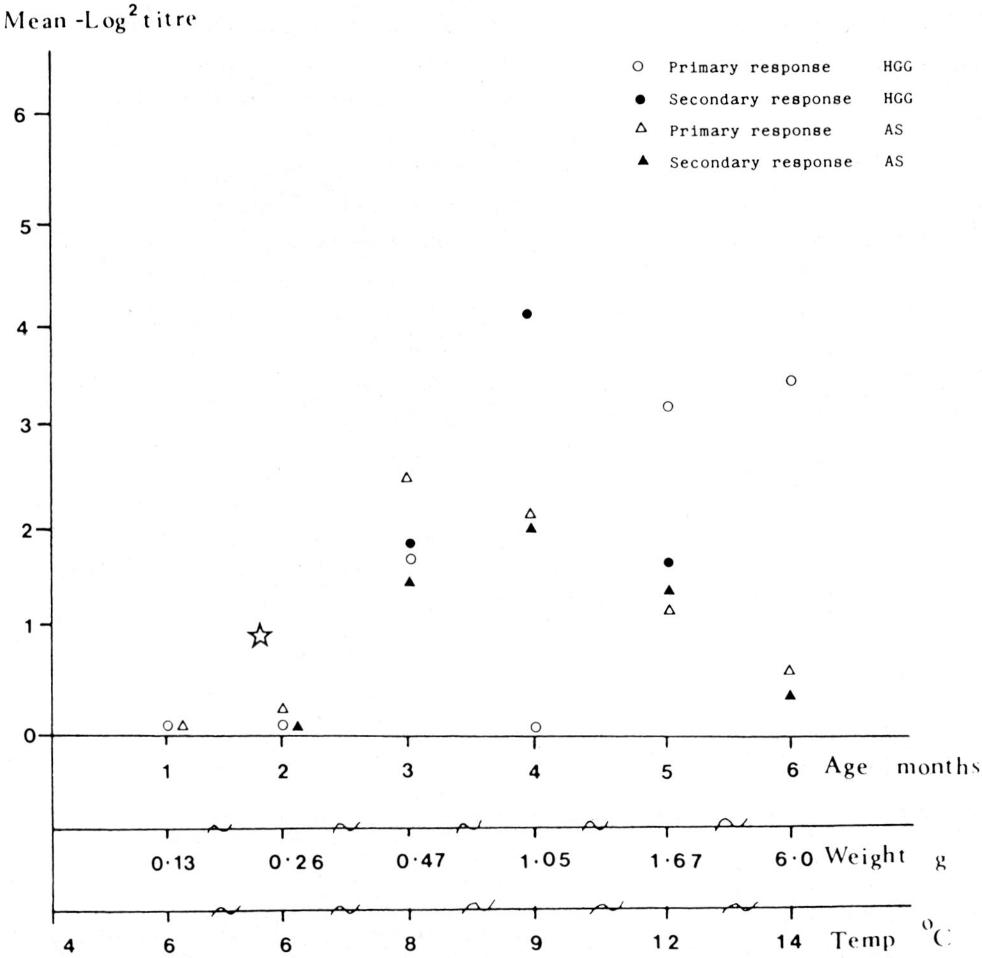

Fig. 3. Ontogeny of humoral immunity in rainbow trout

ceased to be effective when the operation was performed as late as 3 months. Apart from Sailendri's (1973) observation in 2 month old *Tilapia*, previous work on fish thymectomy has been confined to adults. Jayaraman et al. (1979) found that short term adult thymectomy in *Tilapia* reduced the response to sheep erythrocytes (a thymus dependent antigen), whilst leaving unaltered the response to polyvinylpyrrolidone. In carp immunised 4 weeks after thymectomy, Secombes (1981) found that serum antibody levels to *A. salmonicida* were elevated compared to sham operated fish at day 7 of the response and then returned to normal levels, whereas in trout, thymectomy had no effect on the response to AS though both the primary and secondary responses to HGG were elevated. Adult *Tilapia* which were left for one year after thymectomy could still respond to bovine serum albumin (Sailendri, 1973). The role of the thymus and the existence of 'helper' and 'suppressor' cell equivalents in the fish humoral immune response needs further investigation in both the adult and young stage.

ACKNOWLEDGEMENTS

This work was funded under a Royal Society of Edinburgh Research Fellowship. I wish to thank Mr William Leschen for his care in maintaining the experimental animals, and for Kathy McKenzie for typing the manuscript.

REFERENCES

Dorson, M., 1974. Production d'anticorps précipitants anti-dinitrophénol chez les alevins de truite arc-en-ciel (*Salmo gairdneri*) immunisés á l'âge d'une mois. C.R. Acad. Sci. Paris, 278: 3151-3152.

Dunier, M., 1975. Absence of anamnestic antibody response to DNP-haemocyanin and DNP-Ficoll in rainbow trout. In: M.J. Manning and M.F. Tatner (Editors), Fish Immunology. Fisheries Society of Great Britain Symposium. Academic Press, London, pp.171-184.

Etlinger, H.M., Chiller, J., and Hodgins, H.O., 1979. Evolution of the lymphoid system. IV. Murine T-independent but not T-dependent antigens are very immunogenic in rainbow trout (*Salmo gairdneri*). Cell. Immunol., 47: 400-406.

Jayaraman, S., Mohan, R., and Muthukkaruppan, V.R., 1979. Relationship between migration inhibition and plaque forming cell responses to sheep erythrocytes in the teleost, *Tilapia mossambica*. Develop. Comp. Immunol., 3:67-75

Johnson, K.A., Flynn, J.K., and Amend, D.F., 1982. Onset of immunity in salmonid fry vaccinated by direct immersion in *Vibrio anguillarum* and *Yersinia ruckeri* bacterins. J. Fish Dis., 5: 197-206.

Khalifa, K.A., and Post, G., 1976. Immune response of advanced rainbow trout fry to *Aeromonas liquefaciens*. Prog. Fish. Cult., 38: 66-68.

Lamers, C.H.J., and de Haas, M.J.H., 1985. Bath vaccination and development of immunological memory in carp (*Cyprinus carpio* L.). In: M.J. Manning and M.F. Tatner (Editors), Fish Immunology. Fisheries Society of Great Britain Symposium. Academic Press, London, pp.231-232.

Manning, M.J., and Mughal, M.S., 1985. Factors affecting the immune responses of immature fish. In: A.E. Ellis (Editor), Fish and Shellfish Pathology. Academic Press, London, pp.27-40.

Mughal, M.S., and Manning, M.J., 1985. Antibody responses of young carp, *Cyprinus carpio*, and grey mullet, *Chelon labrosus*, immunized with soluble antigen by various routes. In: M.J. Manning and M.F. Tatner (Editors), Fish Immunology. Fisheries Society of Great Britain Symposium. Academic Press, London, pp.313-326.

Paterson, W.D., and Fryer, J.L., 1974. Immune response of juvenile coho salmon (*Oncorhynchus kisutch*) to *Aeromonas salmonicida* cells administered intraperitoneally in Freund's complete adjuvant. J. Fish. Res. Bd Can., 31: 1751-1755.

Sailendri, K., 1973. Studies on the development of lymphoid organs and immune responses in the teleost *Tilapia mossambica* (Peters). PhD Thesis, Madurai University, India.

Secombes, C.J., 1981. Comparative studies on the structure and function of teleost lymphoid organs. PhD Thesis, University of Hull, U.K.

Tatner, M.F., and Horne, M.T., 1983. Susceptibility and immunity to *Vibrio anguillarum* in post hatching rainbow trout fry, *Salmo gairdneri* Richardson 1836. Develop. Comp. Immunol., 7: 465-472.

Tatner, M.F., and Horne, M.T., 1984. The effects of early exposure to *Vibrio anguillarum* vaccine on the immune response of the fry of rainbow trout, *Salmo gairdneri* Richardson. Aquaculture, 41: 193-202.

Tatner, M.F., and Manning, M.J., 1983. Growth of the lymphoid organs in rainbow trout, *Salmo gairdneri* Richardson, from one to fifteen months of age. J. Zool. Lond., 199: 503-520.

Tatner, M.F., and Manning, M.J., 1985. The ontogenetic development of the reticuloendothelial system in the rainbow trout, *Salmo gairdneri* Richardson. J. Fish Dis., 8: 35-41.

Van Loon, J.J.A., van Oosterom R., and van Muiswinkel, W.B., 1981. Development of the immune system in carp. In: J.B. Solomon (Editor), Aspects of Developmental and Comparative Immunology, Vol. 1. Pergamon Press, Oxford, pp.469-470.

Veterinary Immunology and Immunopathology, 12 (1986) 107—116
Elsevier Science Publishers B.V., Amsterdam — Printed in The Netherlands

ONTOGENY OF GUT-ASSOCIATED LYMPHOID TISSUE (GALT) IN THE DOGFISH SCYLIORHINUS CANICULA L.

S. HART, A.B. WRATHMELL and J.E. HARRIS

Dept. Biol. Sci., Plymouth Polytechnic, Drake Circus, Plymouth PL4 8AA, UK

ABSTRACT

Hart, S., Wrathmell, A.B. and Harris, J.E., 1986. Ontogeny of gut-associated lymphoid tissue (GALT) in the dogfish Scyliorhinus canicula L. Vet. Immunol. Immunopathol., 12: 107-116.

Cartilaginous fish occupy a fundamental position in vertebrate phylogeny and it is likely that this group has retained some of the ancestral immune mechanisms. The ontogeny of GALT has received little attention in elasmobranchs and this study correlates this development with morphological differentiation, development of other lymphoid organs, exposure to seawater and transition from yolk dependence to exogenous food as a source of nutrient. GALT was first represented by individual lymphocyte-like and macrophage-like cells in the lamina propria. In later stages accumulations and intraepithelial leucocytes were recorded prior to hatching. The size of accumulations and the number of lymphocyte and macrophage-like cells infiltrating the lamina propria and epithelium increased in fish as they became dependent upon an exogenous diet. Although GALT developed after the thymus and lymphoid-like tissue in the kidney and at approximately the same time as the epigonal, Leydig and spleen, the source of cells populating the gut is unknown. Plasma cells and granulocytes were not observed in the developing fish until 6 months post-hatch after which the fish had a similar GALT distribution and content to the adult fish.

INTRODUCTION

Scyliorhinus canicula L., order Elasmobranchii, class Chondricythes, is a member of a primitive group of fishes that occupy a fundamental position in vertebrate phylogeny. Chondricythes are the most primitive vertebrate group with a clearly defined thymus (Zapata, 1983), and it is considered that within this group of animals a form of immunity exists which is not different in principle from that of mammals (Marchalonis, 1977).

Studies have been undertaken on the nature of elasmobranch immunoglobulin (Kobayashi et al., 1984); on lymphocyte function (Warr, 1981); phagocytic activity of blood leucocytes (Parish, 1981); general immune function (Zapata, 1983) and on the morphology of the lymphomyeloid tissues (Fange, 1984). There is, however, a paucity of information on mucosal immunology in the cartilaginous fishes. Some work has been undertaken on gut-associated lymphoid tissue (Dreszwina, 1905; Jacobshagen, 1915; Kondesa, 1956; Fichtelius et al., 1968; Zapata, 1977; Tomonaga et al., 1984b and Hart et al., 1985).

0165-2427/86/$03.50 © 1986 Elsevier Science Publishers B.V.

In this study, the ontogenesis of gut-associated lymphoid tissue in fish 1-2 months post-fertilization to 6 months post-hatch has been investigated and confined to studying changes in the spiral intestine, for in the adult this part of the gut harbours the majority of this tissue (Hart et al., 1985).

MATERIALS AND METHODS

Eggs were collected from pregnant adult fish (600-1000g). The egg cases were kept in circulating seawater at 12-14°C under a diurnal light regime from December 1984 to July 1985. Fish were removed from the egg cases or collected after hatching and fixed in neutralised 10% formal-saline, in elasmobranch buffer (Hayle, 1965), at 4°C for 48 hours. Twenty fish between stages 1-4 (see Fig. 1); four at 30 days and four at 6 months were analysed.

Whole fish or specific tissue samples were dehydrated, infiltrated with alcohol and embedded in methacrylate resin (TAAB). Semi-thin (1 um) sections were cut and material stained with methylene blue, Giemsa, Periodic acid Schiffs (PAS) and methyl green pyronine.

The infiltration of leucocytes into the gut epithelium was quantified by a stereological technique using a Werbel 2 graticule (Graticules Ltd). The degree of infiltration was expressed as a percentage of the epithelial volume occupied by the leucocytes.

RESULTS

The development of GALT in the spiral intestine was correlated with the development of the gut and major lymphoid organs, the ventilation of the eggs by seawater and transition from a dependence upon the yolk sac to an exogenous diet (Figs. 1 and 2). The four major developmental stages, their approximate age, and size and morphological appearance are illustrated in Fig. 1.

At stage 1 (Fig. 1) the tissue destined to become the spiral valve was present as an outpushing of the gut (Figs. 2 and 3) and the anterior gut was totally occluded. Partial occlusion is demonstrated in Fig. 4. Development of the thymus and lymphoid-like tissue around the kidney had begun by mid-Stage 1 (Fig. 1). Stage 2 was reached when the fish had developed external gills (Fig. 1). Ventilation of the eggcase by seawater did not occur until approximately one third of the way through stage 2. The sprial valve had begun to develop (Fig. 5) but, in the early part of stage 2 GALT was absent and the anterior of the gut was still occluded. At the end of Stage 2 (Fig. 1) the spiral valve had undergone considerable development (Figs. 2 and 6) and was compatible with the adult spiral valve (Fig. 7). It could be differ-

STAGE	GUT DEVELOPMENT (NOT TO SCALE)	LYMPHOID TISSUE AND ORGANS					
		GALT	THYMUS	KIDNEY	SPLEEN	EPIGONAL	LEYDIG
STAGE 1	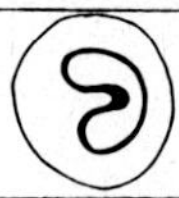	ABSENT	✓	✓	ABSENT	ABSENT	ABSENT
STAGE 2	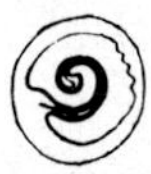	"	✓	✓	"	"	"
		✓	✓	✓	✓	✓	✓
		✓	✓	✓	✓	✓	✓
STAGE 3	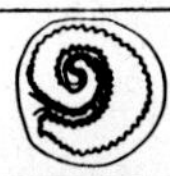	✓	✓	✓	✓	✓	✓
STAGE 4	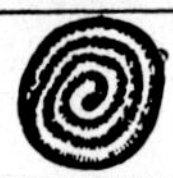	✓	✓	✓	✓	✓	✓

Fig. 1. The major developmental stages of the dogfish.

STAGE AND APPROXIMATE AGE	DEVELOPMENTAL FEATURES	SCHEMATIC REPRESENTATION OF STAGES (NOT TO SCALE)
STAGE 1 1-2 MONTHS	ALBUMIN COATED STAGE. 1 - 2 CM LONG	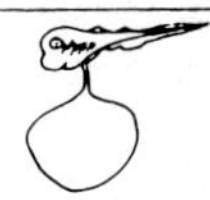
STAGE 2 2-5 MONTHS	EXTERNAL GILL STAGE. 2 - 5 CM LONG	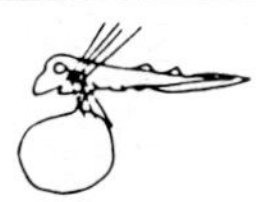
STAGE 3 5-7 MONTHS	INTERNAL YOLK SAC STAGE. 5 - 10 CM LONG	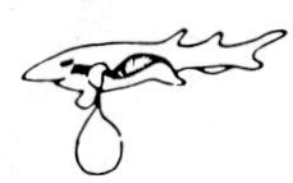
STAGE 4 POST-HATCH UP TO 3-4 WEEKS	POST-HATCH STAGE. 16 CM LONG	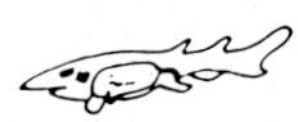

Fig. 2. Initial development of gut-associated lymphoid tissue (GALT) in the dogfish.

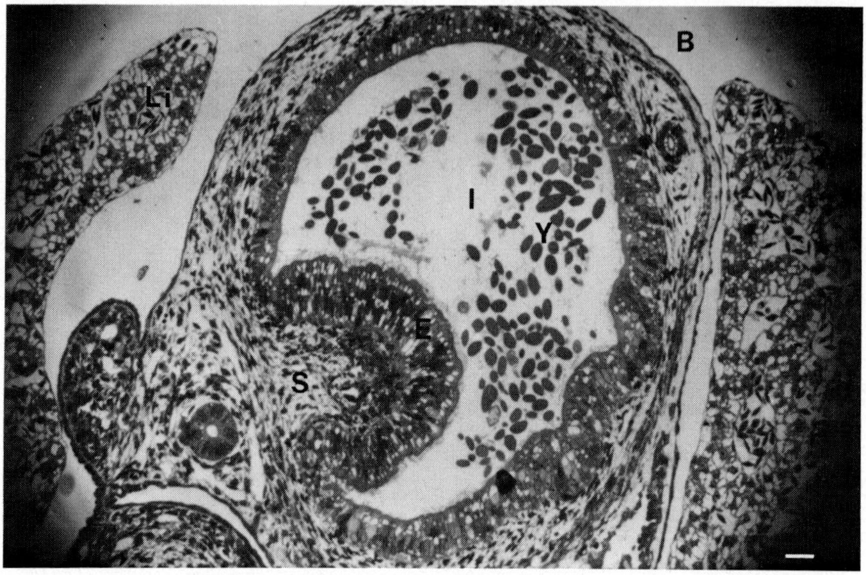

Fig. 3. Early developmental stage of the spiral valve in a Stage 1 fish. Note the yolk platelets. Bar = 100 μm. I = intestine; S = spiral valve; Y = yolk platelets; E = epithelium; Li = liver; B = body cavity.

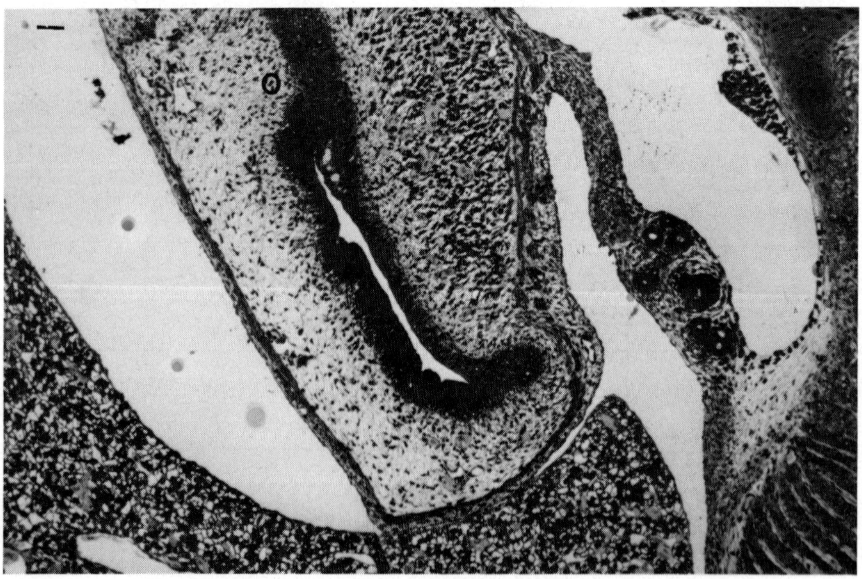

Fig. 4. A partial gut occlusion. Bar = 100 μm. O = occluded tissue.

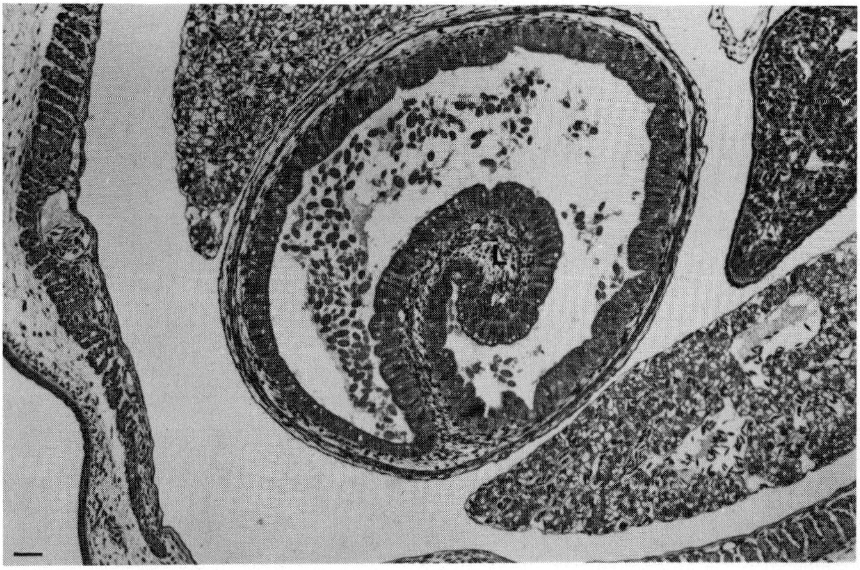

Fig. 5. Spiral valve showing the first coil development. Bar = 100 μm. L = lamina propria.

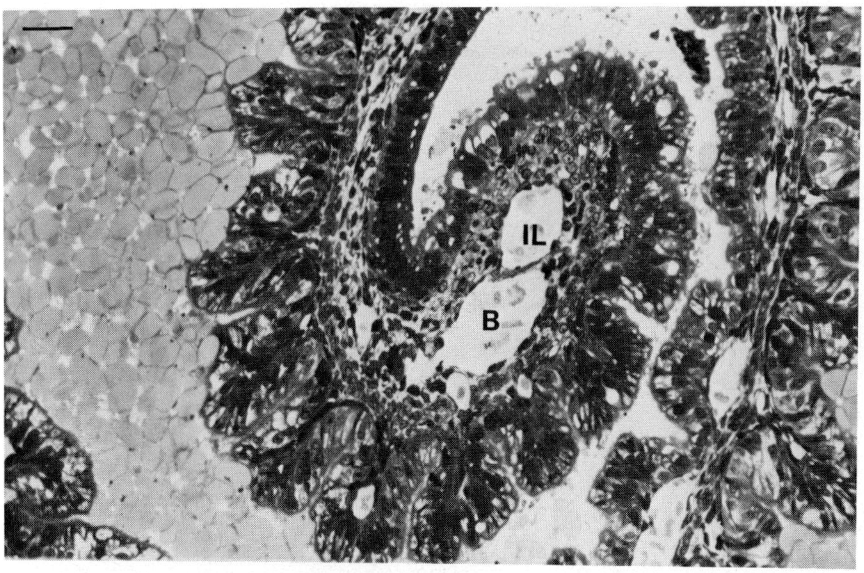

Fig. 6. Spiral valve showing the epithelium thrown into folds at Stage 3. Bar = 100 μm. F = intestinal fold; B = blood vessel; IL = intralaminal leucocyte.

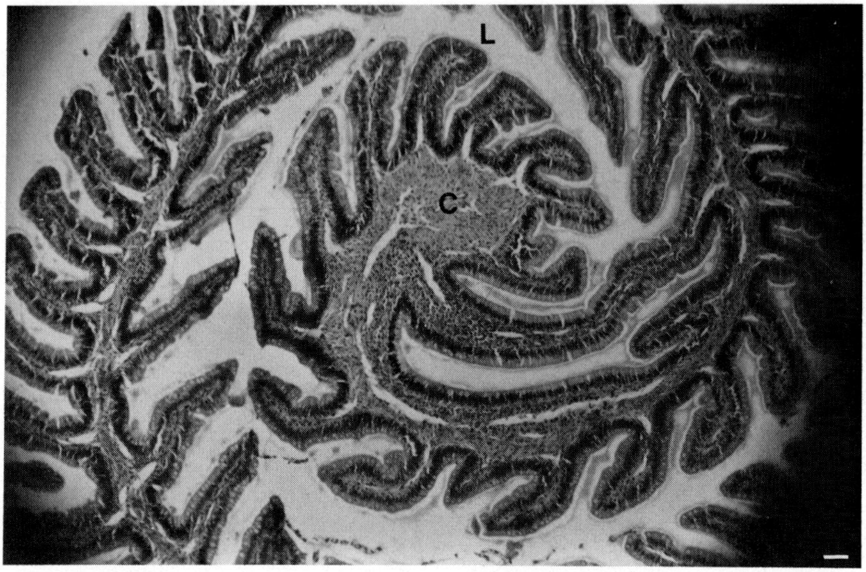

Fig. 7. Fully differentiated spiral valve tissue of a 1-year old fish. Bar = 100 μm. C = connective tissue; L = lumen.

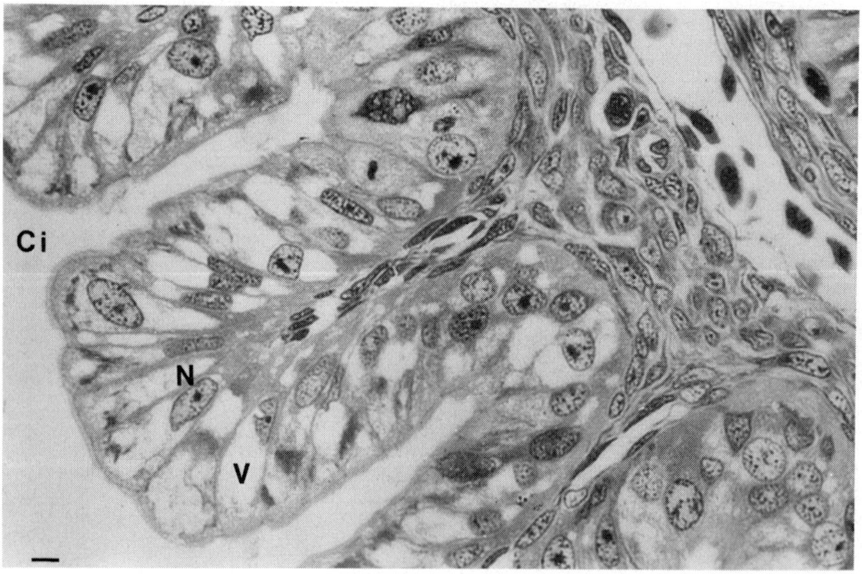

Fig. 8. A fold in the intestine showing vacuolar epithelial cells. Bar = 80 μm. V = vacuolated epithelial cell; N = nucleus; Ci = cilia.

entiated from the adult, however, as the intestinal folds were small and the epithelial cells vacuolated in appearance (Fig. 8). The gut is no longer occluded at this stage and lymphocyte-like and PAS positive macrophage-like cells were present in the lamina propria (Fig. 9). The leydig, epigonal and spleen had also begun to develop by this stage (Fig. 2). Stage 3 was characterised by the absence of external gills and the development of the internal yolk sac. Stage 4 was free swimming but still possessed an internal yolk sac. Stages 3 and 4 differed from previous stages as intraepithelial lymphocyte-like and macrophage-like cells were recognised (Fig. 10), and accumulations of predominately lymphocyte-like and macrophage-like cells were observed in the lamina propria of the central core of the spiral (Fig. 11). These accumulations increased in size as the fish aged. The development of the intraepithelial leucocyte population is recorded in Fig. 12. This depicts a relatively uniform increase in the volume of epithelium occupied by leucocytes from the stages 3 and 4 to the adult. Granular cells and plasma cells were not observed in the mucosae of fish examined approximately one month after hatch. However, by six months granulocytes were observed in the mucosa and plasma cells in the lamina propria.

DISCUSSION

Gut-associated lymphoid tissue was present in the dogfish in the latter part of stage 2. First, as individual lymphocyte-like and macrophage-like cells in the lamina propria and later in stages 3 and 4 as accumulations in the lamina propria and as intraepithelial leucocytes. By six months all the cell types described in adult GALT (Hart et al., 1985) were present.

Precursors to GALT appeared after the thymus had differentiated and lymphoid-like cells had appeared in the developing kidney. The spleen, Leydig organ and epigonal tissue differentiated at approximately the same time. It is impossible to decide from histological studies from which organ or cells, developing GALT originated. The origin of most cells in the intraepithelial tissue of mammals is also unclear. Some appear to be derived from precursors in Peyers patches which migrate via the mesenteric lymph nodes to the lamina propria and intraepithelial compartment. Thymectomy reduces the intra-epithelial cell population by 40-50%. Most granulated intraepithelial leucocytes are, however thymus-independent (Ernst et al., 1985).

While the development of GALT has been mapped from embryonic, through neonatal, to mature stages in <u>S. canicula</u>, the role of antigens in this process is unknown. In mammals, the location and distribution of leucocytes is independent of antigen (Ferguson and Parrot, 1972; Husband and Gowans,

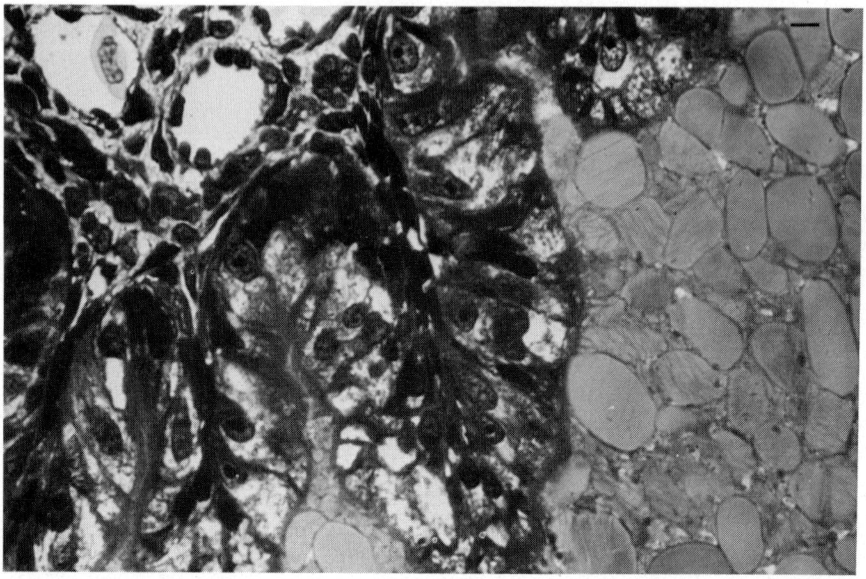

Fig. 9. Intestinal fold surrounded by yolk platelets. Bar = 10 µm.

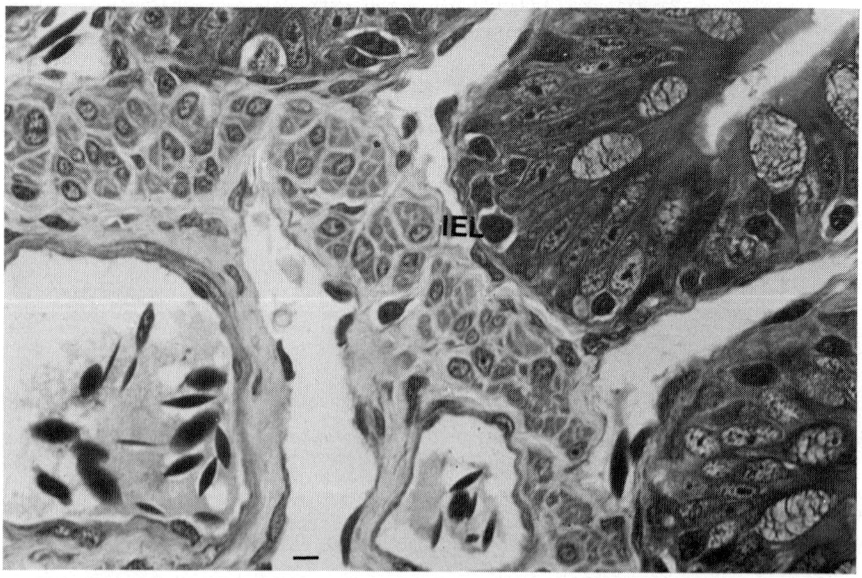

Fig. 10. Base of an intestinal fold infiltrated by leucocytes in a stage 3 fish. Bar = 10 µm.
IEL = intraepithelial leucocytes.

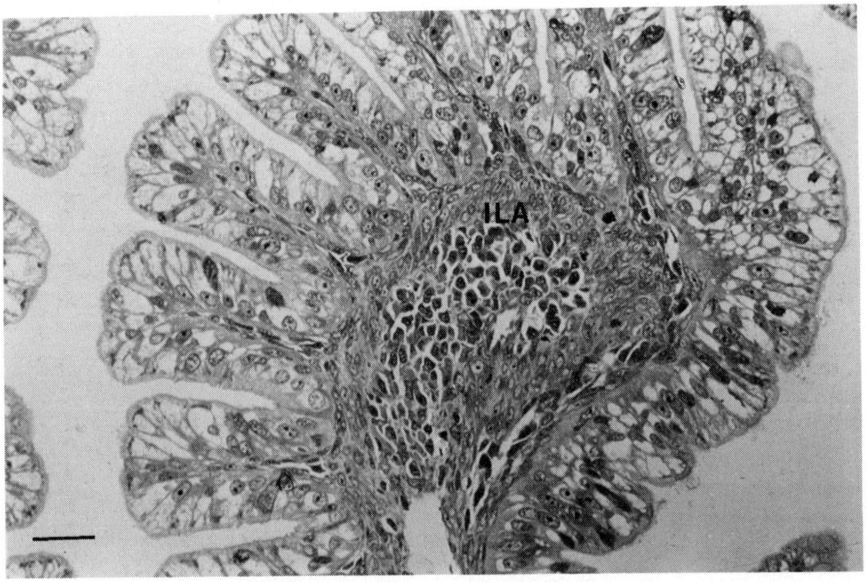

Fig. 11. Intralaminal accumulation of macrophage-like and lymphocyte-like cells at the core of the spiral valve in a stage 3 fish. Bar = 100 μm. ILA = intralaminal accumulations.

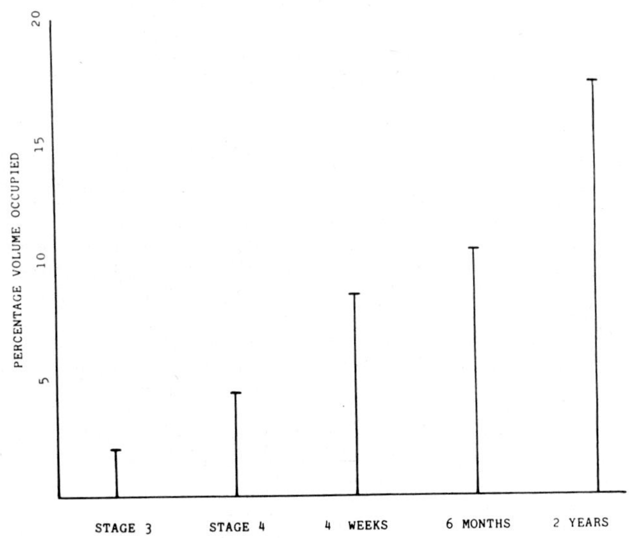

Fig. 12. The percentage of epithelial volume occupied by leucocytes.

1978) but the numbers of cells will increase in the presence of antigen (Ferguson, 1977). The role of antigens in the development of GALT in elasmobranchs is further complicated as the developing embryo is exposed to seawater, which is likely to contain antigens, from the middle of stage 2, whereas the murine model, for example, will develop in a sterile womb until parturition.

The epithelial cells of the spiral valve appear to have a particular vacuolar-like appearance when the fish is dependent upon the yolk sac for nutrients. A preliminary experiment has indicated that the epithelial cells at this stage will absorb carbon particles. This mechanism was not evident in the adult gut. We are currently investigating when this mechanism is lost, and whether it correlates with a transition to an exogenous diet.

REFERENCES

Drezwina, A., 1905. Contribution at l'etude du tissue lymphoide des Ichthyopsides. Archs. Zool. exp. gen., 4: 145-338.

Ernst, P.B., Befus, A.B., and Bienenstock, J., 1985. Leucocytes in the intestinal epithelium: an unusual immunological compartment. Immunol. Today, 6: 50-55.

Fange, R., 1984. Lymphomyeloid tissues in fishes. Vidensk. Meddr dansk naturh. Foren., 145: 143-162.

Ferguson, A., 1977. Intraepithelial lymphocytes of the small intestine. Gut, 18: 921-937.

Ferguson, A., and Parrot, D.M.V., 1972. The effect of antigen deprivation on thymus-dependent and thymus-independent lymphocytes in the small intestine of the mouse. Clin. exp. Immunol., 12: 477-488.

Fichtelius, K.E., Finstad, J., and Good, R.A., 1968. Bursa equivalents of bursaless vertebrates. Lab. Invest., 19: 339-351.

Hale, L.J., 1965. Biological Laboratory Data. Methuen, London. pp. 132.

Hart, S., Harris, J.E., and Wrathmell, A.B., 1985. Gut-associated lymphoid tissue (GALT) in the dogfish *Scyliorhinus canicula* L.; a light microscopic study (submitted for publication).

Husband, A.J. and Gowans, J.C., 1978. The origin and antigen dependent distribution of IgA-containing cells in the intestine. J. exp. Med. 148: 1146-1160.

Jacobshagen, E., 1915. Zur Morphologie des Spiraldarms. Anat. Anz., 48: 188-254.

Kobayashi, K., Tomonaga, S., and Kajii, T., 1984. A second class of immunoglobulin other than IgM present in the serum of cartilaginous fish, the skate *Raja kenajei* : Isolation and Characterisation. Mol. Immunol., 21: 397-404.

Kondesa, A., 1956. A phylogenetic survey of haemocytopoietic tissues in submammalian vertebrates. Bull. Yamaguchi med. Sch., 4: 1-35.

Marcholonis, J.J., 1977. Immunity in Evolution. Harvard University Press, Cambridge (Mass.), 316 pp.

Parish, N.M., 1981. A study of the structure, distribution and function of phagocytic cells in the immune system of fish. Ph.D. thesis, Plymouth Polytechnic, Plymouth, U.K.

Tomonaga, S., Kobayashi, K., Kajii, T., and Awaya, K., 1984. Two populations of immunoglobulin-forming cells in the skate *Raja kenojei*: their distribution and characterisation. Dev. Comp. Immunol., 8: 801-812.

Warr, G.W., 1981. Evolution of the lymphocyte. Immunol. Today, 2: 63-68.

Zapata, A., 1977. Estructura des los arganos linfoides y linformieloides de Peces. Ph.D. thesis, Universidad Compatense de Madrid, Madrid, Spain.

Zapata, A., 1983. Phylogeny of the fish immune system. Bull. Inst. Pasteur, 81: 165-186.

Veterinary Immunology and Immunopathology, 12 (1986) 117–126
Elsevier Science Publishers B.V., Amsterdam — Printed in The Netherlands

STRUCTURE AND FUNCTION OF THE MELANO-MACROPHAGE CENTRES OF THE GOLDFISH *Carassius auratus*

M.P. HERRAEZ and A.G. ZAPATA

Departamento de Morfología Microscópica. Facultad de Biología. Universidad de León, León 24071 (Spain)

ABSTRACT

Herráez, M.P. and Zapata, A.G., 1986. Structure and function of the melano-macrophage centres of the goldfish *Carassius auratus*. Vet. Immunol. Immunopathol., 12: 117-126.

We have studied the melano-macrophage centres (MMCs) of *Carassius auratus* as well as the changes they undergo in different experimental conditions. The MMCs of the spleen contain brown and yellow pigments, but dark pigments abound in those of the kidney. They occur in association with splenic ellipsoids and scattered throughout the renal parenchyma. Histochemical tests demonstrated small amounts of lipids and basic proteins, abundant neutral mucopolisaccharids and differences between the spleen MMCs and those of the kidney, specially regarding the presence or absence of haemosiderins and melanins. Electron microscopy shows them to consist of phagocytes containig degenerated debris, sometimes surrounded by a discontinuous layer of flat reticular cells. The MMCs of the spleen and kidney trap carbon material 48 hours after injection of Indian ink. Primary and -more so- secondary immunization with SRBC produces a net increase in number and size of MMCs. Treatment with phenylhydrazine produces a notable and fast increase of the MMCs in both organs. After 5 days the MMCs degenerated and erythroblasts restored the erythroid population. Apparently , MMCs represent non-specific means of phagocytosis related to different physiological processes.

INTRODUCTION

Pigment-containing cells are a constant feature of the lympho-haemopoietic tissues of fish, which in most teleosts form the so-called melano-macrophage centres (MMCs) (Agius, 1980; Zapata, 1983). These structures are aggregations of closely packed macrophages containing heterogeneous inclusions, the most frequent of which are melanin, haemosiderin and lipofucsin (Agius and Agbede, 1984). Morphology and content of MMCs vary in different conditions, such as after bleeding (Grover, 1968; Yu et al., 1971), with vitamin-deficient or rancid diets (Blazer and Wolke, 1983), starvation (Agius and Roberts, 1981; Agius, 1983; Agius and Agbede, 1984), age (Brown and George, 1985), and disease processes (Roberts, 1975). MMCs have been related to age pigments (Roberts, 1975; Brown and George, 1985), to tissue breakdown (Agius, 1979; Agius and Roberts, 1981; Moccia et al., 1984) and to defence mechanisms (Ellis et al.,

0165-2427/86/$03.50 © 1986 Elsevier Science Publishers B.V.

1976; Ferguson, 1976; Ellis 1980; Secombes and Manning, 1980; Agius, 1981; Secombes et al., 1982; Fulop and McMillan, 1984; Lamers, 1985). Despite all these studies our knowledge of the significance of MMCs is scant. In this regard, we have analyzed the structure of MMCs of the spleen, pro- and mesonephros as well as their quantitative and qualitative variations under several experimental conditions in the goldfish, Carassius auratus. Our results suggest that the MMCs might represent ways of reacting non-specifically to different physiological conditions.

MATERIALS AND METHODS

Spleen, pro- and mesonephros of goldfish, 6-10 gm. in weight, were routinely processed for light and electron microscopy. Histochemical techniques were applied to study of carbohydrates, lipids, proteins, pigments and enzymes (acid alkaline phosphatase and endogenous peroxidase). The capacity of the MMCs to trap carbon particles was tested 6 and 48 hours after intraperitoneal and intramuscular injection of a 1% solution of Indian ink in water. Fishes received intraperitoneal immunizing injections of 0.1 ml. of a 25% solution of SRBC in PBS. Quantitative and morphological changes in the MMCs were tested at 5, 7, 14 and 21 days for both primary and secondary immunization. The second challenge with the immunogen was effected 40 days after the first injection. In other experiments, fishes underwent a single injection of 0.5 mg. of phenylhydrazine in 0.1 ml. of PBS. The organs were analyzed by light and electron microscopy at 12 and 24 hours, 5, 6 and 7 days.

RESULTS

The MMCs occurred in the spleen of C. auratus as irregular yellowish-brown clusters of phagocytic cells, the largest of which showed an incomplete capsule and were associated with the blood vessels. Lymphoid cells were also related to the MMCs, although the lymphoid tissue was scantly developed. In the kidney the MMCs were randomly distributed throughout the lympho-haemopoietic tissue. In addition to the yellowish-brown pigments, the kidney MMCs contained black melanin pigments, more abundant in the pronephros than in the mesonephros. Histochemical analysis demonstrated a high heterogeneity in the content of the MMCs. In short, they showed traces of lipids, neutral mucopolysaccharides and traces of basic proteins. Lipofucsin was demonstrated by the Schmorl's method but not whith the more selective Nilo blue reagent. Melanins were strongly positive in the MMCs of the kidney and very slightly in those of the spleen. Perl's reaction was positive in all three organs, confirming ulrastructural evidence of the presence of erythrocyte debris. Finally, acid phosphatase showed a slight reactivity in some centres but not alkaline phosphatase or endogenous peroxidase.

Ultrastructural analysis confirmed the organization of MMCs. Numerous phagocytic cells occurred in a network of reticular cells joined together by desmosomes. These cells also formed a non-continuous capsule sometimes in continuity with the endothelial cells of the sinusoids or with the reticular cells of the splenic parenchyma. The organization is similar in the MMCs of the pro- and mesonephros. Phagocytic cells in the MMCs appeared as single, isolated cells with eccentric nuclei and cytoplasm completely filled with cell debris. The phagocytic content was very heterogeneous; large degenerated cells -mainly granulocytes and erythrocytes- were phagocytosed, as well as crystalline inclusions, lipofucsin, lipid deposits and melanin granules. Remarkably, nerve endings were found among the macrophages of the MMCs. In addition there occurred smaller, non-encapsulated aggregates of macrophages with abundant phagocytosed material, distributed randomly among the elements of the lymphoid parenchyma.

Six hours after intraperitoneal or intramuscular injection of an Indian ink solution, carbon particles appeared phagocytosed into the macrophage cytoplasm of the splenic ellipsoids. In the kidney, sinusoidal lining cells contained abundant carbon particles. 48 hous after intraperitoneal injection carbon was present in the MMCs in the spleen but not in those of the kidney. In the latter organ, blood sinusoids still showed the engulfed carbon. By contrast, 48 hours after intramuscular injection, the MMCs of the kidney did exhibit carbon particles, but in the spleen these occured mainly in the ellipsoids, only a few scattered MMCs containing traces. In all locations, carbon deposits were intracellular as demonstrated by electron microscopy.

Changes in the lymphoid tissues occurred in both after primary and secodary immunization, mainly after 7 and 14 days. In the spleen (see Table 1), increased lymphoid tissue appeared associated with ellipsoids and MMCs. In the kidney, numerous lymphocytes appeared among the renal tubules. However there was no correlation between antibody titres and number and/or size of the MMCs. Thus, fishes with the highest levels of circulating antibodies did not necessarily show high numbers of MMCs.

After primary immunization, the area occupied by the MMCs in relation to the total area of the histological section selected increased from the 5th day, reaching peaks at 14 and 21 days (no significant differences between both values). By contrast all control fish showed a similar ratio, significantly different to that of of the immunized animals. The ratio of MMCs/total area of histological section also increased in comparison with the controls, peaking at 14 days and then decreasing. However the mean size of the MMCs increased from the 7th day, suggesting that the decrease in the number of the MMCs, 21 days after immunization, was due to their increased size. In short, there were significant differences in the number and size of the splenic MMCs between con trol and immunized fish. Their number increased rapidly at 5 and 7 days, while the size of the MMCs became very prominent at 14 and 21 days. After secondary immunization, the total area of the MMCs increased from the 5th day peaking at 14 days with a slight drop at 7 days. No significant differences occurred at 14 and 21 days. A great increase occurred in the number of MMCs, which reached its maximum registered level at 14 days, decreasing thereafter to the values observed at 7 days. The mean size decreased after the 5th day with a small increase at 21 days. These results suggest that the secondary immunization induces an increase in the number of MMCs but not in their size.

TABLE 1

Morphometrical changes in the MMCs of the spleen after primary and secondary immunization with SRBC.

Immunization	Days after 1st immunization	A		N		M	
		$\bar{x}$	σ_{n-1}	$\bar{x}$	σ_{n-1}	$\bar{x}$	σ_{n-1}
PBS (day 0)	5	0.046	0.003	11.04	0.23	4.16	0.18
	7	0.049	0.002	12.51	0.19	3.98	0.21
	14	0.042	0.007	12.70	0.98	3.30	0.20
	21	0.045	0.010	12.08	5.61	3.81	0.86
SRBC (day 0)	5	0.062	0.004	20.47	0.79	2.91	0.34
	7	0.075	0.006	24.67	2.28	3.03	0.18
	14	0.098	0.012	27.51	2.60	3.55	0.19
	21	0.092	0.006	21.20	2.88	4.28	0.51
Immunization	**Days after 2nd immunization**	**A**		**N**		**M**	
		$\bar{x}$	σ_{n-1}	$\bar{x}$	σ_{n-1}	$\bar{x}$	σ_{n-1}
PBS (day 0) + PBS (day 40)	5	0.053	0.004	17.70	0.63	2.99	0.14
	7	0.054	0.003	18.59	0.79	2.96	0.31
	14	0.054	0.004	19.25	0.83	2.80	0.16
	21	0.047	0.002	14.81	0.02	3.20	0.13
PBS (day 0) + SRBC (day 40)	5	0.073	0.008	20.86	0.26	3.52	0.43
	7	0.073	0.003	23.44	1.52	3.15	0.05
	14	0.081	0.020	24.36	4.16	3.37	0.50
	21	0.089	0.007	21.04	0.09	4.24	0.04
SRBC (day 0) + SRBC (day 40)	5	0.098	0.002	23.12	2.10	4.38	0.57
	7	0.090	0.007	25.61	2.36	3.57	0.26
	14	0.123	0.030	35.04	1.70	3.56	1.31
	21	0.105	0.010	28.58	3.98	3.73	0.56

A Total area of MMCs/Total area of the histological section
N Number of MMCs/Total area (mm^2) of the histological section
M Mean size of the MMCs ($mm^2 \times 10^{-3}$)
$\bar{x}$ Mean
σ_{n-1} Standard deviation

The ratio total area of MMCs/total area of the histological section increased rapidly in the pronephros of immunized fishes (see Table 2). Five and 7 days after immunization, this ratio was very high compared with that of the controls, becoming even higher at 14 days and then decreasing to the level of the 5th day. In contrast, a progressive decrease took place in the number of MMCs after the 5th day, being specially notable between 14 and 21 days, but their size increased until the 14th day to diminish again to the value of 7 days. Apparently, the effects of immunization on the MMCs of the pronephros are faster than on those of the spleen. The secondary immunization elicited an enormous increase in the total area of the pronephric MMCs. However, The numbers of MMCs increased rapidly until the 7th day and then remained constant without differing significantly from the values obtained after the primary immunization. In any case, the low numbers of MMCs in this condition are explained by the large increase in the mean size of MMCs in all four stages studied. Pronephros seem to show the greatest quantitative modifications in the MMCs, specially after secondary immunization.

TABLE 2

Morphometrical changes in the MMCs of the pronephros after primary and secondary immunization with SRBC.

Immunization	Days after 1st immunization	A		N		M	
		$\bar{x}$	σ_{n-1}	$\bar{x}$	σ_{n-1}	$\bar{x}$	σ_{n-1}
PBS (day 0)	5	0.014	0.003	7.64	0.40	1.83	0.32
	7	0.015	0.002	8.17	0.71	1.84	0.35
	14	0.026	0.004	7.57	0.34	3.50	0.40
	21	0.018	0.006	7.79	0.32	2.39	0.96
SRBC (day 0)	5	0.048	0.004	13.91	0.32	3.49	0.36
	7	0.054	0.003	12.69	1.01	4.34	0.58
	14	0.060	0.006	12.91	0.72	4.81	0.20
	21	0.044	0.006	10.40	1.01	4.25	0.38

Immunization	Days after 2nd immunization	A		N		M	
		$\bar{x}$	σ_{n-1}	$\bar{x}$	σ_{n-1}	$\bar{x}$	σ_{n-1}
PBS (day 0) + PBS (day 40)	5	0.052	0.002	15.35	0.65	3.39	0.32
	7	0.040	0.001	14.03	0.80	2.95	0.001
	14	0.043	0.003	16.63	0.30	2.55	0.19
	21	0.047	0.009	16.25	1.99	2.96	0.42
PBS (day 0) + SRBC (day 40)	5	0.065	0.007	19.51	0.04	3.29	0.30
	7	0.048	0.001	13.27	2.31	3.71	0.44
	14	0.062	0.009	14.95	0.56	4.24	0.56
	21	0.069	0.009	17.95	2.05	3.83	0.11
SRBC (day 0) + SRBC (day 40)	5	0.060	0.007	14.51	1.97	4.19	0.27
	7	0.077	0.010	16.89	1.72	4.64	0.56
	14	0.097	0.010	16.60	0.61	5.89	0.63
	21	0.124	0.010	16.29	3.51	7.66	0.80

TABLE 3

Morphometrical changes in the MMCs of the mesonephros after primary and secondary immunization with SRBC.

Immunization	Days after 1st immunization	A		N		M	
		$\bar{x}$	σ_{n-1}	$\bar{x}$	σ_{n-1}	$\bar{x}$	σ_{n-1}
PBS (day 0)	5	0.033	0.001	14.44	0.79	2.33	0.01
	7	0.031	0.004	13.26	2.39	2.44	0.07
	14	0.030	0.008	9.75	1.73	3.25	1.15
	21	0.031	0.001	12.48	2.43	2.67	0.50
SRBC (day 0)	5	0.049	0.006	13.79	1.17	3.57	0.20
	7	0.051	0.010	15.91	2.38	3.19	0.39
	14	0.078	0.007	17.89	1.64	4.40	0.28
	21	0.074	0.007	16.09	1.31	4.42	0.51
Immunization	**Days after 2nd immunization**	**A**		**N**		**M**	
		$\bar{x}$	σ_{n-1}	$\bar{x}$	σ_{n-1}	$\bar{x}$	σ_{n-1}
PBS (day 0) + PBS (day 40)	5	0.040	0.010	13.16	3.32	3.29	1.52
	7	0.036	0.004	13.88	0.67	2.62	0.19
	14	0.036	0.006	12.75	0.35	2.82	0.58
	21	0.037	0.007	13.21	2.29	2.95	0.98
PBS (day 0) + SRBC (day 40)	5	0.058	0.020	15.34	5.11	3.68	0.58
	7	0.043	0.006	11.04	0.40	3.95	0.73
	14	0.073	0.010	16.37	1.68	4.54	1.02
	21	0.062	0.007	16.65	0.65	3.76	0.08
SRBC (day 0) + SRBC (day 40)	5	0.057	0.007	13.05	1.20	4.44	0.19
	7	0.082	0.010	17.83	1.12	4.73	0.95
	14	0.080	0.010	18.82	1.78	4.28	0.66
	21	0.090	0.010	14.88	0.37	6.12	0.72

The area occupied by the MMCs in the mesonephros increased after primary immunization at 7 days, peaking at 14 and 21 days (see Table 3). On the other hand, the number of MMCs increased progressively until the 14th day, although at 5 days there were no significant differences with the control fish, after which the number decreased. Moreover, the size of the centres increased from the 5th day, reaching peaks at 14 and 21 days. The process is slower than in the pronephros and spleen with few changes at 5 and 7 days but remaining important still at 21 days. Fish receiving a second dose of SRBC showed a rapid and large increase in the total area of MMCs, which persisted after 21 days. The differences at 14 and 21 days were significant in comparison with control animals receiving PBS in both immunizations, or PBS first and SRBC in the second challenge. The number of MMCs increased until the 14th day but then underwent a sharp decrease.

On the other hand the mean size of the MMCs remains constant until the 14th day, peaking remarkably after 21 days. This result explains the fall in the number of the MMCs after 14 days. Therefore after secondary immunization there is, in the mesonephros, a faster response than after the first immunization, when important differences appeared only after 14 or 21 days.

Ultrastructural analysis confirmed these quantitative differences and demonstrated the role of the macrophages of the splenic ellipsoids and that of the phagocytic reticular cells of the kidney in SRBC-trapping, and the massive presence of engulfed erythrocytes and crystalline inclusions in the MMCs. In the first days after primary and secondary immunization, ellipsoidal macrophages and phagocytic reticular cells contained more or less degraded remains of engulfed erythrocytes in their cytoplasm. These cells migrated presumably to the neighbouring MMCs, were the accumulations of degraded erythrocytes with giant crystalline inclusions reached a notable size. In some fish, however, 14 or 21 days after immunization ellipsoids and/or sinusoidal lining cells contained debris of erythrocytes and/or crystalline inclusions. On the other hand, the large MMCs found after secondary immunization sometimes underwent processes of encystment.

Phenylhydrazine was used as a tool to analyze the changes affecting the MMCs in a rapid and massive erythrocyte destruction. Twelve hours after treatment, the number and individual size of the MMCs increased enormously. At 24 hours the greater part of all three organs was occupied by very large, pale MMCs. At 5 days some MMCs appeared encysted and containd melanin. From the 5th day, the MMCs seemed to undergo a process of degeneration which culminated on the 6th and 7th days with the appearance of numerous small groups of two or three pale cells wich electron microscopy confirmed as degenerated macrophages from the MMCs. Ultrastructure of these giant MMCs showed numerous macrophages completely filled with remains of degenerated erythrocytes, mainly consisting of haemosiderin and crytalline inclusions. At 4 or 5 days, numerous macrophages could be seen containing several engulfed erythrocytes, and the crystalline inclusions were more frequent. From then on, numerous erythroblasts started the recovery of the erythroid population.

DISCUSSION

The histological organization of the MMCs in *C. auratus* agrees with that described for other teleosts (Agius, 1980; Agius and Agbede, 1984; Fulop and McMillan, 1984). All authors describe MMCs as aggregations of phagocytic cells with abundant cell debris, associated with the vascular system and surrounded by a capsule. According to our observations, lipofucsin, crystalline inclusions, probably representing haematoidin and/or haemosiderin, and fragments of erythrocytes and granulocytes are the most frequent contents of the MMCs. Some authors considered that the remains present in the MMCs are mainly concerned with the destruction of erythrocytes (Graf and Schlüns, 1979; Fulop and McMillan,1984) while others (Agius and Agbede, 1984), considered lipofucsin, coming from degraded mitochondria, the most widespread pigment; and in some conditions and/or species, melanins are the most abundant (Agius and Agbede, 1984). In any case, all authors have pointed out the heterogeneity of the pigments in fish MMCs.

Our results suggest conclusively a role for MMCs in the trapping of antigenic and non-antigenic material. The role of splenic ellipsoids and sinusoidal cells of the kidney as points for an initial trapping of carbon as demonstrated in our study has been found repeatedly (Lamers, 1985). From this location free macrophages migrate to the MMCs where they apparently accumulate. This phenomenon was also reported by Ellis et al. (1976). Whether the carbon-laden macrophages move to pre-existant MMCs (Mori, 1980) or form new aggregates (Ellis et al., 1976) is a matter of discussion, probably dependent on the amount of engulfed material and the number of MMCs present. Electron microscopy demonstrated that carbon-trapping was an intracellular process. Other authors (Lamers, 1985) however, have suggested an intra- and extracellular localization. On the other hand differences in the carbon-trapping of the kidney and spleen in relation to the route of injection -intraperitoneal or intramuscular- might represent the facility of movement of the particles to one or other organ.

The antigen-trapping changes in the MMCs after SRBC-immunization suggest a role for them in antigen-binding. Erythrocytes appear first in the cytoplasm of the macrophages of the splenic ellipsoids and of the endothelial cells of the kidney. An extracellular deposition was never found, as in the case of soluble antigens (Ellis, 1980; Secombes and Manning, 1980). In contrast, an intracellular localization has been described for A. hydrophila, a cellular antigen like SRBC (Lamers, 1985). Our results suggest also that macrophages in spleen or phagocytic-reticular cells in the kidney might transport the engulfed erythrocytes to MMCs. Lamers (1985) was, however, unable to demonstrate this antigenic transport in the case of A. hydrophila. Apparently, therefore, antigens processed by macrophages accumulated finally in the MMCs over long periods, suggesting a phylogenetic relationship to the germinal centres of higher vertebrates, despite their evident morphological differences.

On the other hand, a relationship between MMCs and iron metabolism has been suggested (Grover, 1968; Yu et al., 1971; Agius, 1979). Agius (1979) concluded that under conditions of starvation and in diseased fish, a markedly increased deposition of ferric iron occurred in the splenic centres. Our results using phenylhydrazine confirm this relationship. The induction of a fast and massive anaemia produces a rapid increase in the number and size of MMCs. These MMCs accumulate huge amounts of altered erythrocytes and after 5 days degenerate, coincident with the appearance of erythroblasts for the recovery of the erythroid population, suggesting a certain relationship between the need for iron in erythropoiesis and the disappearance of MMCs. In summary, present results sug gest that MMCs represent a non-specific system related to various physiological processes including, among others, processing of antigenic and non-antigenic material and the catabolism of erythroid tissue.

ACKNOWLEDGMENTS

Authors thank SCIG (León) for their magnificient assistance in these difficult moments.

REFERENCES

Agius, C., 1979. The role of melano-macrophage centres in iron storage in normal and diseased fish. J. Fish Dis., 2: 337-343.

Agius, C., 1980. Phylogenetic development of melano-macrophage centres in fish. J. Zool. (Lond.), 191: 11-31

Agius, C., 1981. The effects of splenectomy and subsequent starvation on the storage of haemosiderin by melano-macrophages of rainbow trout Salmo gairdneri Richardson. J. Fish Biol., 18: 41-44.

Agius, C., 1983. On the failure to detect haemosiderin in the melano-macrophages of the dogfish Scylorhinus canicula (L.) after prolonged starvation. Experientia, 39: 64-67.

Agius, C. and Agbede, S.A., 1984. An electron microscopical study on the genesis of lipofucsin, melanin and haemosiderin in haemopoietic tissues of fish. J. Fish Biol., 24: 471-488.

Agius, C. and Roberts, R.J., 1981. Effects of starvation on the melano-macrophage centres of fish. J. Fish Biol., 19: 161-169.

Blazer, V.S. and Wolke, R.E., 1983. Ceroid deposition, retinal degeneration and renal calcium oxalate crystals in cultured clown fish, Amphiprion ocellaris. J. Fish Dis., 8: 135-138.

Brown, C.L. and George, C.J., 1985. Age dependent accumulation of macrophage aggregates in the yellow perch, Perca fluviatilis (Mitchell). J. Fish Dis., 8: 135-138.

Ellis, A.E., 1980. Antigen trapping in the spleen and kidney of the plaice Pleuronectes platessa L.. J. Fish Dis., 3: 413-426.

Ellis, A.E., Munroe, A.L.S. and Roberts, R.J., 1976. Defence mechanisms in fish. 1. A study of phagocytic system and the fate of intraperitoneally injected particulate material in the plaice (Pleuronectes platessa L.). J. Fish Biol. 8: 67-78.

Ferguson, H.W., 1976. The relationship between ellipsoids and melano-macrophage centres in the spleen of turbot (Scophthalmus maximus). J. Comp. Pathol., 86: 377-380.

Fulop, G.M.I. and McMillan, D., 1984. Phagocytosis in the spleen of the sunfish Lepomis sp. J. Morphol., 179: 175-195.

Graf, R. and Schlüns, J., 1979. Ultrastructural and histochemical investigation of the terminal capillaries in the spleen of the carp (Cyprinus carpio L.) Cell Tissue Res., 196: 289-306.

Grover, J.H., 1968. Haemosiderins in bluegill spleens. Trans. Am. Fish. Soc., 97: 48-50.

Lamers, C.H.J., 1985. The reaction of the immune system of fish to vaccination. Ph.D. Thesis. University of Wageningen. Holland.

Mori, M., 1980. Studies on the phagocytic system in goldfish. I. Phagocytosis of intraperitoneally injected carbon particles. Fish Pathol., 15: 25-30.

Moccia, R.D., Hung, S.S.O., Slinger, S.J. and Ferguson, S.W., 1984. Effect of oxidized fish oil, vitamin E and ethoxyquin on histopathology and haematology of rainbow trout, Salmo gairdneri Richardson. J. Fish Dis., 7: 269-282.

Roberts, R.J., 1975. Melanin-containing cells of teleost fish and their relation to disease. In: W.E. Ribelin and G. Migali (Editors), The Pathology of Fishes. University of Wisconsin Press, Madison, pp. 399-428.

Secombes, C. and Manning, M.J., 1980. Comparative studies on the immune system of fishes and amphibians: Antigen localization in the carp *Cyprinus carpio*. J. Fish Dis., 3: 399-412.

Secombes, C.J., Manning, M.J. and Ellis A.E., 1982. Localization of the immune complex and heat-aggregated immunoglobulin in the carp *Cyprinus carpio* L.. Immunology, 47: 101-105.

Yu, M.L., Kiley, C.W., Sarat, D.A. and Perlmuter A., 1971. Regulation of haemosiderin to erythropoiesis in the blue gourami, *Trichogaster tricopterus*. J. Fish Res. Board Can., 28: 47-48.

Zapata, A., 1983. Phylogeny of the fish immune system. Bull. Inst. Pasteur, 81: 175-186.

Veterinary Immunology and Immunopathology, 12 (1986) 127—140
Elsevier Science Publishers B.V., Amsterdam — Printed in The Netherlands

ULTRASTRUCTURAL OBSERVATIONS ON PERITONEAL EXUDATE CELLS FROM THE STRIPED BASS

J.E. BODAMMER

National Marine Fisheries Service, Northeast Fisheries Center, Oxford, Maryland 21654 , USA

ABSTRACT

Bodammer, J.E., 1986. Ultrastructural observations on peritoneal exudate cells from the striped bass. Vet. Immunol. Immunopathol., 12: 127-140.

An ultrastructural study was conducted of the principal cells recovered from the peritoneal exudate of striped bass (*Morone saxatilis*) injected with killed *Bacillus cereus*. The most frequently observed cells were identified as macrophages, eosinophils, and neutrophils on the basis of comparing their structure with that reported for other fish species and higher vertebrates. All three of the types of cells were phagocytic; however, the numbers of bacteria engulfed were limited. Like other studies of this type in fish, the peritoneum of the striped bass proved to be a good source of cells for morphological investigations of phagocytosis.

INTRODUCTION

Because of a serious decline in striped bass (*Morone saxatilis*) populations along the east coast of the United States (U.S. Department of Commerce and U.S. Department of the Interior, 1984), they have been intensively studied in recent years. Despite this interest, however, little is presently known about their immunological defense mechanisms. Except for the recent findings by Stave and Roberson (1985) and Stave et al. (1983, 1984) on the chemiluminescent behavior of kidney derived phagocytes, only general information regarding the blood and hemopoietic system is available for this species (Groman, 1982). The purpose of this report is to provide a brief, but reasonably detailed, description of the principal cell types recovered from the peritonea of young striped bass after intraperitoneal injection of killed bacteria (*Bacillus cereus*). Tentative identification of these cells was made by comparing their cytological characteristics with those of other fish species and indicated that macrophages, eosinophils, and neutrophils were the major cell types present.

METHODS

The six, pond-reared, striped bass used in this study ranged in length from 28 to 35 cm, had a mean hematocrit of 36% (range 30-45%), and were maintained

0165-2427/86/$03.50 © 1986 Elsevier Science Publishers B.V.

before (7 days) and during the study in three, running water (12 ‰ salinity), 100 liter aquaria at 12-13°C. Prior to removing the peritoneal cells by lavage with sterile, Dulbecco's phosphate buffered saline (PBS) at a pH of 7.4, four of the fish were injected intraperitoneally with formalized *Bacillus cereus* that were washed and suspended (1-2 × 10^8 cells/ml) in PBS. The injection schedule and recovery of peritoneal cells for all fish was as follows: (a) Two fish received no bacteria and their peritoneal cells were collected immediately by washing with 2.0 ml of PBS; (b) two fish received 0.5 ml each of the bacterial suspension and the cell containing exudate was collected in 1.5 ml PBS after 45 minutes; and (c) two fish received 0.5 ml and 0.75 ml each of the bacterial solution at a 30-minute interval and the cells were collected in 1.0 ml PBS after 60 minutes. The exudate cells from both fish in each group were pooled after collection. All fish were sacrificed by a blow to the head prior to removing the cells from the peritoneum.

The cells were fixed in cold (0-4°C), 2% glutaraldehyde in 0.1 M phosphate buffer at a pH of 7.4. The cells were then washed several times in the same buffer, and post-fixed at room temperature in 1% osmium tetroxide in 0.1 M phosphate buffer (pH 7.4) for 1 hour. Prior to dehydration, the cells were stained with aqueous uranyl acetate (Terzakis, 1968). The cells were then dehydrated in a graded series of ethanols, followed by propylene oxide, and embedded in Spurr (1969) low viscosity medium. Thick sections (1-2 μm) were stained with toluidine blue dye and examined with a Zeiss[1] photomicroscope. Thin sections (60-90 nm) were stained with alcoholic uranyl acetate and lead citrate before examination with a Zeiss[1] EM 9 S2 electron microscope.

RESULTS

Electron microscopic observation of peritoneal cells from inoculated fish failed, despite the test organism's large size, to reveal any appreciable number of intracellular or surficially adherent bacteria. In addition, activated cells, demonstrating a hyaline ectoplasm, ruffles, lamellipodia, and other surface modifications (Stossel, 1974; Polliack and Gordon, 1975; Hoffstein et al., 1982), were present in all fishes regardless of treatment. The numbers of activated cells and the extent of their surface modifications appeared to be greater in fishes injected with bacteria. Because of these observations, it is not possible to provide a description of the sequence of events which occurs during phagocytosis (Stossel, 1974; Yin and Stossel, 1982).

---

[1]Reference to trade names does not imply endorsement by the National Marine Fisheries Service.

Macrophages

Macrophages were spherical in shape (M, Fig. 1) with a prominent, round nucleus near their centers; their cytoplasm was often divided into a dense endoplasm and hyaline ectoplasm. The cells varied in size (8.75-12.5 μm diam.) and dramatic increases in breadth were noted for those cells having extensively modified surfaces and/or large digestive vacuoles. Their nuclei (N, Fig. 2) were heterochromatic around their margins and within scattered islands throughout the nucleoplasm. Frequently, a nucleolus was observed. The endoplasm of the cells contained filaments, membrane profiles of rough and smooth endoplasmic reticulum, a Golgi complex, and large distinctive mitochondria (M, Figs. 2, 3). Common to both regions of the cytoplasm were many vesicles, lysosome-like bodies, autophagic vacuoles (AV), multivesicular bodies (MVB), and glycogen (Figs. 2, 3). The ectoplasm was best observed in areas where the cell's surface had been modified to form lamellipodia or ruffles (L, R, Fig. 2). The hyaline cytoplasm in these regions was composed mainly of vacuoles (V, Fig. 2) that probably resulted from infoldings of the plasmalemma, smooth or coated vesicles (CV, Fig. 2), fine filaments, and glycogen. The phagocytic capability of these cells is illustrated in Figures 2 and 3 where bacteria are present in phagolysosomes.

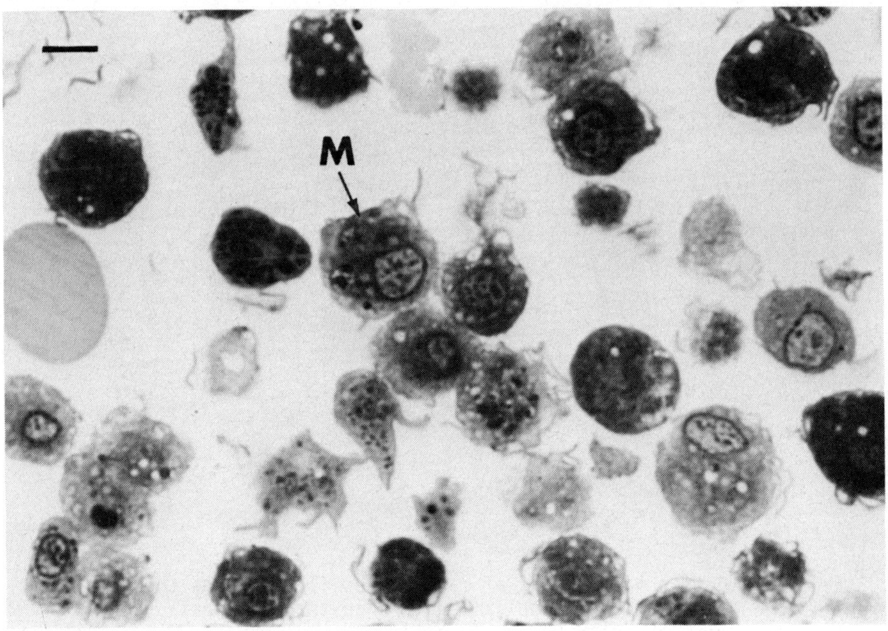

Fig. 1. Photomicrograph of several macrophages (M) in a group demonstrating their variable size and surface modifications. ×1600.

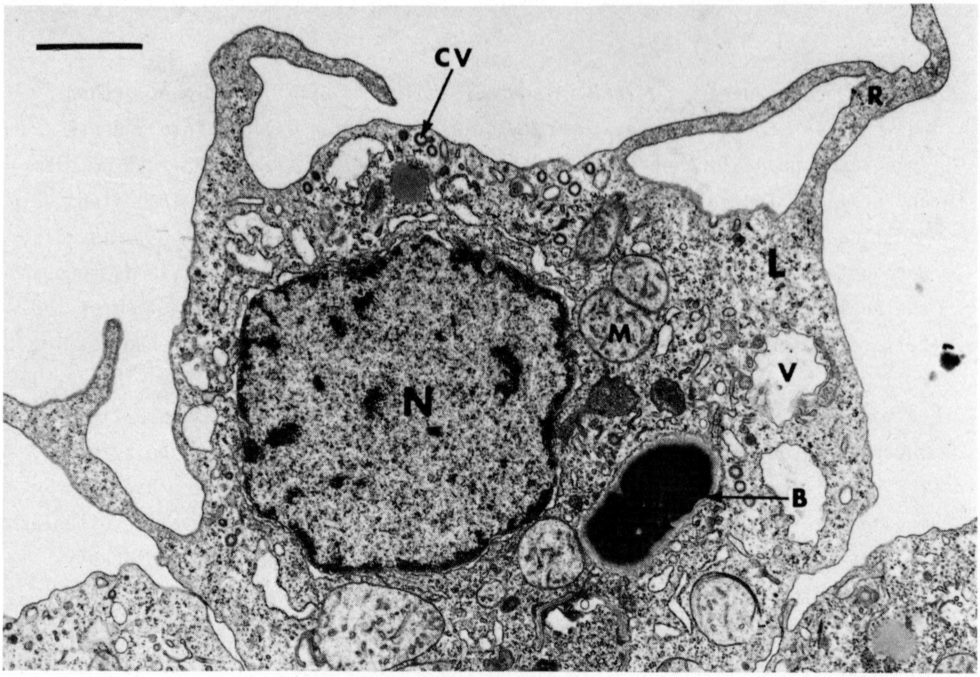

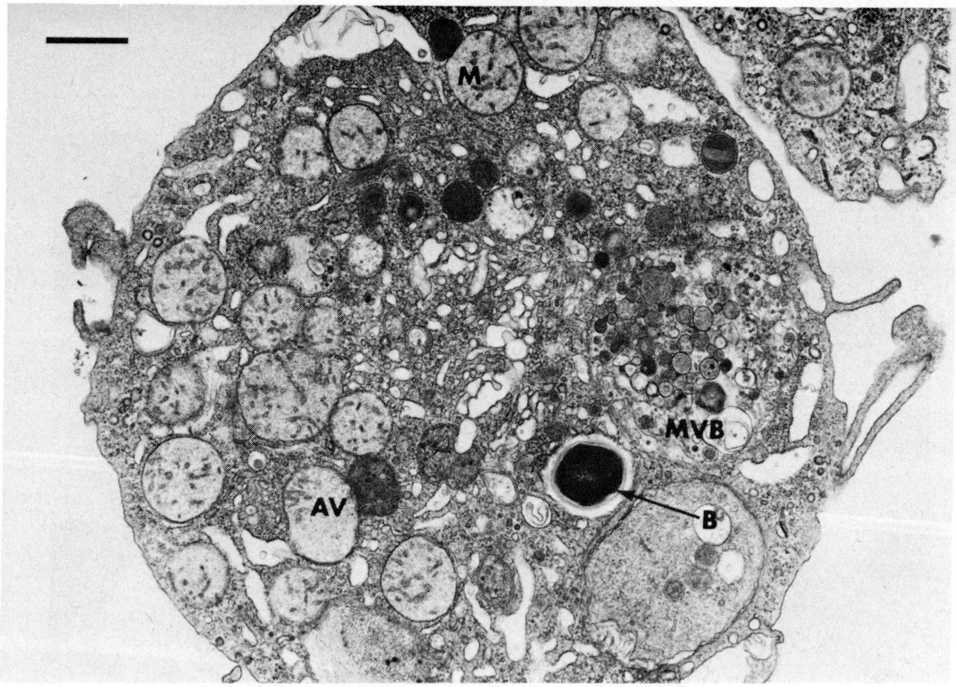

Figs. 2 and 3. Electron micrographs of macrophages illustrating the fine structure of the endoplasm and ectoplasm and phagocytized bacteria (B). (N = nucleus; M = mitochondria; AV = autophagic vacuole; MVB = multivesicular body; L = lamellipodium; R = ruffles; CV = coated vesicles; V = vacuoles.) Fig. 2, ×13,920; Fig. 3, ×10,670.

<u>Eosinophils</u>

The eosinophils (E, Fig. 4) were oval in form, had an eccentrically positioned nucleus, and were approximately 15 by 9 µm in size. They were easily recognized by their large, densely stained, irregularly shaped granules (Figs. 5, 6). The granules appeared to be either smooth or lightly stippled (granular). Their nuclei (N, Fig. 5) had patches of heterochromatin around their borders and distributed throughout the nucleoplasm. A small nucleolus was infrequently observed. In those instances where the surface of the cell was modified to form a lamellipodium (L, Fig. 5), a distinct ectoplasm contained mainly fine filaments and glycogen. The endoplasm of the cell (Figs. 5, 6) was composed of granules, small vesicles, many profiles of tubular, smooth endoplasmic reticulum, a modest amount of rough endoplasmic reticulum, and a prominent Golgi complex (GC, Fig. 5). The oval mitochondria (M, Fig. 5) were dispersed throughout the cell. The presence of the test bacterium within a developing phagosome (Fig. 6) or found more deeply within the cells confirmed that they were phagocytic.

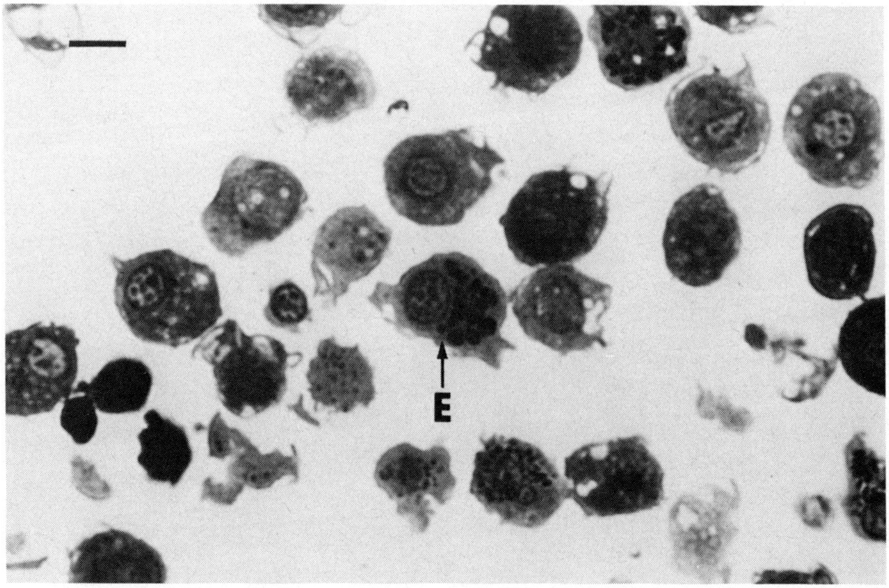

Fig. 4. Photomicrograph of an eosinophil (E) showing the typical large granules found in these cells and their characteristically eccentric nuclei. ×1500.

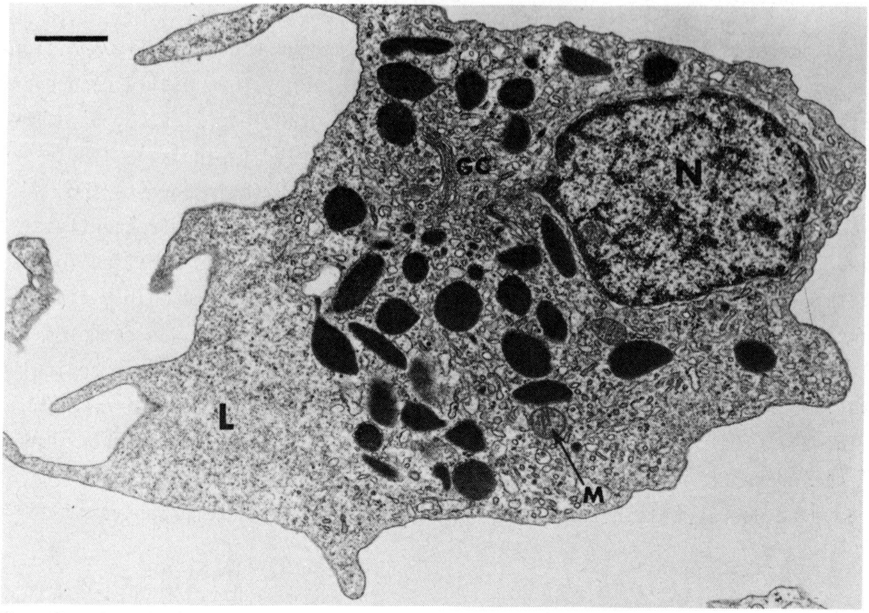

Fig. 5. An electron micrograph of an eosinophil showing the cell's granules, Golgi complex (GC), nucleus (N), mitochondria (M), and lamellipodium (L). ×10,670.

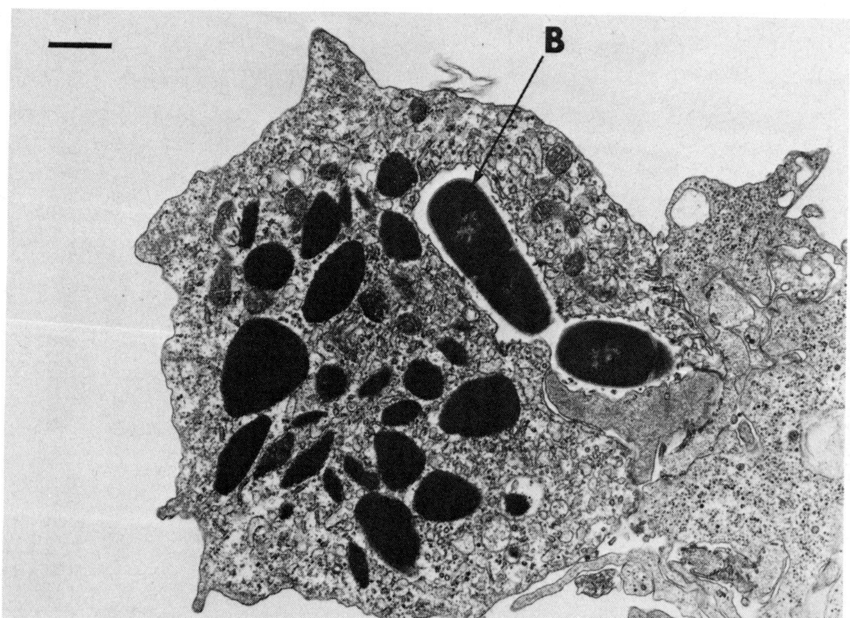

Fig. 6. An electron micrograph of a portion of an eosinophil featuring the engulfment of a bacterium (B) within a phagosome. ×9600.

Neutrophils

As shown in Figures 7, 8, and 10, these cells were pleomorphic, had a slightly oval nucleus, and contained spherical granules within their cytoplasm. Measurements on cells like those in Figure 7 indicated that they were approximately 9 μm in width and 12 μm in length. Their nuclei (N, Figs. 8, 10) did not contain a nucleolus, and the heterochromatin was distributed peripherally or in dispersed patches throughout the nucleoplasm. The endoplasm of these cells contained granules (Figs. 8, 10) which varied both in size (.21-.53 μm diam.) and density, oval mitochondria (M, Fig. 8), a Golgi complex (GC, Fig. 10), profiles of rough and smooth endoplasmic reticulum membranes, smooth surfaced tubules, vesicles, and glycogen (G, Fig. 10). A more detailed examination of their granules showed that their contents were stippled, smooth, or striate in appearance. In some cells, the apparent loss of granule contents (extraction) revealed an underlying filamentous (Fig. 9) substructure which could have provided, depending on the plane of section, the stippled or striate appearance described. The hyaline cytoplasm observed around the periphery of these cells was most noticeable in surface projections such as lamellipodia (L) or ruffles (R) as shown in Figures 8, 9, and 10. In these regions, the cell was devoid of organelles except for small vesicles, fine filaments, and glycogen. Bacteria (B, Fig. 10) observed within these cells indicated that phagocytosis had occurred.

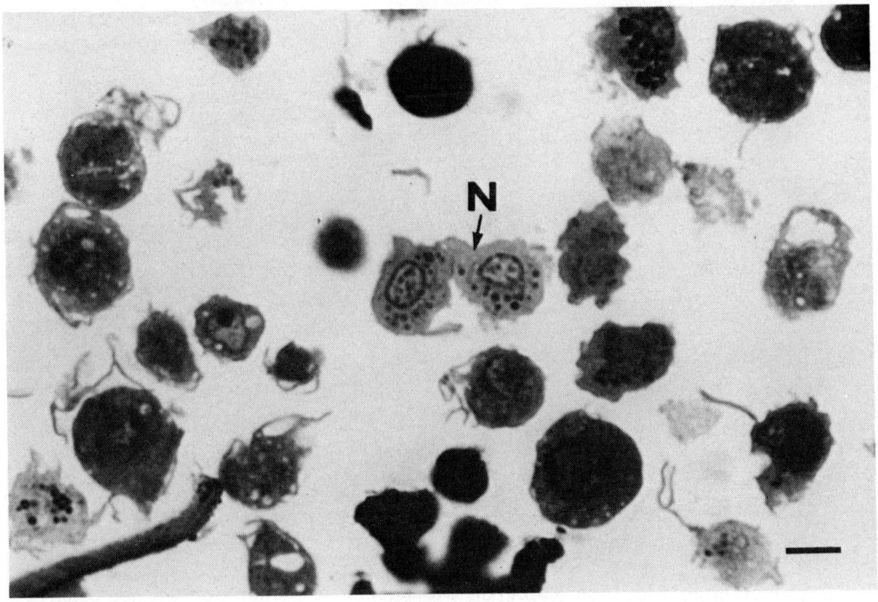

Fig. 7. Photomicrograph of two neutrophils (N) adjacent to each other and demonstrating their non-lobulate nuclei and spherical granules. ×1380.

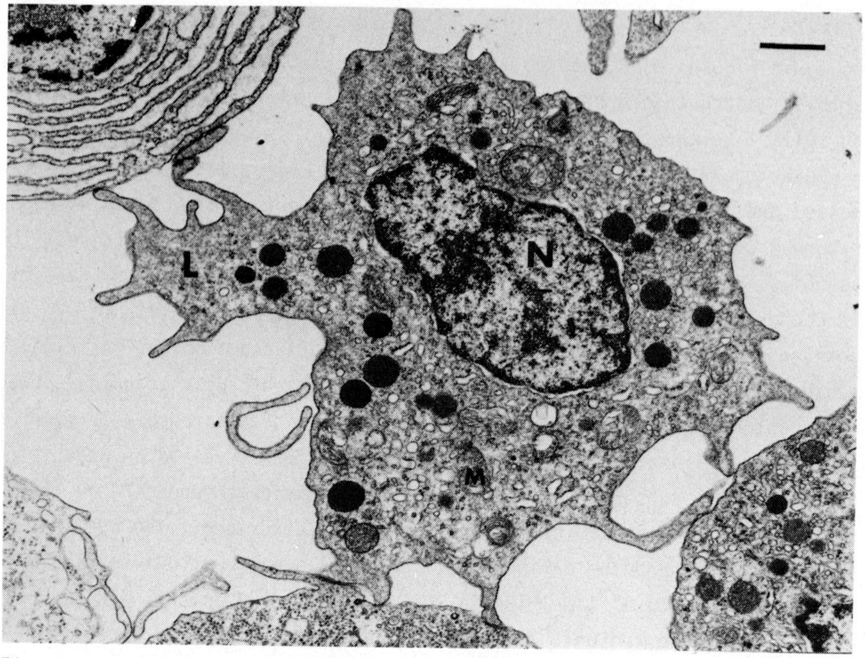

Fig. 8. An electron micrograph of a neutrophil having a highly modified surface showing both ruffles and a lamellipodium (L) plus the typical dense granules found in these cells. (N = nucleus; M = mitochondria.) ×9600.

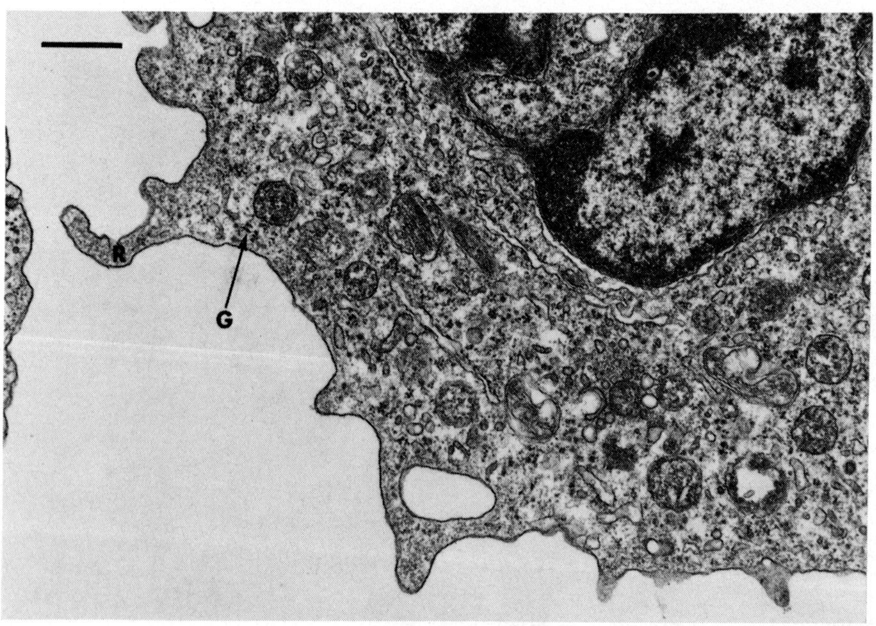

Fig. 9. A higher magnification electron micrograph of a portion of neutrophil cytoplasm showing the filamentous substructure of the granules, small aggregates of glycogen (G), and ruffles (R). ×23,750.

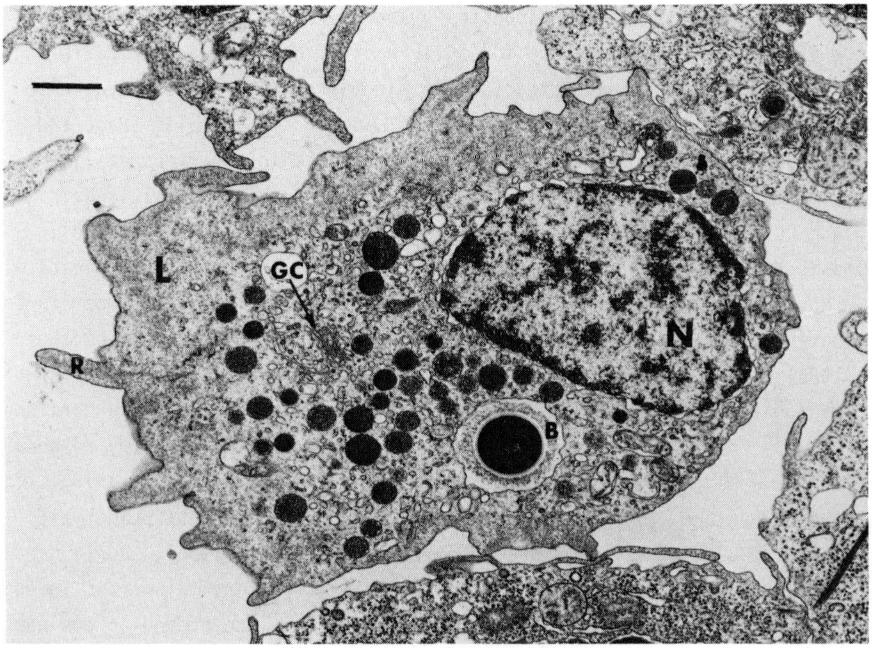

Fig. 10. An electron micrograph of a neutrophil containing a bacterium (B) and illustrating a large lamellipodium (L), ruffles (R), an active Golgi complex (GC), and numerous spherical granules of varying size and density. (N = nucleus.) ×10,670.

DISCUSSION

The modest phagocytic response observed for the striped bass peritoneal cells may have been due to such factors as temperature, concentration of bacteria, the use of formalin fixed cells, response time, or failure to opsonize the test organism, all of which are important to studying cellular defense mechanisms in fish (Fujii, 1981; Griffin, 1983; Stave et al., 1983, 1984; Sakai, 1984; Scott et al., 1985). The finding that resident peritoneal cells from injected fish often appeared to be activated is without present explanation; however, a subsequent discussion of striped bass neutrophils in this report will consider this problem in more detail.

In keeping with Ellis' (1977) terminology for fish, the agranular, phagocytic cells observed in the peritoneum of striped bass are interpreted as being macrophages. The salient features, derived from studies on mammals (Bessis, 1973; Stossel, 1974; Polliack and Gordon, 1975) that assisted in the identification of these cells were the apparent loss of granules during the transition from blood-borne monocyte to peritoneal macrophage; the presence of lysosome-like bodies, autophagic vacuoles, and multivesicular bodies within their cytoplasm;

the division of the cell into an organelle-rich endoplasm and hyaline ectoplasm bearing ruffles and lamellipodia; and the presence of vesicles and small vacuoles suggestive of a cell involved in pinocytosis and secretion (both functions well described for macrophages). Except for their lack of granules and/or differences in nuclear morphology, the ultrastructure of the macrophages was comparable to the monocytes found in the peripheral blood of *Lampetra fluviatilis* (Page and Rowley, 1983) where lytic enzymes were demonstrated within the lysosome-like vesicles, *Pleuronectes platessa* (Ferguson, 1976), *Scyliorhinus canicula* L. (Morrow and Pulsford, 1980), and *Ictalurus punctatus* (Cannon et al., 1980b). Phagocytosis has been demonstrated for cells from the last three fish species listed. Most significant cytologically, macrophages from striped bass peritonea were comparable to those of peritoneal macrophages from *P. platessa* (MacArthur et al., 1984) which were shown to be phagocytic for bacteria and oyster glycogen.

Both the presence and role of eosinophils in fish blood are poorly understood (Ellis, 1977). In mammals, eosinophils participate in the inflammatory response and are known to be phagocytic (Bessis, 1973; Sanderson and De Souza, 1979). Recent studies of them in elasmobranchs indicate that they are not phagocytic (Hyder et al., 1983), or are weakly so (Morrow and Pulsford, 1980). Rowley and Page (1985), however, have reported that eosinophils from larval lampreys ingest bacteria but fail to engulf colloidal carbon. The cells interpreted as eosinophils in this study engulfed the test bacteria and their fine structure was similar to that of eosinophils in the blood of *Carassius auratus* (Davies and Haynes, 1975), *Catostomus commersoni* (Lester and Desser, 1975), *Scyliorhinus canicula* (Morrow and Pulsford, 1980), *Salmo gairdneri irideus* (Bielek, 1980), and larval *Lampetra* sp. (Rowley and Page, 1985). Like the granules found in the eosinophils from the species mentioned above, those from the cells in striped bass lacked the crystalline substructure commonly found in eosinophil granules in mammals (Bessis, 1973). Thus far, a definitive intragranular crystal has only been reported in eosinophils from the nurse shark, *Ginglymostoma cirratum* (Hyder et al., 1983). The potentially lytic capabilities of these granules in fish eosinophils, and their relationship to the granulocytes of higher vertebrates have been suggested by Rowley and Page's (1985) demonstration of acid phosphatase within them, and Bielek's (1981) observation that they contain peroxidase. The striped bass eosinophils were differentiated from basophils on the basis that the latter are not believed to be phagocytic either in fish (Ellis, 1977) or in mammals (Bessis, 1973).

To mammalian hematologists, the neutrophil is known as an actively phagocytic and mobile cell that responds rapidly to the presence of antigens and/or other inflammatory agents (Bessis, 1973; Stossel, 1974). For students of fish hematology, however, the identification and function of this cell has been a difficult and controversial subject (Ellis, 1977). There have been recent and important advances of our understanding of neutrophils in fish. Known also as polymorphonuclear leukocytes, it is presently accepted that their nuclei show varying degrees of lobulation depending on the species (Ellis, 1977), or on their state of maturation (Bielek, 1980; Page and Rowley, 1983). Their typical oval or elongate granules are normally of one type for a given species and generally present an internal structure that is either striate (Ferguson, 1976; Bielek, 1980; Cannon et al., 1980b; Hyder et al., 1983) or crystalline (Davies and Haynes, 1975; Lester and Desser, 1975; Bielek, 1980; Page and Rowley, 1983). Like the nucleus, variations in granule structure within neutrophils of a particular species may depend upon the maturity of the cell (Bielek, 1980; Page and Rowley, 1983). Phagocytosis by fish neutrophils both *in vivo* (Morrow and Pulsford, 1980; MacArthur et al., 1984; Miyazaki and Plumb, 1985) and *in vitro* (Fujii, 1981; Griffin, 1983; Hyder et al., 1983; Sakai, 1984) has been demonstrated. Additionally, cytochemical studies conducted on their granules have shown they contain peroxidase (Ellis, 1976; Cannon et al., 1980a; Bielek, 1981) and both acid phosphatase and β-glucuronidase (Page and Rowley, 1983).

When compared to the neutrophils studied by the authors cited above, those from the striped bass examined herein, because of their simple, round or oval nuclei and spherically shaped granules which were often uncondensed or lacked definitive striae, appeared to be immature cells (promyelocytes, myelocytes) as described in other fish species (Bielek, 1980; Page and Rowley, 1983) or in mammals (Bessis, 1973). Observation of peripheral blood neutrophils from striped bass (Bodammer, unpublished observations) showed that they possessed a horseshoe or bilobed nucleus and oval or elongate granules in which the striae were clearly visible. Comparing the data herein with observations on peritoneal neutrophils from the plaice, *Pleuronectes platessa* (MacArthur et al., 1984), the cells of both species are phagocytic; however, those from the plaice have nuclear (i.e., bilobed) and granule (i.e., elongate or oval) characteristics of mature cells. If this study of striped bass leukocytes had been conducted on hemopoietic tissues or peripheral blood, the occurrence of immature cells would have been expected. As Bessis (1973) has mentioned, however, mammalian granulocytes leave the hemopoietic tissues normally as mature cells prior to entering the blood and/or body cavities. Regrettably, the peripheral blood of the fish used in this study was not examined. Consequently, it is not possible to state whether these fish had neutrophilia as a consequence of stress or disease (Bessis, 1973; Ellis, 1977). Additionally, the appearance of activated cells and/or debris containing macrophages in the non-injected fish suggests that the latter were compromised in some way at the time the experiment was conducted. This could have served as a source or stimulus for the immature neutrophils that were recovered.

CONCLUSION

The data presented herein have demonstrated that the striped bass peritoneum contains macrophages, eosinophils, and neutrophils, all of which were shown to phagocytose killed bacteria (*Bacillus cereus*). This study constitutes the first ultrastructural description of blood cells in this species and indicates that the cells are comparable in structure to those described for other fish. Additionally, this report extends the significance of other recent studies (Murray and Fletcher, 1976; MacArthur et al., 1984; Sakai, 1984) and attests to the usefulness of the fish peritoneum as a source of leukocytes for the future study of cellular mediated immunity.

ACKNOWLEDGMENTS

I wish to thank Dr. R.A. Robohm, National Marine Fisheries Service, Milford, Connecticut, for the bacteria. The critical review of Dr. R.A. Murchelano and editorial assistance of Mrs. J. Swann were very much appreciated. In addition, I wish to thank Ms. J.T. Wade for technical assistance.

REFERENCES

Bessis, M., 1973. Living Blood Cells and Their Ultrastructure. Springer-Verlag, Berlin, 767 pp.

Bielek, E., 1980. Electron microscopical studies of blood cells in teleosts. III. Granulocytes. Zool. Jb. Anat. 103: 105-121.

Bielek, E., 1981. Developmental stages and localization of peroxidatic activity in the leucocytes of three teleost species (*Cyprinus carpio* L.; *Tinca tinca* L.; *Salmo gairdneri* Richardson). Cell Tiss. Res. 220: 163-180.

Cannon, M.S., Mollenhauer, H.H., Cannon, A.M., Eurell, T.E. and Lewis, D.H., 1980a. Ultrastructural localization of peroxidase activity in neutrophil leukocytes of *Ictalurus punctatus*. Can. J. Zool. 58: 1139-1143.

Cannon, M.S., Mollenhauer, H.H., Eurell, T.E., Lewis, D.H., Cannon, A.M. and Tompkins, C., 1980b. An ultrastructural study of the leukocytes of the channel catfish, *Ictalurus punctatus*. J. Morphol. 164: 1-23.

Davies, H.G. and Haynes, M.E., 1975. Light- and electron-microscope observations on certain leukocytes in a teleost fish and a comparison of the envelope-limited monolayers of chromatin structural units in different species. J. Cell Sci. 17: 263-285.

Ellis, A.E., 1976. Leucocytes and related cells in the plaice *Pleuronectes platessa*. J. Fish Biol. 8: 143-156.

Ellis, A.E., 1977. The leucocytes of fish: a review. J. Fish Biol. 11: 453-491.

Ferguson, H.W., 1976. The ultrastructure of plaice (*Pleuronectes platessa*) leucocytes. J. Fish Biol. 8: 139-142.

Fujii, T., 1981. Antibody-enhanced phagocytosis of lamprey polymorphonuclear leucocytes against sheep erythrocytes. Cell Tiss. Res. 219: 41-51.

Griffin, B.R., 1983. Opsonic effect of rainbow trout (*Salmo gairdneri*) antibody on phagocytosis of *Yersinia ruckeri* by trout leukocytes. Dev. Comp. Immunol. 7: 253-259.

Groman, D.B., 1982. Histology of the Striped Bass. Am. Fish. Soc. Monogr. 3, Bethesda, Maryland, 116 pp.

Hoffstein, S.T., Korchak, H.M., Smolen, J.E. and Weissmann, G., 1982. Early consequences of neutrophil activation and their association with degranulation. In: M.L. Karnovsky and L. Bolis (Editors), Phagocytosis--Past and Future. Academic Press, New York, pp. 47-65.

Hyder, S.L., Cayer, M.L. and Pettey, C.L., 1983. Cell types in peripheral blood of the nurse shark: an approach to structure and function. Tissue & Cell 15: 437-455.

Lester, R.J.G. and Desser, S.S., 1975. Ultrastructural observations on the granulocytic leucocytes of the teleost *Catostomus commersoni*. Can. J. Zool. 53: 1648-1657.

MacArthur, J.I., Fletcher, T.C., Pirie, B.J.S., Davidson, R.J.L. and Thomson, A.W., 1984. Peritoneal inflammatory cells in plaice, *Pleuronectes platessa* L.: effects of stress and endotoxin. J. Fish Biol. 25: 69-81.

Miyazaki, T. and Plumb, J.A., 1985. Histopathology of *Edwardsiella ictaluri* in channel catfish, *Ictalurus punctatus* (Rafinesque). J. Fish Dis. 8: 389-392.

Morrow, W.J.W. and Pulsford, A., 1980. Identification of peripheral blood leucocytes of the dogfish (*Scyliorhinus canicula* L.) by electron microscopy. J. Fish Biol. 17: 461-475.

Murray, C.K. and Fletcher, T.C., 1976. The immunohistochemical localization of lysozyme in plaice (*Pleuronectes platessa* L.) tissues. J. Fish Biol. 9: 329-334.

Page, M. and Rowley, A.F., 1983. A cytochemical, light and electron microscopical study of the leucocytes of the adult river lamprey, *Lampetra fluviatilis* (L. Gray). J. Fish Biol. 22: 503-517.

Polliack, A. and Gordon, S., 1975. Scanning electron microscopy of murine macrophages. Lab. Invest. 33: 469-477.

Rowley, A.F. and Page, M., 1985. Ultrastructural, cytochemical and functional studies on the eosinophilic granulocytes of larval lampreys. Cell Tiss. Res. 240: 705-709.

Sakai, D.K., 1984. Opsonization by fish antibody and complement in the immune phagocytosis by peritoneal exudate cells isolated from salmonid fishes. J. Fish Dis. 7: 29-38.

Sanderson, C.J. and De Souza, W., 1979. A morphological study of the interaction between *Trypanosoma cruzi* and rat eosinophils, neutrophils and macrophages *in vitro*. J. Cell Sci. 37: 275-286.

Scott, A.L., Rogers, W.A. and Klesius, P.H., 1985. Chemiluminescence by peripheral blood phagocytes from channel catfish: function of opsonin and temperature. Dev. Comp. Immunol. 9: 241-250.

Spurr, A.R., 1969. A low-viscosity epoxy resin embedding medium for electron microscopy. J. Ultrastruct. Res. 26: 31-43.

Stave, J.W. and Roberson, B.S., 1985. Hydrocortisone suppresses the chemiluminescent response of striped bass phagocytes. Dev. Comp. Immunol. 9: 77-84.

Stave, J.W., Roberson, B.S. and Hetrick, F.M., 1983. Chemiluminescence of phagocytic cells isolated from the pronephros of striped bass. Dev. Comp. Immunol. 7: 269-276.

Stave, J.W., Roberson, B.S. and Hetrick, F.M., 1984. Factors affecting the chemiluminescent response of fish phagocytes. J. Fish Biol. 25: 197-206.

Stossel, T.P., 1974. Phagocytosis. New Engl. J. Med. 290: 717-839.

Terzakis, J.A., 1968. Uranyl acetate, a stain and a fixative. J. Ultrastruct. Res. 22: 168-184.

U.S. Department of Commerce and U.S. Department of the Interior, 1984. Emergency striped bass research study, report for 1982-1983. Washington, D.C., 37 pp.

Yin, H.L. and Stossel, T.P., 1982. The mechanism of phagocytosis. In: M.L. Karnovsky and L. Bolis (Editors), Phagocytosis--Past and Future. Academic Press, New York, pp. 13-24.

Veterinary Immunology and Immunopathology, 12 (1986) 141—151
Elsevier Science Publishers B.V., Amsterdam — Printed in The Netherlands

PRONEPHRIC LEUCOCYTES OF *Cyprinus carpio*: ISOLATION, SEPARATION AND CHARACTERIZATION

CHRISTOPHER J. BAYNE[1]

Dept of Experimental Animal Morphology and Cell Biology, The Agricultural University, Wageningen, The Netherlands

ABSTRACT

Bayne, C.J., 1986. Pronephric leucocytes of *Cyprinus carpio*: Isolation, separation and characterization. Veterinary Immunology and Immunopathology, 12: 141-151.

Since the teleost pronephros is an important source of diverse immunocytes, suspensions of pronephric cells from young adult carp have been characterized. In freshly prepared suspensions, adherent, spreading cells (macrophages?) constituted <3% of the total population. Granulocytes and lymphocytes were co-dominant (<80%) leucocyte types. Continuous Percoll density gradient centrifugation yielded discrete subpopulations with these ρ values and cytological characteristics:

Fraction	I & II	ρ = 1.055 - 1.070	thrombocytes, monocytes, macrophages, and lymphocytes.
Fraction	III	ρ = 1.080 - 1.090	granulocytes, type 1.
Fraction	IV	ρ = 1.105 - 1.110	erythrocytes and granulocytes, type 2.
Fraction	V	ρ = 1.118 - 1.125	granulocytes, type 3.
Fraction	VI	ρ = 1.140 - 1.150	granulocytes, type 4.

Granulocyte motility increased markedly over the first 24 hr *in vitro*, and was enhanced by components washed from intact yeast. The subtypes of granulocytes were distinguishable by not only the ρ values, but also on the basis of cell size, ultra-structure of the granules, and their histochemical and phagocytic characteristics. After simultaneous *in vivo* injection of *Bacillus megaterium* (Gram + ve), *Aeromonas hydrophila* (Gram - ve) and *Saccharomyces cerevisiae* (yeast), individual pronephric leucocytes were found capable of phagocytosing all three types of particle. Granulocytes which had phagocytosed *B. megaterium* were slower than macrophages in their ability to kill the bacteria. Encounter with *B. megaterium* or *S. cerevisiae in vitro* elicited a clumping reaction which involved mostly the larger leucocytes [granulocytes]. Both adherent cells and non-adherent cells were phagocytic *in vitro*.

---

[1]Present Address: Department of Zoology, Oregon State University, Corvallis, Oregon 97331, USA.

0165-2427/86/$03.50 © 1986 Elsevier Science Publishers B.V.

INTRODUCTION

The teleost pronephros, or head-kidney, is a pivotal component of the immune system. In addition to being the major site of production of erythroid, lymphoid and myeloid cells (Smith et al., 1970), it traps antigens (Ellis et al., 1976), and its lymphoid cells secrete antibody (Smith et al., 1967). Effectors of cell-mediated immunity are also located in the pronephros: for example, nonspecific cytotoxic cells (NCC) have been isolated from this organ (Graves et al., 1984). Furthermore the pronephros has been found to be a good source of macrophages (Braun-Nesje et al, 1982). The presence of melanomacrophage centers (Agius, 1981) supports the contention that all the cellular elements essential for antigen trapping, processing and presentation are present here. Indeed, the failure of splenectomy to depress the humoral immune response of teleosts has been interpreted as meaning that the pronephros may well be able to complete all phases of an immune response independently of other lymphoid organs (Ferren, 1967).

Investigations utilizing pronephric cells *in vitro* have tended to focus on one or another cell type or function, and it has been unclear to what extent any one subpopulation dominates. To provide information on the subpopulations of the adult carp pronephros, its cells have been separated by density gradient centrifugation and characterized with respect to cytological, behavioral, some cytochemical, and functional (phagocytic) properties. The myeloid cells are as numerous as the lymphoid cells, and the diversity of granulocytes is notable.

MATERIALS AND METHODS

Fish.

Male and female carp, weighing 90 - 200g, were raised at 20±1° C in a recirculating system. The pelleted food was K20 (Trouw & Co, Putten, The Netherlands). Prior to surgery, fish were anaesthetized in MS222 (Sandoz).

Cell Cultures.

Fish were bled by syringe as completely as possible (*ca.* 2-3 ml.) from the caudal circulation to reduce the blood volume in the pronephros, then surface sterilized with 70% alcohol. Using sterile technique, the tissue overlaying the pronephros of each side was removed, and the organ was freed of neighboring tissues and placed in 2ml ice-cold tissue culture medium with heparin (TCM-hep). Both head kidneys were placed on a nylon net. Using a syringe plunger, and accompanied by 4ml ice-cold TCM-hep added dropwise, the cells were expressed and washed through into a siliconized glass container on ice.

Cell suspensions from the two organs were pooled in siliconized tubes and centrifuged at 250-400g for 10min at 4° C. The cells were resuspended in fresh TCM-hep if density gradient centrifugation was to follow, or in TCM without heparin if cells were to be placed directly into culture. Counts of living and dead cells were made with trypan blue and hemacytometers.

Media.

TCM was RPMI-1640 supplemented with 5% fetal calf serum, 1% pooled carp serum (PCS), 2mM L-glutamine and 10%(v/v) distilled water. TCM-hep was the same, with heparin added to 10 I.U. per ml. When bovine serum albumin fraction V was added, it was dissolved in medium, and filter sterilized.

Density gradient centrifugation.

Percoll (Pharmacia) was mixed 9:1 with 10X Hanks Balanced Salt Solution. This Percoll-SIP was made to 80, 60 and 54% with TCM-hep. Such mixtures (10ml each) were spun in a fixed angle rotor at 30,000g for 25 - 30min at 4° C to generate continuous density gradients which were monitored using colored beads, with calibrated ρ values, from Pharmacia. Suspensions of pronephric cells (1 - 3 x 10^7 cells total in 2 - 3 ml) were gently layered on top of gradients, then the tubes were spun in a swing-out rotor at 350g for 30min at 4° C.

Microscopy.

Cells obtained from Percoll gradients were washed in TCM. For phase contrast and UV microscopy live cells were used. Acridine Orange (50 or 100μg/ml TCM) vital staining was for one minute followed by a brief rinse in TCM. To ensure maximum retention of cells, they were first allowed to settle on to poly-L-lysine (100μg/ml, 30 min) treated, rinsed coverslips.

For cytochemistry, cells were left to settle for 30 min onto poly-l-lysine coated glass in a moist box, then the atmosphere over the cells was saturated with formaldehyde vapor for at least another 30min. Periodic acid-Schiff positive material, peroxidase (diamino-benzidine) and acid phosphatase were detected following standard procedures.

Phagocytosis.

Yeast (*Saccharomyces cerevisiae*), *Bacillus megaterium* and *Aeromonas hydrophila* were heat-killed then labelled with rhodamine isothiocyanate (RITC) or with fluorescein ITC by incubation with these dyes (75µg/ml) in 500mM carbonate buffer, pH9.5, followed by rinsing in 10% FCS in TCM to remove unbound dye. The microbes were added to cells for _in vitro_ phagocytosis, or injected _in vivo_ 2hr before fish were killed for pronephric cell preparation.

RESULTS

Cell types and abundance.

Pronephric cell suspensions included monocytes, macrophages, lymphocytes, plasma cells, granulocytes, erythrocytes (RBC) and an occasional thrombocyte probably due to residual blood in the organ. Stem cells and developmental stages of erythroid, myeloid and lymphoid lines are considered to be part of the population; in this study identification of immature stages was not attempted. One typical preparation consisted of 45% small leucocytes (predominantly lymphocytes), 47% large leucocytes (monocytes, macrophages and granulocytes) and 8% RBC. When the numbers of cells obtained from fish weighing 75 - 208g were plotted against fish weight (Fig. 1), it appeared that about 10^8 cells were obtainable over the entire weight range. A regression analysis found the relationship to be:
No. of cells = 0.04 x wt(g) + 4.18 (r^2 = 0.26). This marginally significant

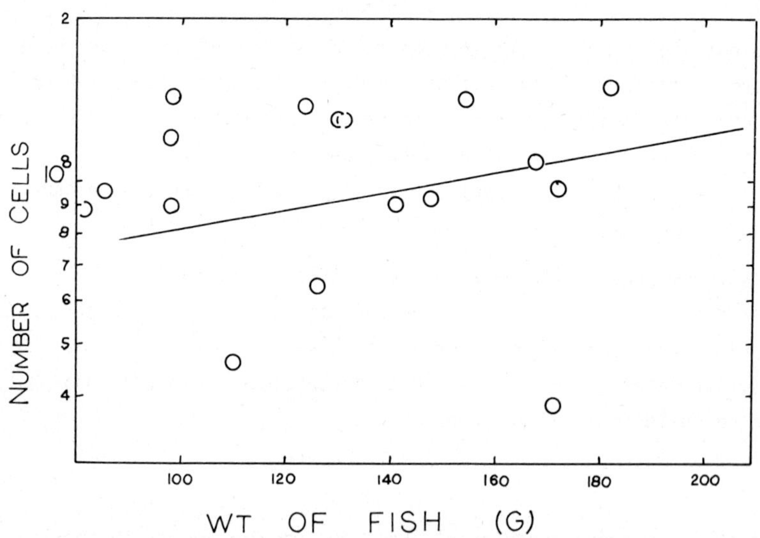

Figure 1. Relationship between weight of carp and the number of cells in suspensions obtained from both pronephroi.

relationship ($0.01 < p < 0.05$) means that there is a small increase in cell yield with increase in body weight. An impression was gained that the healthiest-looking fish had smaller-than-average head kidneys.

In 15 runs over 3 months the cells separated consistently into 6 bands ("fractions") in continuous gradients of Percoll. The two uppermost bands were diffuse and difficult to collect separately, though separation on a 54% Percoll gradient made this easier. Similarly, bands 5 and 6, which were denser than RBC, lay close together in 60% Percoll and were separated better in 80% gradients. Table I lists the subpopulations and some of their characteristics, and Fig. 2 shows their relative abundances. An ultrastructural study of the cells will be published separately (Temmink and Bayne, in preparation).

Lymphocytes constituted slightly less than 50% of the cells. They have been characterized structurally (Davina et al., 1980), and were typical vertebrate lymphocytes. Macrophages. From studies in salmonids (Braun-Nesje et al, 1982) it was anticipated that macrophages would be numerous in the head kidney; yet in 4 separate preparations, cells with size and behavioral traits typical of macrophages constituted only 1 - 3% of the total population. These were counted within an hour of the cell suspensions being prepared; possibly higher numbers may have been seen if macrophages were counted after longer *in vitro*.

Granulocytes. These were found in four distinct ρ-value populations. Eosinophils, neutrophils, basophils and heterophils have been reported in carp blood (Hofte et al., 1984). We distinguish 3 types of pronephric granulocyte on the basis of granule ultrastructure (Temmink and Bayne, loc. cit.). The 'type 1' granulocyte (ρ= 1.080 - 1.090) is by far the most abundant non-lymphoid leucocyte ($>2 \times 10^7$ per fish). It is negative for PAS and acid phosphatase, but contains peroxidase, and phagocytoses *Bacillus megaterium*.

The type 2 granulocyte (ρ= 1.105 - 1.110) always moved isopycnically with RBC. Their granules correspond with those ascribed by J. Lehmann (pers. comm) to basophils. Their staining reactions to PAS (+ve), peroxidase (-ve) and acid phosphatase (+ve) are all distinctive from those in the type 1 cell; however type 2 cells also engulfed *B. megaterium*.

Those granulocytes with densities greater than RBC (types 3 and 4) were few in number; yet their large diameters (a few µm more than other granulocytes) caused them to produce bands in Percoll visible to the naked eye.

Cell behavior and function.

Observations were made on populations of cells not separated on Percoll. Macrophages rapidly attached to and spread on glass. In plastic

TABLE I. Cells from the Pronephros of Carp, Separated on the Basis of Density, Presented with Certain Characteristics of the Subpopulations.

FRACTION #	ρ value	Cell Types Present	Sizes* (µm)	Phagocytosis	PAS	Peroxidase	Acid Phosphatase
I & II	1.055-1.070	Monocyte	9-14	+ve	-ve	-ve	+ve?
		Macrophage	10-15	+ve	-ve	-ve	+ve?
		Thrombocyte	3-13	-ve?	-ve	-ve	-ve
		Lymphocyte	5-10	-ve	-ve	-ve	-ve
III	1.080-1.090	Granulocyte, type 1	n.d.	+ve	-ve	+ve	-ve ?
IV	1.105-1.110	Erythrocyte	10-13	-ve	-ve	+ve	-ve
		Granulocyte, type 2	n.d.	+ve?	+ve	-ve	+ve
V	1.118-1.125	Granulocyte, type 3	n.d.	-ve	40%+ve (V and VI)	-ve?	+ve
VI	1.140-1.150	Granulocyte, type 4	n.d.	-ve		n.d.	+ve

n.d. = not done
? = uncertain designation
* = measurements of cells from peritoneal cavity

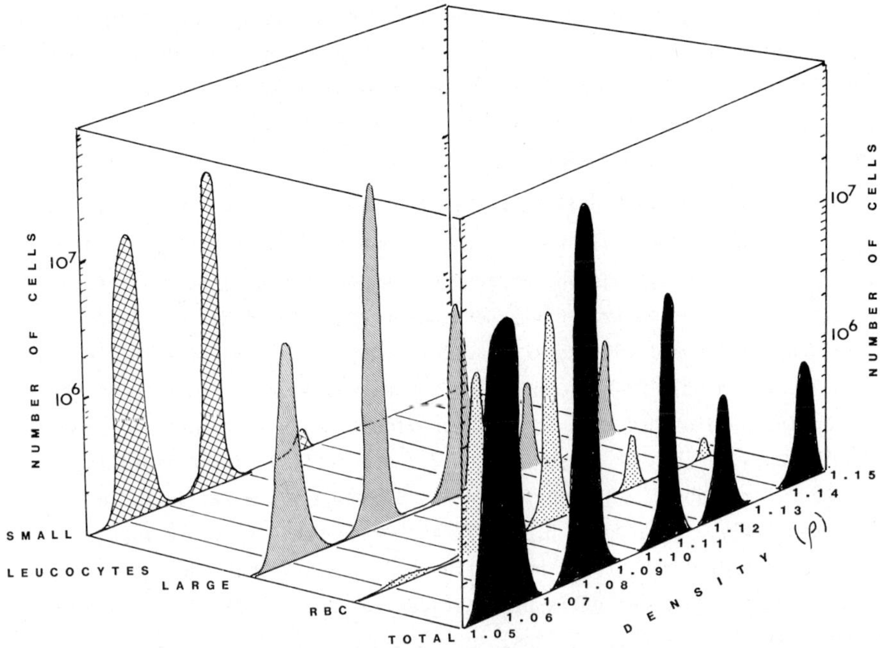

Figure 2. Pronephric cells of carp: numbers of cells in fractions separated on the basis of density. Total cells, small and large leucocytes, and RBC are shown separately for each of the distinct ρ value sub-populations.

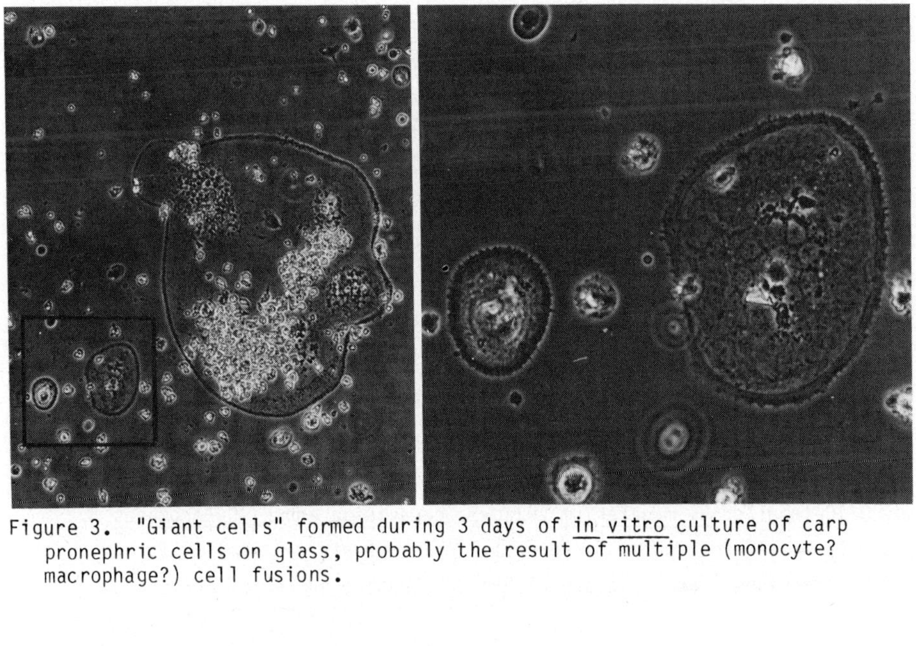

Figure 3. "Giant cells" formed during 3 days of in vitro culture of carp pronephric cells on glass, probably the result of multiple (monocyte? macrophage?) cell fusions.

culture wells or on glass coverslips, over a period of days, there appeared giant multinucleate cells (Fig. 3) similar to those observed in other teleost species (Secombes, 1985). Since coverslips washed 1 hr after set-up were seen to have giant cells two days later, it is assumed that these were the result of monocyte and macrophage fusions.

Granulocytes were not motile when first placed in culture, but after 24hr or more many of them (probably type 1) became ameboid. Their motility was studied by time-lapse micrography of both newly prepared cell suspensions and ones prepared 2 d previously. Cells were observed in (a) RPMI-1640 + 5%FCS, 1%PCS, 2mM glutamine and 10% distilled water, in (b) the same plus 1% BSA fraction V, and in (c) TCM-hep containing substances washed from live yeast. (This undefined medium had been observed previously to elicit ameboid movement of granulocytes.) A higher proportion of 2 d old cells exhibited motility during the 2.5 min observation period: 46%, 33.5% and 49% moved while in a, b and c respectively, compared to 8.3%, 27% and 22% respectively for younger cells. The rate of movement was not influenced by BSA V, but appears to have been increased in the older cells by yeast-derived substances: $\bar{x}$ = 1.15μm/min per moving cell (n = 45 observations) in 'c' versus 0.75μm (n=74) in 'a' and 0.62μm (n=46) in 'b'.

Cell adhesion to plastic was influenced by BSA V. Freshly prepared pronephric cells were suspended in RPMI-1640 + 5% PCS, 2mM L-glutamine, penicillin-G (100 i.u./ml) and Streptomycin (100 μg/ml) (controls), or in the same plus BSA V (10.0, 3.3 or 1.0 mg/ml). Aliquots (4×10^6 cells) were placed into the wells of a 24 well culture plate. After 1hr at 29° C in 6% CO_2 in air, non-adherent cells were removed and the remaining cells were counted. In control wells (n = 10) there were $26.5 \pm 2.7 \times 10^3$ cells, whereas in the BSA-containing wells (2 at each concentration) there were 64.6×10^3 cells at 10mg/ml, 70.6×10^3 at 3.3 mg/ml, and 58.3×10^3 at 1.0 mg/ml. These numbers are 0.66%, 1.62%, 1.76%, and 1.46% respectively of the original cell number added. Thus even 1 mg/ml BSA V enhanced plastic-adherence of some pronephric cells (thought to be macrophages).

Subjective observations suggest that encounter with foreign cells (*Bacillus megaterium* or *Saccharomyces cerevisiae*) elicits clumping of leucocytes. These appeared to be mostly larger, non-glass adherent cells i.e. granulocytes.

Pronephric cells prepared from fish injected previously with a mixture of dead, RITC-labelled *B. megaterium*, RITC-*S. cerevisiae* and FITC-*Aeromonas hydrophila* were fractionated in Percoll. Phagocytosis was limited to the cells of fractions I and II along with a substantial number of cells from fraction III i.e. fractions with the monocytes, macrophages and type 1 granulocytes. Lymphocytes and types 3 and 4 granulocytes did not contain microbes. In the pooled cells of fractions I and II, some of the macrophages contained phagocytosed microbes, but more of the phagocytes were non-spreading, round cells of medium size (larger than lymphocytes), probably monocytes. The mononuclear phagocytic activity of this organ (Lamers and Pilarzyk, 1982) may be predominantly a function of the more mature monocytes. Acridine Orange vital staining could be used to quantify monocytes in fractions I and II since lysosomes, distinctive of the monocytes and macrophages, fluoresced red, which distinguised these cells from the co-occuring lymphocytes.

In one preliminary experiment cell suspensions were also made from spleens and trunk kidneys of 2 yeast-injected fish. Phagocytic activity was much more prevalent in head and trunk kidney cells than in spleen cells.

In vitro phagocytosis experiments using pre-separated pronephric cell populations showed again that cells of fractions I and II, larger than lymphocytes, were the dominant phagocytes. Day-old cells were more phagocytic than freshly-prepared cells (for *B. megaterium* at least). As with the *in vivo* experiments, phagocytes were indiscriminate; some contained both *B. megaterium* and *A. hydrophila*. To ascertain the relative contributions of adherent (A, monocyte and macrophage-type) cells and of non-adherent (non-A, granulocyte) cells to phagocytosis, live *B. megaterium* were added to tissue culture wells containing coverslips and unfractionated cell populations. The coverslips (with A cells) and the non-A cells were processed separately through Acridine Orange. (The non-A cells were placed in Cunningham-type chambers for UV microscopy.) Using the fluorescent color shift from green to red as an indicator of killing of *B. megaterium* (Pantazis and Kinkes, 1979), data were obtained on the number of phagocytes and the numbers of live and dead bacteria. Both A and non-A cells were phagocytic. However, whereas the A cells readily killed the bacteria (about 50% intracellular bacteria killed after 30min of co-incubation), the non-A cells were less effective at killing; after 1.5hr only 10 - 25% of phagocytosed *B. megaterium* had been killed. These large, non-adherent leucocytes lacked red-fluorescing organelles (probably lysosomes) which were characteristic of the adherent cells.

DISCUSSION

Phagocytosis is both a primary defensive mechanism and the first step in the generation of specific humoral immunity towards particulate antigens. In endothermic vertebrates, non-specific defences against microbial pathogens are a highly complex orchestration of myeloid cell potentials. The at least equally diverse spectrum of potential pathogens encountered by aquatic animals, and the diversity of cell types constituting the internal defense systems of teleosts indicate a high likelihood that similarly complex mechanisms will be found to occur in these animals. The two functionally distinct phagocyte subpopulations found in carp probably parallel the mononuclear and polymorphonuclear phagocytes of mammals. Type 1 granulocytes contained granules which resembled in ultrastructure those of mammalian eosinophils. The cells had abundant peroxidase, and were phagocytic (Temmink and Bayne, loc. cit.). It would be premature, however, to conclude that type 1 granulocytes of carp are homologs of the mammalian eosinophil. It should be expected that the division of labor between immunocytes may differ subtley in teleosts and mammals.

Granulocytes in fish have been variously reported to be phagocytic (Weinreb and Weinreb, 1969; reviewed by Rijkers, 1980) or not (Ellis, 1976; McKinney et al., 1977). The 'maturation' of ameboid potential observed in my _in vitro_ work may be the basis for this difference; granulocytes in healthy, unprimed fish may have very low phagocytic capacity, and this may be enhanced in stimulated fish. The _in vitro_ acquisition of ameboid and phagocytic capacities parallels the activation of cytotoxic potential reported by others (Graves et al, 1984). We appear to find that, like macrophages, certain granulocytes of the teleost require activation before their defensive armamentum is fully effective. The nature of the activating stimulus and the process of activation need to be determined; foreign proteins (e.g. FCS - Graves et al, 1984) may be one stimulus.

Among questions raised by this study, the functions of the large, high density granulocytes (types 3 and 4) are particularly intriguing. These were not phagocytic; possibilities include these cells being blast stages of other leucocytes, or the so-called NCC (Graves et al., 1984).

Though hemopoiesis is one of the functions of the versatile cyprinid pronephros, it appears not to be predominant; early ontogenetic stages of blood cells were not much in evidence in cell suspensions made from the head kidneys of young, adult carp.

Studies of cell cooperation profit from methods to separate cell types prior to reconstitution. The continuous density gradient methods used here provide a very easy means to this end.

ACKNOWLEDGEMENTS

I thank the Netherlands-America Commission for Educational Exchange for a Fulbright Award, and the Agricultural University, Wageningen, The Netherlands for a fellowship. John Groten provided encouragement throughout this work and data on cell sizes. Anja and Nico Taverne did the histochemistry. Hans Temmink's electron micrographs revealed details of granule structure. Willem van Muiswinkel, Egbert Egberts and Ellen Harmsen provided facilities, support and encouragement. Mary Yui and Craig Flory gave critical comments on an earlier draft of this paper.

REFERENCES

Agius, C., 1981. Preliminary studies on the ontogeny of the melano-macrophages of teleost haemopoietic tissues and age-related changes. Dev. Comp. Immunol., 5: 597-606.

Braun-Nesje, R., Kaplan, G. and Seljelid, R., 1982. Rainbow trout macrophages in vitro: morphology and phagocytic activity. Dev. Comp. Immunol., 6: 281-291.

Davina, J.H.M., Rijkers, G.T., Rombout, J.H.W.M., Timmermans, L.A.M. and van Muiswinkel, W.B., 1980. Lymphoid and non-lymphoid cells in the intestine of Cyprinid fish. In: J.D. Horton (Editor), Development and Differentiation of Vertebrate Lymphocytes. Elsevier/North Holland, Amsterdam, pp. 129-140.

Ellis, A.E., Munroe, A.L.S. and Roberts, R.J., 1976. Defence mechanisms in fish. I. A study of the phagocytic system and the fate of intraperitoneally injected particulate material in the plaice (Pleuronectes platessa L.). J. Fish Biol., 8: 67-78.

Ferren, F., 1967. Role of the spleen in the immune response of teleosts and elasmobranchs. J. Fla. Med. Assoc., 54: 434-437.

Graves, S.S., Evans, D.L., Cobb, D. and Dawe, D.L., 1984. Nonspecific cytotoxic cells in fish (Ictalurus punctatus). I. Optimum requirements for target cell lysis. Dev. Comp. Immunol., 8: 293-302.

Hofte, B.B.T., Lehmann, J. and Sturenberg, F.-J., 1984. Untersuschungen zum Blutbild gesunder und an der "Infektiosen Bauchwassersucht" erkrankter Karpfen (Cyprinus carpio L.). Fisch und Umwelt 13: 71-87.

Lamers, C.H.J. and Pilarczyk, A., 1982. Immune response and antigen localization in carp (Cyprinus carpio) after administration of Yersinia ruckeri O-antigen. Dev. Comp. Immunol. Suppl. 2: 107-114.

McKinney, E.C., Smith, S.B., Haines, H.G. and Sigel, M.M., 1977. Phagocytosis by fish cells. J. Reticuloendothel. Soc., 21: 89-95.

Pantazis, C.G. and Kniker, W.T., 1979. Assessment of blood leucocyte microbial killing by using a new fluorochrome microassay. J. Reticuloendothel. Soc., 26: 155-170.

Rijkers, G.T., 1980. The immune system of Cyprinid fish. Ph.D. Thesis, Agricultural University, Wageningen, The Netherlands, pp. 176.

Secombes, C.J., 1985 The in vitro formation of teleost multinucleate giant cells. J. Fish Dis. 8:in press.

Smith, M., Potter M. and Merchant, B., 1967. Antibody-forming cells in the pronephros of the teleost Lepomis macrochirus. J. Immunol., 99: 876-882.

Smith, A.M., Wivel, N.A. and Potter, M., 1970. Plasmacytopoiesis in the pronephros of the carp (Cyprinus carpio). Anat. Rec., 167: 351-370.

Weinreb, E.L. and Weinreb, S., 1969. A study of experimentally induced endocytosis in a teleost. 1. Light microscopy of peripheral blood cell response. Zoologica N.Y., 54: 25-34.

Veterinary Immunology and Immunopathology, 12 (1986) 153—161
Elsevier Science Publishers B.V., Amsterdam — Printed in The Netherlands

LYMPHOID ORGANS IN STURGEONS (ACIPENSERIDAE)

R. FÄNGE

Department of Zoophysiology, P.B. 25059, S-40031, Göteborg (Sweden)

ABSTRACT

Fänge, R., 1986. Lymphoid organs in sturgeons (Acipenseridae). Vet. Immunol. Immunopathol., 12: 153-161.

Lymphoid (lymphomyeloid) tissues in sturgeons (hybrid sturgeon, *Huso huso* x *Acipenser ruthenus*, and white Pacific sturgeon, *A. transmontanus*) were investigated by dissection, histology and transmission electron microscopy. The main lymphomyeloid tissues are the thymus, the spleen, the anterior part of the kidney, the meningeal myeloid tissue, the pericardial tissue and lymphoid masses of the intestine, especially in the spiral valve. The kidney is the main hemopoietic tissue. The meningeal tissue is bone marrow-like (myeloid), mainly granulopoietic, but it also contains lymphoid elements. The pericardial tissue is predominantly lymphoid. The pericardial tissue has a lymph node-like appearance. It seems to be the site of interaction between lymphocytes and vascular endothelium. The thymus contains cortex and medulla. The spleen, as in higher vertebrates, is differentiated into white and red pulp. The highly diversiform and well developed lymphoid tissues of sturgeons may serve as basis of efficient immune mechanisms.

INTRODUCTION

Chondrosteans (sturgeons, paddlefish) possess several primitive features and are supposed to be phylogenetically related to extinct ancestors of teleostean fishes. Sturgeons have a reputation for longevity and large body size, and within this group the largest now living fishes are to be found. Long-living fishes like sturgeons presumably have to survive many attacks of microbes, virus and parasites and ought to have developed efficient defense mechanisms to a large extent based upon leucocyte-producing tissues. Already long ago investigators put attention to some rather unique lymphomyeloid structures, which are situated in the meninges of the central nervous system and in the pericardium of the heart of sturgeons (meningeal tissue: Drzewina, 1905, Scharrer, 1944; pericardial tissue: Hertwig, 1873,Drzewina, 1905, Scatizzi, 1933). Several other lymphomyeloid tissues have been studied in sturgeons and

0165-2427/86/$03.50 © 1986 Elsevier Science Publishers B.V.

paddlefish (thymus: Sokolova, 1912, Good et al., 1966. Spleen: Clawson et al., 1966. Kidney: Drzewina, 1905, Downey, 1909, Georgi and Beedle, 1978. Intestine: Weisel, 1973. Liver: Drzewina, 1905). Ivanova (1983) examined the hematology of different species of sturgeons. The present paper summarizes some results of a reinvestigation of lymphomyeloid structures in sturgeons.

MATERIALS AND METHODS

Preliminary observations were made on young specimens of hybrid sturgeons (*Huso huso* x *Acipenser ruthenus*) with body weight of 70-170 g. The main part of work was done on about 20 specimens of the Pacific white sturgeon (*Acipenser transmontanus*). The body weight of those varied between 60.8 g and 33.2 kg. Small-sized sturgeons of both species had been hatchery raised. White sturgeons heavier than about 10 kg were caught in the wild by hook and line.

Methods were dissections and naked eye observations, histological routine technique and, occasionally, transmission electron microscopy. Histological material was fixed in 10% formalin. Paraffin sections were stained with eosin-haematoxylin, Mallory or May-Grünwald-Giemsa (MGG). After air-drying blood smears and imprints were fixed 15 min in abs methanol and stained with MGG. If not otherwise stated the observations were on white sturgeons.

RESULTS

Thymus

A well developed thymus was found in 1/2 year old sturgeons (body weights 70-300 g), and in a sturgeon of unknown age (caught wild) weighing 12.5 kg. In one 2 1/2 year old sturgeon the size of the thymus in relation to the body weight was less than in younger individuals (Table I). (According to Sokolova (1912) the thymus persists in the European sturgeon, *A. sturio*, until two or three years age). The thymus is lobulated and contains cortex and medulla (Fig. 1). Lymphocytes, reticular cells, myoid cells, mucous cells and macrophages were identified in the histological sections but no Hassall's corpuscles. Imprints (hybrid sturgeon): small lymphocytes (4-7 μm), medium lymphocytes (7-10 μm), large

Lymphocytes (lymphoblasts)(10-17 μm), erythrocytes and scattered granulocytes are found.

Spleen

The spleen constitutes about 0.24% of the body weight(Table I). It is surrounded by a capsule of connective tissue and cubical peritoneal epithelium. The parenchyma consists of white and red pulp. The white pulp forms follicle-like periarterial masses containing lymphocytes, granulocytes (eosinophils)and scattered macrophages. The eosinophilic granulocytes occur mainlyat the periphery of the periarterial masses forming almost a marginal zone towards the red pulp. Ellipsoidal arterioles are well developed and are not surrounded by lymphoid tissue but by red pulp. Imprints (hybrid sturgeon): large numbers of small lymphocytes, a small number of blast cells (10-17 μm), erythrocytes and granulocytes are found.

Kidney

The kidney of sturgeons consists of both excretory and lymphoid tissue (Georgi and Beedle, 1978). Lymphoid, or rather hemopoietic, tissue is found mainly in the anterior part of the kidney. Imprints (hybrid sturgeon) show numerous blast cells (13-20 μm), medium-sized lymphocytes (12 μm), granulocytes, macrophages and erythrocytes. Cells with intensely basophilic cytoplasm and an eccentric large nucleus look like plasma cells but are difficult to distinguish from large blast cells. Mitotic stages of blast cells are frequent.

Pericardial tissue

The heart of the hybrid sturgeon was covered by a nodular tissue, but in two very small specimens this was poorly developed. The same tissue is associated with the heart of the white sturgeon. In large individuals of this species the heart is covered by a several mm thick layer of whitish or reddish nodes. The general appearance of the heart (Fig. 2) is closely similar

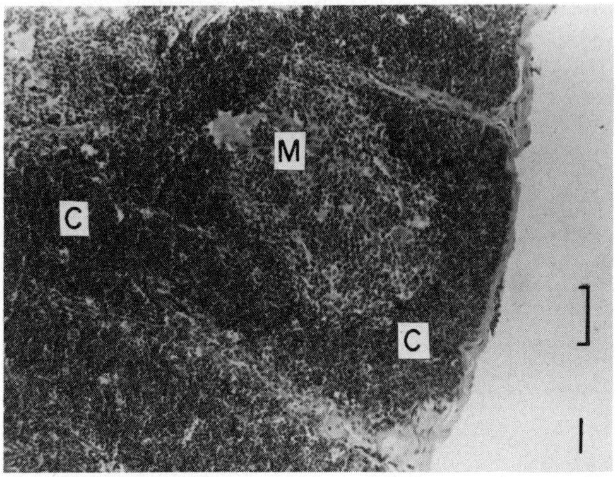

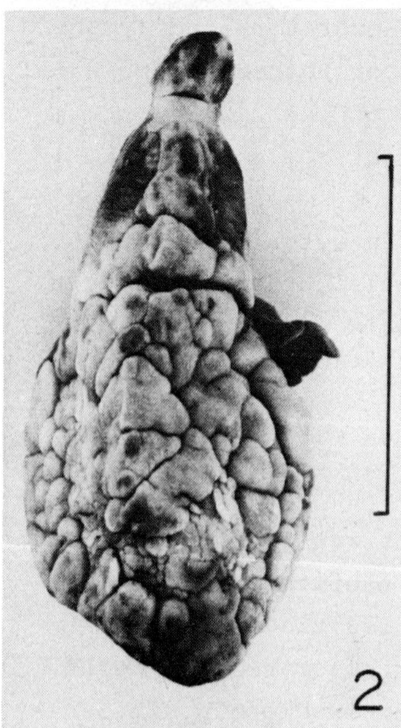

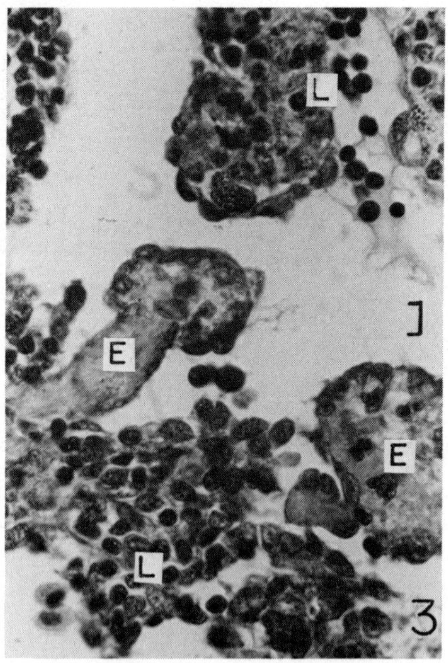

Fig. 1. *Acipenser transmontanus*, body weight 192.7 g. Histological section through the thymus. Haematoxylin-eosin. C, cortex; M, medulla. Bar = 100 μm.
Fig. 2. *A. transmontanus*, body weight 31 kg. Heart, ventral view. Bar = 5 cm.
Fig. 3. *A. transmontanus*. Histological section through the pericardial tissue. E, endothelium; L, lymphocytes. Bar = 10 μm.

to that of the adult European sturgeon (*Acipenser sturio*) as described by Hertwig (1873). The nodules or lobes of the pericardial organ are subdivided into smaller compartments separated from one another by connective tissue. Each compartment contains an irregular cell mass surrounded on all sides but one by a sinus filled with blood or lymph. At one side the cell mass joins the wall of the compartment. The cell mass consists of lymphocytes, reticular cells,granulocytes and scattered macrophages. It is penetrated by small arteries. The cell mass is covered by the endothelium of the blood sinus. In histologic and in electron microscopic sections lymphocytes are observed, which are in the process of migrating through or between the endothelial cells. The endothelial cells have a swollen appearance with a light cytoplasm (Fig. 3). The pericardial tissue is supplied with blood from coronary and mammary arteries (Hertwig, 1873), but details of microcirculation have never been clarified. The tissue may be drained by veins and a kind of lymph vessels (Kampmeier, 1969).

Small lymphocytes are found everywhere within the central cell mass and the connective tissue walls of the compartments. In certain areas of the cell mass and the connective tissue lymphocytes form dense aggregations. These lymphocytic accumulations have more diffuse borders than the lymphoid follicles or germinal centres of mammals and birds, but according to Drzewina (1905) the pericardial organ of sturgeons resemble fairly well avian lymph nodes in its structure. Imprints (hybrid sturgeon): small lymphocytes (4-7 μm), medium lymphocytes (7-10 μm) and lymphoblasts (10-17 μm) are common.Eosinophils occur in groups. Clusters of detached endothelial cells look like multinucleate cells in imprint preparations stained with MGG.

Meningeal tissue

The grayish or pinkish tissue is situated within the cranial cavity in a saddlelike manner above the hind part of the brain and the anterior part of the spinal cord. It extends ventrolaterally on each side between the central nervous system and the nervus vagus. Histological sections show lobes separated by irregular blood- or lymphfilled sinuses. The lobes contain loosely packed free cells interspersed with connective tissue, small arteries and nerve bundles. About half of the free cells have a cytoplasm which stains eosinophilic with eosin-haematoxylin. Imprints (hybrid sturgeon): heterophilic and eosinophilic granulocytes, promyelocytes, small lymphocytes, medium lymphocytes, large lymphocytes and blast cells, erythrocytes and small numbers of immature erythrocytes. A few blast cells show mitotic figures.

Intestine

The lamina propria contains large numbers of lymphocytes. Several follicle-like accumulations of lymphocytes are found in histological sections through the thickened margin of the spiral valve.

Blood cells

The blood morphological findings agree well with those of Ivanova (1983) on other species of sturgeons. Four lines of blood cells may be recognized in blood smears (hybrid sturgeon, white sturgeon): erythrocytes, granulocytes, lymphocytes and other nongranulated cells with basophilic cytoplasm, spindle cells. Immature red cells (polychromatic with a round nucleus) occur but are rare in the peripheral blood. Heterophilic (neutrophilic) and eosinophilic granulocytes may have unsegmented, bilobed, threelobed or fourlobed nuclei. Spindle cells (thrombocytes) are oval or fusiform.

Total amount of lymphomyeloid tissues

TABLE I
Body weight, weight of lymphomyeloid tissues in per cent of body weight, and age of six specimens of the white sturgeon (*Acipenser transmontanus*).

Body weight (g)	Age (years)	Thymus (%b.w.)	Meningeal tissue (%b.w.)	Spleen (%b.d.)
179	1/2	0.09	0.07	0.36
193	1	0.09	0.09	0.24
259	1/2	-	0.08	0.26
309	1/2	0.08	0.07	0.18
4300	2 1/2	0.04	0.06	0.12
33200	unknown	-	0.08	0.28
Mean values		0.08	0.08	0.24

Isolated tissues were weighed (Table I). The sum of the mean percentual weight of the thymus, the spleen and the meningeal tissue was about 0.4. The anterior part of the kidney, the pericardial tissue (organ) and the lymphoid tissue of the intestine were difficult to isolate and weigh. A rough estimation by the eye indicated that their total weight was approximately 0.2% of the body weight. Thus the total weight of major lymphomyeloid tissues in the white sturgeon may be about 0.6% of the body weight.

DISCUSSION

Lymphoid and myeloid (hemopoietic) tissues are connected into a lymphomyeloid complex by migrating lymphocytes and stem cells (Yoffey, 1985). The total weight of this tissue complex in sturgeons, about 0.6% of the body weight, is of about the same magnitude as in cartilagenous fishes (Fänge, 1977). In sturgeons the anterior kidney, the spleen and the meningeal tissue are both myeloid and lymphoid, while lymphoid functions may predominate in the thymus, the pericardial tissue and the intestinal spiral valve.

A meningeal myeloid tissue occurs in chondrosteans and holosteans (Scharrer, 1944), and somewhat similar structures may also be found in a brachiopterygian (*Polypterus*: Waldschmidt, 1887) and in certain elasmobranchs (Vialli, 1933).The meningeal tissue of sturgeons is mainly granulopoietic. It resembles functionally lymphomyeloid tissues of elasmobranchs (Leydig and epigonal organs) and holocephalans, and in part also the head kidney of teleosts, and the hemopoietic bone marrow of higher vertebrates (Fänge, 1984).

In sturgeons the anterior part of the kidney probably is the main site of erythropoiesis, but blood cells other than erythrocytes may also originate in the kidney.

Migration of lymphocytes through a specialized endothelium may be of functional importance in the pericardial tissue. Lympho-endothelial interactions within mammalian lymph nodes are supposed to be associated with production of substances, that cause lymphocyte accumulation (Baldwin III, 1982). The presence of lymphocytes and plasma cells in the pericardial tissue (Clawson et al., 1966) suggests that it has immune functions. The lymphoid tissue of the intestine, especially the extensive lymphocytic accumulations in the spiral valve, may have relationship to infections or parasitic attacks (Weisel, 1973).

Sturgeons are commercially important, are being kept in hatcheries in some parts of the world, and several aspects of their biology has been studied in recent years (Doroshov, 1985), but so far little is known about their immune responses. Probably in many respects they are similar to the paddlefish (*Polyodon spathula)*, which is closely related to sturgeons. The paddlefish may be described as a specialized plancton-feeding sturgeon. The paddlefish has efficient production of antibodies (Finstad and Good, 1966; Acton et al., 1971) and complement (Legler et al., 1967).

ACKNOWLEDGEMENTS

For material and other help I thank Prof. V. Govirin (Setchenov Inst.,Leningrad,USSR), Ass.Prof. John Simmons and Prof. R. Smith (Deptm. Zoology, UC Berkeley), Prof. S. Doroshov (UC Davis), Dr. R. Buddington (Deptm. Physiology, UCLA), Mr. Sky van Scoy, Mr. Steve Crandall (Rodeo Marina, Rodeo, CA), Mr. G.J.Morlock (Troy's Fish Markets, Portland, Oregon) and Mr. Jim Galbreath (Deptm. Fish and Wildlife, Clackamas, Oregon, USA). Ms. Christina Hagström and Ms. Inger Holmqvist gave expert technical assistance. The work was supported by the Swedish National Science Research Council (Stockholm) and by the Royal Society of Science and Literature (Göteborg, Sweden).

REFERENCES

Acton, R.T., Weinheimer, P.F., Dupree, H.K., Russel, T.R., Wolcott, M., Evans, E.E., Schrohenloher, R.E. and Bennett, J.J., 1971. Isolation and characterization of the immune macroglobulin from the paddlefish, *Polyodon spathula*. J. Biol. Chem., 246: 6760-6769.

Baldwin III, W.M., 1982. The symbiosis of immunocompetent and endothelial cells. Immunology Today, 3: 267-268.

Clawson, C.C., Finstad, J. and Good, R.A., 1966. Evolution of the immune response. V. Electron microscopy of plasma cells and lymphoid tissue of the paddlefish. Lab. Invest. 15: 1820-1847.

Doroshov, S., 1985. Biology and culture of sturgeon Acipenseriformes. In: Recent Advances in Aquaculture (Muir, J.F. and Roberts, R. eds) Vol. 2, pp. 251-274. London: Croom Helm.

Downey, H., 1909. The lymphatic tissue of the kidney of *Polyodon spathula*. Folia Haematologica Lpz, 8: 415-466.

Drzewina, A., 1905. Contribution a l'étude du tissu lymphoide des Ichthyopsidés. Arch.zool. expér. gén. sér.4, 3: 145-338.

Fänge, R., 1977. Size relations of lymphomyeloid organs in some cartilaginous fish. Acta zool. Stockh., 49: 155-161.

Fänge, R., 1984. Lymphomyeloid tissues in fishes. Vidensk. Meddr dansk naturh. Foren., 145: 143-162.

Finstad, J. and Good, R.A., 1966. Phylogenetic studies of adaptive immune responses in the lower vertebrates. In: Phylogeny of Immunity (Smith, R.T., Miescher, P.A. and Good, R.A., eds) pp. 105-117. Gainesville, Florida: Univ. Florida Press.
Georgi, T.A. and Beedle, D., 1978. The histology of the excretory kidney of the paddlefish (*Polyodon spathula*). J. Fish Biol., 13: 587-590.
Good, R.A., Finstad, J., Oollara, B. and Gabrielson, A.E., 1966. Morphologic studies on the evolution of the lymphoid tissues among the lower vertebrates. In: Phylogeny of Immunity (Smith, R.T., Miescher, P.A. and Good, R.A., eds) pp. 149-170. Gainesville, Florida: Univ. Florida Press.
Hertwig, R., 1873. Die lymphoiden Drüsen auf der Oberfläche des Störherzens. Arch.f.Mikr. Anatomie, 9: 62-79.
Ivanova, N.T., 1983. Atlas kletok krovi ryb. Publ. Legkaya i pischchevaya prom. Moscow. 80 pp., 58 Pl. (in russian).
Kampmeier, O.F., 1969. Evolution and Comparative Morphology of the Lymphatic System. Springfield, Ill.: C.C. Thomas.
Legler, D.W., Evans, E.E. and Dupree, H.K., 1967. Comparative immunology: serum complement of freshwater fishes. Trans. Am. Fish. Sic., 96: 237-242.
Scatizzi, I., 1933. L'organo linfomieloide pericardico dello storione. Arch. Zool. Ital., 18: 1-26.
Scharrer, E., 1944. The histology of the meningeal myeloid tissue in the ganoids *Amia* and *Lepisosteus*. Anat. Rec., 88: 291-310.
Sokolova, A. Ja., 1912. K istorii razvitija thymus'a i sterljadi. Mém. Scient. Univ. Imp. Kazan, 79: 1-44 (in russian).
Vialli, M., 1933. Formazioni linfoidi meningee e perimeningee nei Selaci. Bolletino di Zoologia (Ital.), 4: 123-134.
Waldschmidt, J., 1887. Beitrag zur Anatomie des Zentralnervensystem und des Geruchsorgan von *Polypterus bichir*. Anat. Anz. 2: 308-322.
Weisel, G.F., 1973. Anatomy and histology of the digestive system of the Paddlefish (*Polyodon spathula*). J. Morph., 140: 243-255.
Yoffey, J.M., 1985. Cellular migration streams. The integration of the lymphomyeloid complex. Lymphology, 18: 5-21.

Veterinary Immunology and Immunopathology, 12 (1986) 163—174
Elsevier Science Publishers B.V., Amsterdam — Printed in The Netherlands

INFLUENCE OF ROUTE OF ADMINISTRATION ON THE HUMORAL RESPONSE OF CHANNEL CATFISH (*ICTALURUS PUNCTATUS*) TO *YERSINIA RUCKERI*

D.A. NEUMANN and M.R. TRIPP

School of Life and Health Sciences, University of Delaware, Newark, Delaware 19716 (USA)

ABSTRACT

Neumann, D.A. and Tripp, M.R., 1986. Influence of route of administration on the humoral response of channel catfish (*Ictalurus punctatus*) to *Yersinia ruckeri*. Vet. Immunol. Immunopathol., 12: 163-174.

Channel catfish were inoculated intraperitoneally, intramuscularly, or intraesophageally with *Yersinia ruckeri*. Three antigen doses were administered by each route of injection. Four fish from each treatment were sacrificed at 5-day intervals for 40 days. Serum from each individual was tested for antibody activity against *Y. ruckeri* by indirect enzyme-linked immunosorbent assay (ELISA). High titers of anti-*Y. ruckeri* antibody were elicited by all doses (10^5 to 10^9 cells/g of fish) regardless of the route of administration. Mean titers for saline injected fish ranged up to 1:64 for each route of inoculation while mean titers for bacteria injected fish ranged up to 1:4096. Mean titers of 1:128 or greater were observed by day 15 post injection; titers peaked about day 30 and diminished thereafter. Channel catfish were most responsive to the antigen (10^7 to 10^9 cells/g of fish) when administered intramuscularly although lower doses (10^5 to 10^6 cells/g of fish) administered intraperitoneally elicited a substantial response. There was little evidence of dose-dependent responses for any of the routes of immunization. The rapid onset of relatively high serum titers suggests that the fish were mounting a secondary response to *Yersinia ruckeri*.

INTRODUCTION

The efficacy of fish immunization protocols is determined in part by the immunogenicity of the antigen (Harris, 1973; Anderson and Dixon, 1980; Avtalion et al., 1980), the dose (Ingram and Alexander, 1979; Secombes and Manning, 1980; Secombes et al., 1982), and the route of administration (Ingram and Alexander, 1977, 1979). For example, bovine serum albumin (BSA) is poorly antigenic in some species (Clem and Sigel, 1966; Hodgins et al., 1967; Harris, 1973), while modified or aggregated BSA is a satisfactory immunogen for others (Avtalion et al., 1980). Dose effects are such that each species responds

0165-2427/86/$03.50 © 1986 Elsevier Science Publishers B.V.

optimally to a specific concentration of each antigen (Sailendri and Muthukkaruppan, 1975; O'Neill, 1979; Secombes et al., 1982). Schachte (1978) reported that channel catfish (Ictalurus punctatus) produced higher titer antiserum when injected intramuscularly with a bacterin than when it was administered in the food or by bath immunization. Similarly, intravenous injection of sheep red blood cells into carp (Cyprinus carpio) produced a greater response than when similar doses of antigen were injected intramuscularly (Rijkers et al., 1980).

Detection of fish antibody against a specific antigen is influenced by the assay procedure selected to measure the response. Precipitation assays have generally been unsatisfactory when applied to fish immunology (Harris, 1973; Khalifa and Post, 1976; Ingram and Alexander, 1980). Agglutination assays appear most appropriate for particulate antigens (Khalifa and Post, 1976; Ingram and Alexander, 1977; Schachte, 1978) while indirect hemagglutination or complement fixation procedures appear suitable for detecting the humoral response to soluble antigens (Ingram and Alexander, 1977, 1980; Secombes and Manning, 1980). More recently enzyme-linked immunosorbent assay (ELISA) procedures have been used to demonstrate specific antibody activity in fish serum (Roberson, 1981; Smith, 1981; Bortz et al., 1984; Chart et al., 1984).

The present work was initiated to determine the response of channel catfish to varying doses of antigen administered by each of three routes. A particulate antigen, Yersinia ruckeri, was injected intraperitoneally (IP), intramuscularly (IM), and intraesophageally (IE) to assess the influence of the route of administration on the immune response. The humoral response of the fish was assessed by indirect ELISA.

METHODS

Channel catfish weighing 2.5 to 13.4 g were obtained from Kurtz's Fish Hatchery, Elverson, Pennsylvania and were maintained in polyethylene-lined plywood tanks ~1 m square and 0.3 m deep. Each was equipped with an undergravel filter. Automatically regulated fluorescent lighting provided 15 hr of light daily. The tanks were filled with tap water one to two weeks prior to each collection to facilitate temperature stabilization (20-24C), chlorine dissipation, and the establishment of the filter bed.

Fish were held for one to two weeks prior to the initiation of each experiment and were fed a weighed ration of food pellets (Rangen-Ziegler, Gardners, Pennsylvania) at four-day intervals. Feeding was initiated shortly after the fish arrived in the laboratory: the schedule was adjusted such that all fish were fed on the day on which they were inoculated.

A formalin-killed bacterin of Y. ruckeri was provided by Dr. S. G. Newman (Bio-Med Research Laboratories, Inc., Seattle, Washington). The bacterin was diluted in sterile phosphate buffered saline (PBS), pH 7.2, to yield estimated concentrations of 1×10^{9}, 1×10^{10}, and 1×10^{11} cells/ml. Based on the average live weight of fish in each experiment, the delivered antigen concentrations were 2.5×10^{5}, 1.1×10^{6}, or 5.5×10^{6} cells/g of fish for the IP experiment; 1.7×10^{7}, 1.5×10^{8}, or 1.5×10^{9} cells/g of fish for the IM experiment; and 1.5×10^{7}, 1.7×10^{8}, or 1.7×10^{9} cells/g of fish for the IE experiment. For each experiment ~40 fish each were injected with either of the three vaccine concentrations being tested. A similar number of control fish were injected with an identical volume of sterile PBS.

Intraperitoneal injections (0.1 ml) were administered through the abdominal wall. Intramuscular injections (0.05 ml) were made into the left epaxial muscle just below the dorsal fin. Intraesophageal immunizations (0.1 ml) were performed by inserting a 26 gauge needle with a 3 cm extension of surgical tubing through the mouth and into the esophagus. The inoculum was administered after resistance offered by the esophageal folds which occlude the digestive tract had been overcome.

At the initiation of each experiment blood was collected from four uninjected individuals to provide control serum from fish which had been exposed to neither the antigen nor the inoculation procedure. Antigen injected and PBS injected fish were sampled at 5-day intervals for 40 days post injection.

Four fish from each treatment were sacrificed on each sampling day. Each was blotted dry, weighed, and the caudal peduncle severed. Blood from the caudal artery was collected in a sterile test tube which was immediately placed on ice. Samples were refrigerated overnight and then centrifuged at ~5300 RPM for 15 minutes at room temperature. Serum was collected from each sample and stored at -20C until analyzed for antibody activity.

The ELISA procedures were based on those of Voller et al. (1979) and Cumming et al. (1980). A suspension of 1×10^{9} Y. ruckeri cells/ml was prepared in carbonate coating buffer (Voller et al., 1979) and 50 μl aliquots were dispensed into each well of a 96-well Immulon II microtiter plate (Dynatech Laboratories, Inc., Alexandria, Virginia). The plates were incubated for 1 hr at 60C (Cumming et al., 1980) and washed three times with PBS containing 1% Tween 20 (PBST). Serum from each fish was inactivated at 45C for 1 hr and serially diluted in PBS containing 0.05% Tween 20 and 1% BSA (PBST/BSA) and 50 μl of each dilution of each serum sample was placed in separate wells. A pool of negative fish serum was obtained from unimmunized fish and/or from previously tested individuals with titers of 1:16 or less.

Heat inactivated negative fish serum was serially diluted in PBST/BSA and three 50 μl aliquots of each dilution were placed in separate wells on each plate. The plates were covered and incubated overnight at 4C.

Following incubation the plates were processed as indicated in Table 1. All reagents were prepared in PBST/BSA and used in 50 μl aliquots. A mouse monoclonal antibody against channel catfish immunoglobulin, provided as the ammonium sulfate precipitate of mouse ascites fluid by Dr. Norman Miller (University of Mississippi Medical Center, Jackson, Mississippi), was diluted 1:500 for use. Alkaline phosphatase conjugated rabbit anti-mouse immunoglobulin antibody (Sigma Chemical Co., St. Louis, Missouri) was used as a 1:1000 dilution. A 1 mg/ml solution of alkaline phosphatase substrate (Sigma Chemical Co.) was prepared in 10% diethanolamine. After incubation the optical density of the contents of each well was measured and recorded with a MicroElisa Auto Reader (Dynatech Laboratories, Inc.).

In addition to the wells utilized as described above, each plate included multiple control wells. The blank well received antigen and substrate. A conjugate control well received antigen, conjugate, and substrate. A positive control well contained antigen, heat inactivated rabbit anti-*Y. ruckeri* serum, goat anti-rabbit conjugate (Cooper Biomedical, Inc., Malvern, Pennsylvania), and substrate; a negative control well was prepared using heat inactivated normal rabbit serum. For each sampling date, equal volumes of serum from each fish in a given treatment were pooled, diluted 1:2 or 1:4, and placed in antigen coated wells. These wells subsequently received a 1:500 dilution of mouse ascites fluid devoid of anti-catfish antibody activity (negative ascites fluid); this was the control for the mouse monoclonal antibody. Similarly, single wells containing each dilution of negative fish serum were reacted with the negative ascites fluid. Any wells not receiving a specific reagent at any particular step received 50 μl of PBST/BSA.

The titer of each serum was determined by comparing the optical density of each dilution with the optical density of the corresponding dilution of negative fish serum on the same plate. Each negative fish serum dilution was tested in triplicate on each plate and the mean optical density and the 99% confidence intervals for each dilution were determined. A dilution was considered to be positive if its optical density exceeded the corresponding negative fish serum mean plus its 99% confidence value. The titer was taken as the greatest dilution meeting this criteria and which was followed by two consecutive dilutions each of which were below their respective cutoff values.

For the IP experiment the volume of negative serum was insufficient to permit testing at dilutions of 1:8 or less. Cut off values for these dilutions were established by determining the mean optical density and 99%

confidence intervals for each of the three negative serum dilutions (1:16, 1:32, and 1:64) tested on the appropriate plates. Mean values were regressed against the corresponding dilution and the resulting equation was used to estimate the mean optical densities for the untested dilutions. The average confidence value of the three tested dilutions was added to each estimated mean to obtain the cut off value.

TABLE 1
Summary of ELISA incubation times and temperatures used to test channel catfish Ictalurus punctatus) serum for anti-Yersinia ruckeri antibody activity. See text for details.

	Anti-Y. ruckeri
Fish serum incubation	Overnight, 4C
Wash[a]	3X
Mouse anti-catfish immunoglobulin	4 hr, 4C
Wash[a]	3X
Rabbit anti-mouse conjugate	4 hr, 4C
Wash[a]	3X
Substrate	30 min, RT[b]

[a]Washed with phosphate buffered saline containing 1% Tween 20.
[b]Room temperature.

RESULTS

In all experiments the control data indicated that the assays performed satisfactorily (Figs. 1 through 3). Mean optical densities of negative fish serum were low and diminished rapidly with successive dilutions. Negative fish serum reacted minimally with the negative ascites fluid at all tested dilutions thus confirming the specificity of the monoclonal antibody. When negative ascites fluid was reacted with the pools of test serum the optical density values were comparably low. The positive and negative rabbit serum controls demonstrated the suitability of the assay procedure. Direct binding of the conjugate to the antigen coated wells was negligible.

Channel catfish immunized IP or IM with Y. ruckeri elicited high antibody titers regardless of the antigen dose (Figs. 1 and 2). Titers rose rapidly through day 15 and generally persisted at high levels until day 35 post immunization. Uninjected and PBS injected control fish in these experiments exhibited generally low levels ($\leq$1:64) of anti-Y. ruckeri activity. Titers of individual fish within a single treatment group were variable with some individuals exhibiting titers as high as 1:32768. Among fish injected IP the

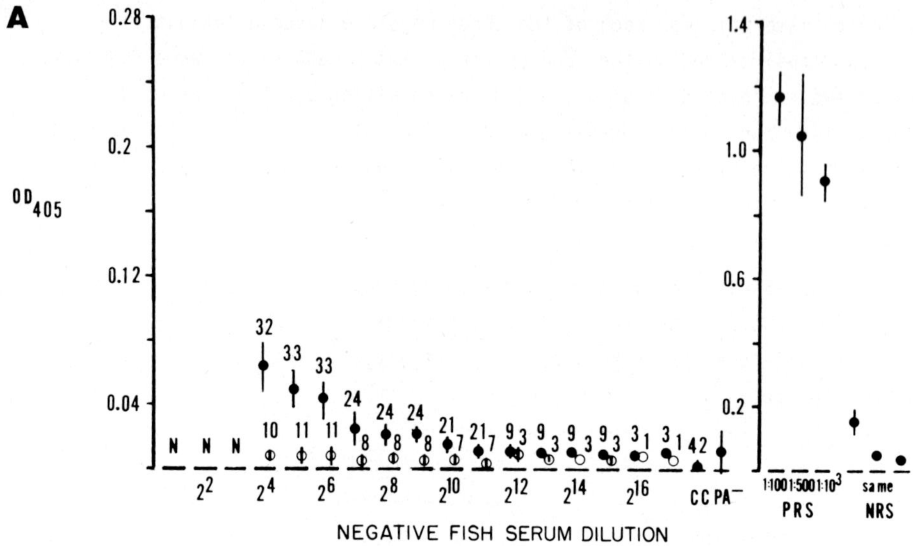

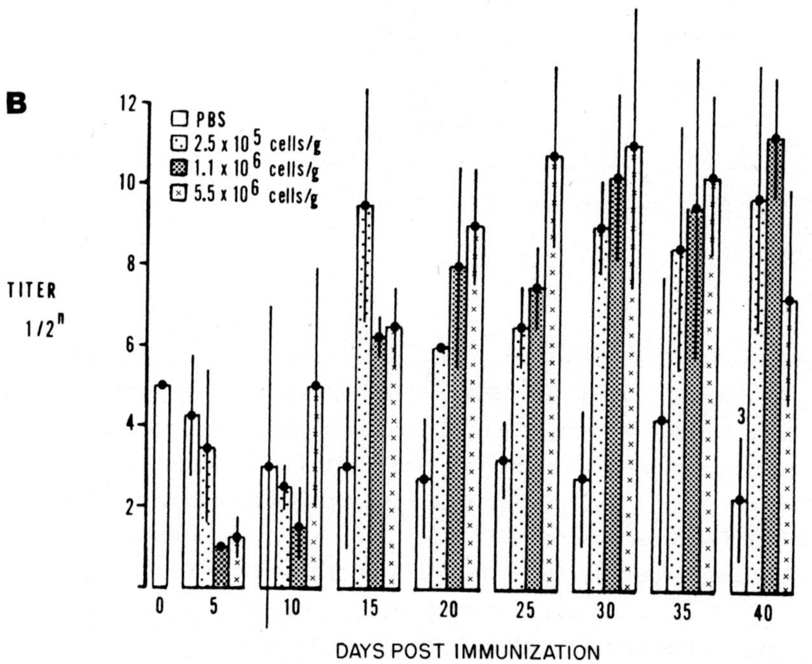

Fig. 1. Humoral immune response of channel catfish (Ictalurus punctatus) to intraperitoneal immunization with three doses of killed Yersinia ruckeri cells. A. Means and standard deviations of optical densities of the various ELISA control samples. Negative fish serum was reacted with mouse monoclonal antibody against catfish immunoglobulin (●) and with negative mouse ascites fluid (○). The number of observations is indicated adjacent to the respective bars; CC - conjugate control, PA - pooled serum reacted with negative ascites fluid, PRS - positive rabbit serum, NRS - negative rabbit serum, N - not tested. B. Means and standard deviations of catfish anti-Y. ruckeri antibody titers. Means are for four observations except where indicated.

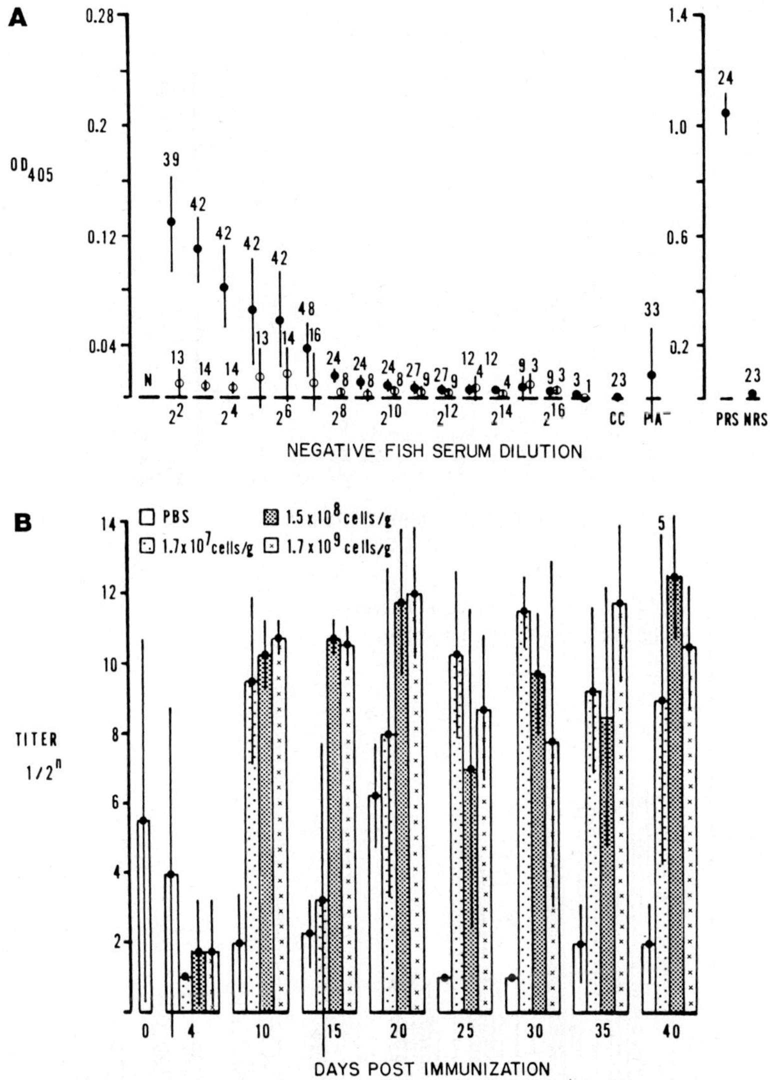

Fig. 2. Humoral immune response of channel catfish (*Ictalurus punctatus*) to intramuscular immunization with three doses of killed *Yersinia ruckeri* cells. A. Means and standard deviations of optical densities of the various ELISA control samples. Negative fish serum was reacted with mouse monoclonal antibody against catfish immunoglobulin (●) and with negative mouse ascites fluid (O). The number of observations is indicated adjacent to the respective bars; CC - conjugate control, PA - pooled serum reacted with negative ascites fluid, PRS - positive rabbit serum, NRS - negative rabbit serum, N - not tested. B. Means and standard deviations of catfish anti-*Y. ruckeri* antibody titers. Means are for four observations except where indicated.

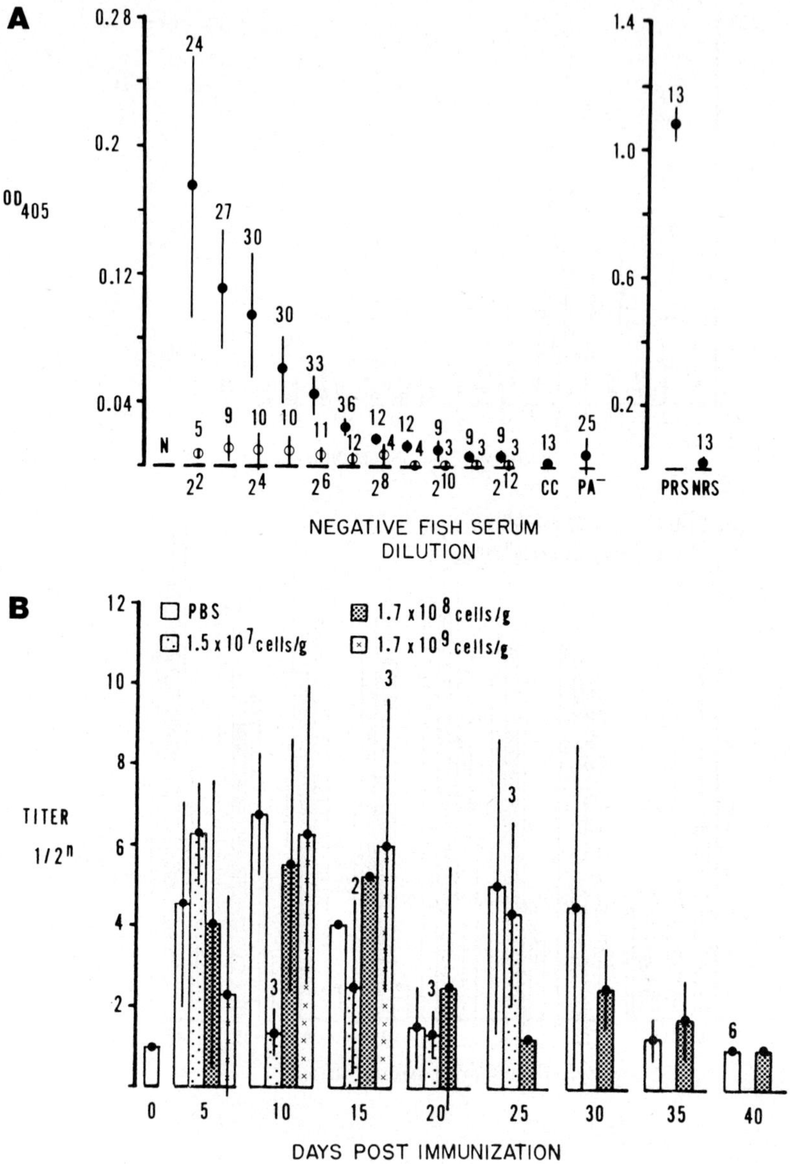

Fig. 3. Humoral immune response of channel catfish (*Ictalurus punctatus*) to intraesophageal immunization with three doses of killed *Yersinia ruckeri* cells. A. Means and standard deviations of optical densities of the various ELISA control samples. Negative fish serum was reacted with mouse monoclonal antibody against catfish immunoglobulin (●) and with negative mouse ascites fluid (O). The number of observations is indicated adjacent to the respective bars; CC - conjugate control, PA - pooled serum reacted with negative ascites fluid, PRS - positive rabbit serum, NRS - negative rabbit serum, N - not tested. B. Means and standard deviations of catfish anti-*Y. ruckeri* antibody titers. Means are for four observations except where indicated.

most efficacious dose was $5.5x10^6$ cells/g of fish while those injected IM responded similarly to each of the three doses. Fish inoculated IE with Y. ruckeri experienced a substantial number of mortalities; no fish receiving $1.7x10^9$ cells/g of fish survived beyond day 15 (67% mortality) while those receiving $1.5x10^7$ cells/g of fish failed to survive beyond day 25 (44% mortality). Surviving fish yielded an ambiguous response (Fig. 3). There were no clear relationships between dose and response for this route of administration. Of the three routes of inoculation the greatest titers were associated with fish receiving IM injections although these fish received greater antigen doses than did the IP immunized fish.

DISCUSSION

The response of individual fish was highly variable as evidenced by the large standard deviations about the mean titers. For example, among fish immunized IM with $1.5x10^8$ Y. ruckeri cells/g of fish and tested on day 25 individual titers ranged from 1:2 to 1:4906. Such broad disparity in the immune response of fishes has been previously noted (Ingram and Alexander, 1977, 1980; Robohm and Sparrow, 1981; Stolen et al., 1984) and this suggests that fish populations may be composed of subpopulations of high responders and low responders. This would be analogous to the situation in mammals and would presumably reflect the genetic makeup of individual fish. Robohm and Sparrow (1981) observed that high responsiveness may be selected for among summer flounders (Paralichthys dentatus) from polluted waters.

Uninjected and PBS injected fish exhibited moderately high titers against Y. ruckeri. It is not clear whether this reflects the presence of specific anti-Y. ruckeri antibody or the presence of cross reacting antibody. Paterson and Fryer (1974) observed high anti-Aeromonas salmonicida endotoxin titers among saline injected coho salmon (Oncorhynchus kisutch) and postulated that it could be due to previous exposure to the bacterium. Although Y. ruckeri is not pathogenic to channel catfish, these fish may encounter, and respond to, this bacterium when it is present in the environment, which may account for the modest titers observed among control fish. These titers might also be associated with cross-reacting antibody in the control sera. Since Y. ruckeri and many other fish pathogens are gram negative rods (Ross et al., 1966; McDaniel, 1979), it is possible that exposure to any of these organisms might induce the production of antibodies which recognize common epitopes. Ourth and Wilson (1982) found that nonimmune channel catfish serum had variable bactericidal activity against gram negative rods, both pathogens and nonpathogens, but was not bactericidal to gram positive organisms. The data reported here suggest that there may be immune cross-reactivity as well.

Fish injected IP or IM with *Y. ruckeri* responded in the typical manner (Avtalion, 1969; Sailendri and Muthukkaruppan, 1975; Ingram and Alexander, 1977, 1980). Titers rose rapidly over the first 15 days with those of immunized fish generally exceeding those of control fish by day 10. By day 35 titers began to diminish, especially among IP injected fish. Dose dependent effects were minimal among the IM injected fish indicating that each dose was equally effective in promoting a strong humoral response. Responses among IP injected fish tended to be lower than those for IM injected animals which reflects the lower doses received by fish in the former treatment. For the IP injected fish titers tended to increase with increasing antigen concentration.

Among channel catfish immunized IE with *Y. ruckeri* there were substantial mortalities in the groups receiving 1.5×10^7 and 1.7×10^9 cells/g of fish. Surviving fish, including PBS injected controls, exhibited erratic and generally low responses. The mortalities appear unrelated to antigen dose since all fish receiving 1.7×10^8 cells/g of fish survived until sampled. This argues against the possibility that the mortalities resulted from endotoxin production associated with digestion of the cells. The absence of mortalities among the PBS injected fish suggests that there was no general malaise among the fish utilized in this experiment. However, the erratic results raise the possibility that the fish used in this experiment may have been immunologically impaired, which might account for the variable responses.

In summary, channel catfish responded strongly when immunized IP or IM with *Y. ruckeri*. Effective doses ranged from 2.5×10^5 to 5.5×10^6 cells/g of fish for those injected IP and from 1.7×10^7 to 1.5×10^9 for those immunized IM. When similar doses were administered IE the response was poor and variable and substantial mortalities occurred. The rapid onset and high titers associated with the response to *Y. ruckeri* suggest that the immunizations stimulated a secondary response. The modest titers detected in the serum of control fish supports this contention. It would be interesting to test this serum against a panel of bacteria isolated from the hatchery environment to determine whether the activity of control fish serum represents specific antibody or cross reacting antibody.

REFERENCES

Anderson, D.P. and Dixon, O.W., 1980. Immunological memory in rainbow trout to a fish disease bacterin administered by flush exposure. In: M.J. Manning (Editor), Phylogeny of Immunological Memory. Elsevier/North Holland Biomedical Press, Amsterdam, pp. 103-111.

Avtalion, R.R., 1969. Temperature effect on antibody production and immunological memory in carp (*Cyprinus carpio*) immunized against bovine serum albumin (BSA). Immunology 17: 927-931.

Avtalion, R.R., Wishkovsky, A., and Katz, D., 1980. Regulatory effect of temperature on specific suppression and enhancement of the humoral immune response in fish. In: M. J. Manning (Editor), Phylogeny of Immunological Memory. Elsevier/North Holland Biomedical Press, Amsterdam, pp. 113-121.

Bortz, B.M., Kenny, G.E., Pauley, G.B., Garcia-Ortigoza, E., and Anderson, D.P., 1984. The immune response in immunized and naturally infected rainbow trout (Salmo gairdneri) to Diplostomum spacthaceum as detected by enzyme-linked immunosorbent assay (ELISA). Develop. Comp. Immunol. 8(4): 813-822.

Chart, H., Pearson, T.W., and Trust, T.J., 1984. Detection of specific fish antibody using an inhibition enzyme-linked immunosorbent assay (inhibition ELISA). J. Immunol. Meth. 68: 19-24.

Clem, L.W. and Sigel, M.M., 1966. Immunological and immunochemical studies on holostean and marine teleost fishes immunized with bovine serum albumin. In: R. T. Smith, P. A. Meischer, and R. A. Good (Editors), Phylogeny of Immunity. University of Florida Press, Gainesville, Florida, pp. 209-217.

Cumming, C.G., Ross, P.W., Poxton, I.R., and McBride, W.H., 1980. Grouping of B-heamolytic streptococci by enzyme-linked immunosorbent assay. J. Med. Microbiol. 13: 459-461.

Harris, J.E., 1973. The immune responses of dace Leuciscus leuciscus (L) to injected antigenic materials. J. Fish Biol. 5: 261-276.

Hodgins, H.O., Weiser, R.S., and Ridgway, G.J., 1967. The nature of antibodies and the immune response in rainbow trout (Salmo gairdneri). J. Immunol. 99: 534-544.

Ingram, G.A. and Alexander, J.B., 1977. The primary immune response to brown trout (Salmo trutta) to injection with cellular antigens. J. Fish Biol. 10: 63-72.

Ingram, G.A., 1979. The immunoglobulin of the brown trout, Salmo trutta, and its concentration in the serum of antigen-stimulated and non-stimulated fish. J. Fish Biol. 14: 249-260.

Ingram, G.A., 1980. The immune response of the brown trout (Salmo trutta) to lipopolysaccharide J. Fish Biol. 16: 181-197.

Khalifa, K.A. and Post, G., 1976. Immune response of advanced rainbow trout fry to Aeromonas liquefaciens. Prog. Fish-Cult. 38(2): 66-68.

McDaniel, D. (Editor), 1979. Procedures for the detection and identification of certain fish pathogens. American Fisheries Society, Bethesda, Maryland, 118 pp.

O'Neill, J.G., 1979. The immune response of the brown trout, Salmo trutta L., to MS 2 bacteriophage: immunogen concentration and adjuvants. J. Fish Biol. 15: 237-248.

Ourth, D.D. and Wilson, E.A., 1982. Bactericidal serum response of the channel catfish against gram-negative bacteria. Develop. Comp. Immunol. 6: 579-583.

Paterson, W.D. and Fryer, J.L., 1974. Immune response of juvenile coho salmon (Oncorhynchus kisutch) to Aeromonas salmonicida cells administered intraperitoneally in Freund's complete adjuvant. J. Fish. Res. Bd. Can. 31: 1751-1755.

Rijkers, G.T., Frederix-Wolters, E.M.H., and van Muiswinkel, W.B., 1980. The immune system of cyprinid fish. Kinetics and temperature dependence of antibody-producing cells in carp (Cyprinus carpio). Immunology 41: 91-97.

Roberson, B.S., 1981. Detection of fish antibody by thin-layer ELISA. In: International Symposium on Fish Biologics: Serodiagnostics and Vaccines, Leetown, West Virginia, USA. Develop. Biol. Standard. 49. S. Karger, Basel, pp. 113-118.

Robohm, R.A. and Sparrow, D.S., 1981. Evidence for genetic selection of high antibody responder in summer flounder (Paralichthys dentatus) from polluted areas. In: International Symposium on Fish Biologics: Serodiagnostics and Vaccines, Leetown, West Virginia, USA. Develop. Biol. Standard. 49. S. Karger, Basel, pp. 273-278.

Ross, A.J., Rucker, R.R., and Ewing, W.H., 1966. Description of a bacterium associated with redmouth disease of rainbow trout (Salmo gairdneri). Can. J. Microbiol. 12: 763-770.

Sailendri, K. and Muthukkaruppan, V., 1975. The immune response of the teleost, Tilapia mossambica to soluble and cellular antigens. J. exp. Zool. 191: 371-382.

Schachte, J.H., Jr., 1978. Immunization of channel catfish, Ictalurus punctatus, against two bacterial diseases. Mar. Fish. Rev. 40(3): 18-19.

Secombes, C.J. and Manning, M.J., 1980. Comparative studies on the immune system of fishes and amphibians: antigen localization in the carp Cyprinus carpio L. J. Fish Dis. 3: 399-412.

Secombes, C.J., Manning, M.J., and Ellis, A.E., 1982. The effect of primary and secondary immunization on the lymphoid tissues of the carp, Cyprinus carpio L. J. exp. Zool. 220: 277-287.

Smith, P.D., 1981. Enzyme-linked immunosorbent assay (ELISA) for detection of Aeromonas salmonicida in diseased fish tissue. In: International Symposium on Fish Biologics: Serodiagnostics and Vaccines, Leetown, West Virginia, USA. Develop. Biol. Standard. 49. S. Karger, Basel, pp. 97-100.

Stolen, J.S., Gahn, T., Kasper, V., and Nagle, J.J., 1984. The effect of environmental temperature on the immune response of a marine teleost (Paralichthys dentatus). Develop. Comp. Immunol. 8(1): 89-98.

Voller, A., Bidwell, D.E., and Bartlett, A., 1979. The enzyme linked immunosorbent assay (ELISA). Dynatech Europe, Guernsey, Great Britain, 125 pp.

Veterinary Immunology and Immunopathology, 12 (1986) 175—180
Elsevier Science Publishers B.V., Amsterdam — Printed in The Netherlands

THE EFFECT OF DOSE, ROUTE, NUMBER OF INJECTIONS AND THE USE OF ADJUVANT ON THE CLEARANCE OF AND IMMUNE RESPONSE TO, HAEMOCYANIN FOLLOWING INJECTION INTO BROWN TROUT (*SALMO TRUTTA*)

G.A. INGRAM and J.B. ALEXANDER

Department of Biological Sciences, University of Salford, Salford M5 4WT, Lancashire, U.K.

ABSTRACT

INGRAM, G.A. and ALEXANDER, J.B., 1986. The Effect of Dose, Route, Number of Injections and the Use of Adjuvant on the Clearance of and Immune Response to, Haemocyanin following Injection into Brown Trout (*Salmo trutta*). Vet. Immunol. Immunopathol., 12: 175-180.

The primary and secondary immune responses were investigated in trout injected with haemocyanin (HCN) intramuscularly (IM) or intraperitoneally (IP), with or without adjuvant. HCN was detected in the blood 30 min after injection and clearance times varied after one injection from 8 to 56 days. Fish given two and three injections cleared the antigen faster.

Precipitins against HCN were first detected 21 to 30 days after injection and were still present on Day 56. However, antibodies detectable by indirect haemagglutination (IHA) and complement fixation (CFA) were initially demonstrated 7 to 21 days after a single injection and highest titres were reached between 33 and 56 days according to the experimental protocol. In fish given two injections, maximum titres were reached between Days 42 and 56 (IM), and Days 50 and 56 (IP). With three injections, maximum CFA and IHA values occurred on Days 62 and 66 respectively in the case of IP, and on Days 103 and 106 respectively with IM. Overall, higher titres were found with IHA than by CFA.

INTRODUCTION

Fish have been used for almost 25 years as models in the study of the phylogeny of the immune system in lower vertebrates. Such investigations have led to the elucidation of cellular and humoral immune mechanisms in many fish species which are similar to the defence reactions which are present in higher vertebrates (Ellis, 1982). Concurrently, development of various methods for the aquaculture of eels, salmon, trout and catfish has progressed (Hildingstam, 1977). Such large scale intensive rearing has resulted in overcrowding stress

0165-2427/86/$03.50 © 1986 Elsevier Science Publishers B.V.

and serious outbreaks of disease which have led to high population mortalities and a reduced economy for the fish farming industry. The diseases have generally been of a viral (Pilcher and Fry, 1980) or bacterial (Sindermann, 1984) aetiology and to a lesser extent caused by fungi and protozoa (Egidius, 1984; Roberts, 1982). To combat such pathogens, attention has focused on the production of appropriate vaccines and vaccination techniques which are applicable to large stocks of fish. These methods have encompassed oral and parenteral immunisation and hyperosmotic infiltration (Post and Vesely, 1983; Ward, 1982), flush exposure (Anderson et al., 1983), spray, shower and direct immersion (Johnson and Amend, 1983; Lamers et al., 1985). Prior to immunisation, various parameters such as dosage, route of inoculation and antigen preparation have been investigated (Ward, 1982). Furthermore, in order to assess the potency of a vaccine or the effectiveness of an immunisation procedure, the 'state of health' of the animal must be examined during the process and the presence of antigen and antibody detected using standard immunological methods.

MATERIAL & METHODS

Brown trout, 1+, length 122 to 315 mm and weight 77 to 307 g, were kept at 12 ^{o}C. The maintainance and transport of the fish were as described by Ingram and Alexander (1977).

The fish were each given a 0.1 ml injection of HCN (Cambridge Bioscience, Cambridge), with or without Freund's complete adjuvant (FCA) either IP or IM. The doses of HCN used were 1, 5, 10 and 20 mg in phosphate buffered saline (PBS) pH 7.4. The animals that received 5 mg HCN, with FCA, were given two or three injections. PBS- and un-injected fish were used as controls.

The isolation of trout serum and the sampling schedules for the control and immunised fish have been described previously (Ingram and Alexander, 1979) and the production of antisera to HCN in rabbits by Ingram and Alexander (1976).

Residual HCN in trout serum was detected by gel diffusion (GD), counter-current electrophoresis (CCE) and single radial immunodiffusion (SRID) as previously described (Ingram and Alexander, 1976, 1979). In the case of SRID, the rabbit anti-HCN antiserum was used at a final concentration of 0.5 ml 100 ml^{-1} in 1% Purified agar (Oxoid Ltd., Basingstoke).

Precipitins were detected by GD and CCE (Ingram and Alexander, 1976). The incubation, processing of plates and scoring system have been reported elsewhere (Ingram and Alexander, 1979, 1980).

The agglutinin titres in trout sera were estimated by IHA (Ingram and Alexander, 1979) and complement-fixing antibodies (CFA) by the complement fixation test (Ingram and Alexander, 1977). For the CFA, HCN was used at a concentration of 0.07 mg ml^{-1} in CFT buffer pH 7.3, guinea pig complement at a dilution of 1:40 and rabbit haemolytic serum at 1:1000. In the case of IHA, sheep erythrocytes were tanned with 0.0025% tannic acid and coated with 2 mg ml^{-1} HCN suspension.

The results were analysed by the Student's t-test for the effect of antigen dose, route of injection, number of injections and the effect of incorporation of the HCN in FCA.

RESULTS

Of the 248 fish examined, antigen was detected in 41%, 4.4% and 1.2% of the sera by SRID, CCE and GD respectively. After a single injection between 14% and 59% of the sera contained detectable HCN by SRID. The %+ varied inversely with the time of first detection and the rate with which the antigen was cleared. In the case of fish given two injections, 19% were positive in the IP+ group; 54% for the IM+. With three injections, these values were 25% and 29% respectively. The time after injection at which antigen was first detected in the serum of the animal varied considerably. When injected IP it was usually present by the time of first bleeding (Day 7), although in some cases it was not detected until the second bleeding (Day 14). Following IM injection, HCN was not detected until at least the second bleeding and in some cases did not appear before Day 35. The disappearance of HCN from the blood depended upon the dose given. After the smaller, single doses of antigen, it was detectable for longer in the case of IM injection than IP. With doses above 5 mg it was normally still present at the end of the experimental period (Day 56).

Precipitins were detected in 23% of the sera by GD and in 39% by CCE. After a single injection, the number of fish with precipitins detectable by CCE varied between 17% and 75%. There appeared to be no correlation between the time of first detection, the route of injection, dose or the rate of clearance from the blood and the % positive. After two and three injections, 76% of the fish injected IM and 83% injected IP showed precipitin activity. All fish which were positive by GD were also positive by CCE.

When the sera were examined by CFT and IHA for the presence of antibodies, the majority of samples were positive compared to the controls. With the exception of the 1 mg groups which contained a lower % of positives, the results for the groups were very similar. The same was also true for the mean titres. The maximum titres detected were 2^{-19} and 2^{-20} for CFA and IHA respectively. When the IHA and CFA titres for each of the IP+ groups were compared with each other, the values were significantly different for the 1 mg group versus the 5, 10 and 20 mg groups ($P<0.005$) and for 5 v 10 and 20 mg ($P<0.02$). In the case of the IM+ groups, significant differences between doses were found for 1 v 5 mg ($P=0.04$) and 5 v 10 mg ($P=0.02$). The effect of dose on the IP- and IM- groups was not significant. Only the IP+ and IM+ routes for the 1 and 5 mg doses of HCN showed significantly different antibody titres (P<0.001). In the case of the use of adjuvant, the 5 mg dose for both IP and IM were different (P<0.01). Only the IM+ route was significantly different when titres from fish that received one injection were compared to those that were given two and three injections (P<0.007). In fish given three injections there were signiificant differences between the IM and IP routes (P<0.005).

DISCUSSION

Neither dose nor adjuvant appeared to have any marked affect upon the time of first detection of HCN. However, a higher percentage of fish had detectable antigen in their sera in the cases of the 10 mg and 20 mg groups and it persisted longer. The use of adjuvant tended to delay the time of first appearance of HCN in the serum, most likely due to its slow release from the emulsion. Similar times of detection of antigen in the blood after IM and IP injections have been found by other workers (O'Neill, 1980; Ferguson et al., 1982) although the rates of antigen clearance have been much higher than in the present study (Page and Rowley, 1984; Russell et al., 1976). The fastest clearances found for trout were 8 days for 5 mg HCN injected IP and 10 days for the same dose injected IM. Other doses took longer. In contrast, dose appeared to have no effect on bacterial clearance from the blood of eels (Kusuda and Ishihara, 1981).

The repeated injection of HCN into brown trout resulted in its more rapid clearance. The results for other fish are variable (Harris, 1973; Russell et al., 1976) and in some fish the repeated injection of antigen even resulted in a slower clearance (Nelstrop et al., 1968). Of the three methods used in the present study to detect HCN, SRID was the most sensitive. Such differences in sensitivity could account for the apparent differences in the rates of clearance of soluble antigens found by the various workers.

CFA and IHA were detected in the majority of injected fish. The times of first detection and maximum titres varied according to the protocol used. CFA values were always lower than those of IHA but the times of first detection were usually the same or only slightly delayed.

The route of injection significantly affected antibody production at low doses of antigen (IP faster than IM). Furthermore for fish given more than two injections, the IM route also gave significantly increased titres. It would appear that the IP route is better than the IM one when adjuvants are used (Ingram, 1978). However, this is not always the case (McCarthy et al., 1983). For both routes, whilst the use of FCA slightly increased the latent period and delayed the time at which the maximum titre occurred, it resulted in increased titres.

The most important factor which affected the immune response to HCN appeared to be the total amount of antigen injected, especially when given IP with adjuvant. The effect of giving the HCN as more than one injection was to increase the titres of both CFA and IHA and to decrease the latent period. Similar results have been reported for other fish (Van Muiswinkel and Cooper, 1982). The multiplicative effect of small doses, different experimental designs and conditions employed complicates any comparison of the results obtained by other workers.

Of the two methods used to detect precipitins, CCE was an order of magnitude more sensitive and was very much faster than GD. Precipitins were detected later than either CFA or IHA and neither route, number of injections nor adjuvant seemed to affect their formation. However, the 5 mg dose stimulated more fish to produce precipitins. The time of first detection was again inversely proportional to the amount of antigen used. The temporal kinetics of precipitin formation is in accordance with the findings of other workers (Harris, 1973; Secombes and Resink, 1984). In teleosts the formation of precipitins seems to depend upon the nature, size and dose of the injected antigen. Fish produce M-immunoglobylins which are poor precipitins and high doses of antigen are often required to stimulate precipitin formation.

REFERENCES

Anderson, D.P., Merchant, B., Dixon, O.W., Schott, C.F. and Lizzio, E.F., 1983. Flush exposure and injection immunization of rainbow trout to selected DNP conjugates. Dev. Comp. Immunol., 7: 261-268.

Egidius, E., 1984. Diseases of salmonids in aquaculture. Helgol. Meeresunters., 37: 547-569.

Ellis, A.E., 1982. Differences between the immune mechanisms of fish and higher vertebrates. In: R.J. Roberts (Editor), Microbial Diseases of Fish. Academic Press, London, pp. 1-29.

Ferguson, H.W., Claxton, M.J., Moccia, R.D. and Wilkie, E.J., 1982. The quantitative clearance of bacteria from the bloodstream of rainbow trout (Salmo gairdneri). Vet. Pathol., 19: 687-699.

Harris, J.E., 1973. The immune response of dace Leuciscus leuciscus (L.) to injected antigenic materials. J. Fish Biol., 5: 261-276.

Hildingstam, J., 1977. Fish farming trends. Vet. Rec., 100: 256-259.

Ingram, G.A., 1978. The immune response of the brown trout (Salmo trutta) to injected antigens. PhD Thesis, University of Salford.

Ingram, G.A. and Alexander, J.B., 1976. The immune response of brown trout (Salmo trutta L.) to injection with soluble antigens. Acta Biol. Med. Ger., 35: 1561-1570.

Ingram, G.A. and Alexander, J.B., 1977. The primary immune reponse of brown trout (Salmo trutta) to injection with cellular antigens. J. Fish Biol., 10: 63-72.

Ingram, G.A. and Alexander, J.B., 1979. The immunoglobulin of the brown trout, Salmo trutta and its concentration in the serum of antigen-stimulated and non-stimulated fish. J. Fish Biol., 14: 249-260.

Ingram, G.A. and Alexander, J.B., 1980. The immune response of the brown trout Salmo trutta to lipopolysaccharide. J. Fish Biol., 16: 181-197.

Johnson, K.A. and Amend, D.F., 1983. Comparison of efficacy of several delivery methods using *Yersinia ruckeri* bacterin on rainbow trout, *Salmo gairdneri* Richardson. J. Fish Dis., 6: 331-336.

Kusuda, R. and Ishihara, S., 1981. The fate of *Edwardsiella tarda* bacteria after intramuscular injection of eels, *Anguilla japonica*. Bull. Jpn. Soc. Sci. Fish., 47: 475-479.

Lamers, C.H.J., de Haas, M.J.H. and van Muiswinkel, W.B., 1985. The reaction of the immune system of fish to vaccination: development of immunological memory in carp, *Cyprinus carpio* L., following direct immersion in *Aeromonas hydrophila* bacterin. J. Fish Dis., 8: 253-262.

McCarthy, D.H., Amend, D.F., Johnson, K.A. and Bloom, J.V., 1983. *Aeromonas salmonicida*: determination of an antigen associated with protective immunity and evaluation of an experimental bacterin. J. Fish Dis., 6: 155-174.

Nelstrop, A.E., Taylor, G. and Collard, P., 1968. Studies on phagocytosis III. Antigen clearance studies in invertebrates and poikilothermic vertebrates. Immunology, 14: 347-356.

Van Muiswinkel, W.B. and Cooper, E.L. (Editors), 1982. Immunology and Immunization of Fish. Pergamon Press, New York.

O'Neill, J.G., 1980. Blood clearance of MS2 bacteriophage in *Salmo trutta*: a paradoxon. Experientia, 36: 1226-1227.

Page, M. and Rowley, A.F., 1984. The reticulo-endothelial system of the adult river lamprey, *Lampetra fluviatilis* (L.): fate of intravascularly injected colloidal carbon. J. Fish Dis., 7: 339-353.

Pilcher, K.S. and Fryer, J.L., 1980. The viral diseases of fish: a review through 1978. Part 1: Diseases of proven viral etiology. CRC Crit. Rev. Microbiol., 7: 287-363.

Post, G. and Vesely, K.R., 1983. Administration of drugs by hyperosmotic immersion or vacuum infiltration or surfactant immersion ineffective for control of intradermally encysted *Ichthyophthirius multifiliis*. Prog. Fish-Cult., 45: 164-166.

Roberts, R.J. (Editor), 1982. Microbial Diseases of Fish. Academic Press, London.

Russell, W.J., Taylor, S.A. and Sigel,M.M., 1976. Clearance of bacteriophage in poikilothermic vertebrates and the effect of temperature. J. Reticuloendothel. Soc., 19: 91-96.

Secombes, C.J. and Resink, J.W., 1984. The immune response of carp, *Cyprinus carpio* L., following injection of antigen-antibody complexes. J. Fish Biol., 24: 193-200.

Sindermann, C.J., 1984. Diseases in marine aquaculture. Helgol. Meeresunters., 37: 505-532.

Ward, P.D., 1982. The development of bacterial vaccines for fish. In: R.J.Roberts (Editor), Microbial Diseases of Fish. Academic Press, London, pp. 47-58.

Veterinary Immunology and Immunopathology, 12 (1986) 181—192
Elsevier Science Publishers B.V., Amsterdam — Printed in The Netherlands

EFFECTS OF DIRECT IMMERSION IN ANTIGEN ON IMMUNOLOGICAL MEMORY IN YOUNG CARP, CYPRINUS CARPIO.

M.S. MUGHAL[1], E.K. FARLEY-EWENS and M.J. MANNING[2]

Biological Sciences Dept., Plymouth Polytechnic, Devon, PL4 8AA, UK

ABSTRACT

Mughal, M.S., Farley-Ewens, E.K. and Manning, M.J., 1986. Effects of direct immersion in antigen on immunological memory in young carp, Cyprinus carpio. Vet. Immunol. Immunopathol., 12: 181-192.

The study asks whether, in fish, antigens encountered early in life can prime the immune system to yield memory responses on subsequent challenge with the same antigen and, if so, whether positive immunity or immunological tolerance is induced.

The direct immersion method of vaccination was used to prime 4 week old carp, Cyprinus carpio, and was compared with priming by injection. Three different forms of antigen were used: the thymus dependent antigen, human gamma globulin (HGG) in soluble and in particulate (latex bound) form; also the putative thymus independent bacterin, formalin-killed Aeromonas salmonicida. The thymus dependent antigens were also used on 9 month old animals.

In 4 week old carp, A. salmonicida vaccine delivered either by direct immersion or intraperitoneally (i.p.) yielded enhanced serum antibody levels and heightened proliferative responses in the lymphoid tissue of the spleen and kidney.

Latex-bound HGG applied by direct immersion was found to partially suppress secondary antibody production while still eliciting enhanced proliferation. The decrease in antibody production following direct immersion priming of young fish with latex-bound HGG was not nearly as marked as the tolerance induced following priming with latex-bound HGG by the i.p. route and, unlike the tolerance induced by the injection route, may possibly still occur in older fish.

When HGG was applied to young carp in soluble form by direct immersion it was ineffective and failed to influence memory induction. This is in contrast to the antibody tolerance, accompanied by an enhanced proliferative response following challenge, which resulted from administration of the soluble antigen by injection in the young fish. The status of the immune system in these antibody-tolerant fish is still far from clear. This highlights the need for further investigation of the role of cell-mediated reactions and local immunity in the immune responses of fish.

---

1 M.S. Mughal's present address is: - Department of Zoology, Government College, Lahore, Pakistan.

2 Correspondence to: - Professor M.J. Manning, Department of Biological Sciences, Plymouth Polytechnic, Plymouth, Devon, PL4 8AA, UK.

0165-2427/86/$03.50 © 1986 Elsevier Science Publishers B.V.

INTRODUCTION

There are advantages to be gained from early vaccination of fish against diseases. To this end, information is required on the maturation of immunocompetence, including the development of immunological memory (anamnesis). Our experiments were designed to determine whether anamnesis could be induced in young fish and, if so, whether the outcome was positive memory, i.e. an enhanced response on secondary encounter with the antigen (the desired effect from vaccination) or tolerance, i.e. the suppression or elimination of immune reactivity. We have been looking at (i) antigen presentation (in solution or carried on particles), (ii) the type of antigen (foreign protein/thymus dependent or bacterial/thymus independent), and (iii) the route of administration, with particular emphasis on the method of vaccination by direct immersion in an antigen bath, compared with vaccination by injection.

Injection procedures provide the most effective method for administering antigens to fish. They have their uses, for example in protecting valuable brood stocks. They are, however, stressful to the fish and inconvenient for the farmer. There may also be a risk of tolerance induction when thymus dependent antigens are injected into immature animals (Secombes, 1981; Van Loon et al., 1981; Mughal, 1984; Mughal and Manning, 1985). More appropriate vaccination techniques for use on a large scale, especially for very small fish, have therefore been sought. This has led to the development of new procedures based on exposure of the fish to vaccines administered externally. One such method is that of direct immersion of the fish in the vaccine. This method has recently been used successfully on young salmonid fish. For example, protective immunity has been bestowed by direct immersion vaccination by Egidius and Anderson, 1979; Johnson et al., 1982a,b: Newman and Majnarich, 1982; Tatner and Horne, 1983a, using bacterial vaccines, and by Wolf and Markiw (1982) using *Tetrahymena thermophilia* protozoa or their sheared cilia (to protect against ichthyophthiriasis). In the work using bacterial vaccines, there were indications that fry can be vaccinated successfully once a critical body weight has been reached. Both vaccine uptake (Tatner and Horne, 1983a) and duration of immunity (Johnson et al., 1982b) appear to depend on the size of the fish.

In older fish (carp) immunized by direct immersion, good secondary antibody responses were obtained when the challenge was given by the same route as the primary immunization, but not when the challenge was administered by a different route. This suggests the existence of a local immune system in fish (Lamers et al., 1985).

In immersion vaccination it appears that the principal route of entry of the antigen is via the gills (Bowers and Alexander, 1981; Smith, 1982; Tatner and Horne, 1983b). The mechanism is not fully understood (see Anderson et al., 1984) but appears to be influenced by the physical form of the antigen. Thus Tatner and Horne (1983b) using a bacterial vaccine found greater uptake of solubilized antigen of small particle size than of whole bacterial cell preparations. With soluble foreign proteins, on the other hand, Smith (1982) showed that attachment of the soluble antigen to a particulate carrier (latex beads) greatly facilitated uptake across the gills.

In the present experiments, secondary antibody production to an immunogenic injection of antigen following priming by direct immersion was compared with that following priming by injection. A comparison was also made between the responses to a thymus dependent antigen (i.e. an antigen for which T-cell help is required in a mammal) and those to a thymus independent bacterial antigen (killed *Aeromonas salmonicida* cells). The thymus dependent antigen was a soluble protein (human gamma globulin) administered either in solution or bound to latex particles.

MATERIALS AND METHODS

Animals

Carp, *Cyprinus carpio*, were obtained from Humberside Fisheries, Skerne, UK and from Priory Fisheries, Kerswell, UK. They were held 10-20 fish per tank of approximate dimensions 35 x 23 x 19 cm containing aerated tap water at 20 ± 2°C. They were fed on powdered Omega no. 2 trout food (Baker, Sudbury, UK) or Mainstream trout diet no. 4 pelleted (B.P. Nutrition, UK), waste material being removed either using sponge filters (Wingate and Golding, Winchester, UK) or by means of a bed of fine gravel approximately 3 cm deep on under gravel filters.

Antigen and antigen administration

HGG, human gamma globulin, Cohn fraction 11, was prepared by dissolving 5mg/ml HGG in 0.85% saline, then diluting to 2.5mg/ml by adding an equal volume of either saline (termed 'HGG in saline') or FCA (Freund's Complete Adjuvant, Difco, Detroit) (termed 'HGG in adjuvant'). For injections the material was administered intra-peritoneally (i.p.) at the rate of 0.01 ml/g body weight (25 µg/g body weight). HGG coated on to latex beads was prepared according to the method outlined in Hudson and Hay (1980) using latex beads of approximately 300nm diameter in a 0.8% suspension (w/v) with 2.5 mg HGG/ml. For injections the dose was again 25 µg HGG/g body weight. For direct immersion immunization, fish were allowed to swim freely for 30 min in a bath containing 5 mg HGG/litre of standing tap water in solution or bound to latex particles. Controls were handled in a similar manner and placed in baths of tap water only, or of uncoated latex suspension.

The bacterial antigen used in these experiments was a formalin-killed Aeromonas salmonicida vaccine (strain 25/77). This was administered in a dose of 10^9 cells/g body weight by i.p. injection or by direct immersion in a bath containing 10^9 cells per litre.

Serum collection and antibody titrations

Fish were bled from the caudal vessels. For small fish, the animal was first killed in MS 222 (Ethyl-m-aminobenzoate, Sigma, St. Louis), the tail was cut off with a sharp razor midway between the ventral fin and the end of the caudal fin. Blood was then collected by capillary action using a drawn out, siliconized capillary tube. For juveniles blood from several fish was pooled (see Figs. 1 and 2) in order to obtain 100 µl of serum for antibody titrations. The serum was used fresh and serum antibody levels determined using the passive haemagglutination technique of Stavitsky (1954) (see Mughal, 1984), for anti-HGG antibody, or by bacterial agglutination for anti-Aeromonas antibody.

Autoradiography

Tritium-labelled thymidine (Radiochemical Centre, Amersham, UK) specific activity 2 Ci/mmol (methyl - 3H) was used as an indicator of lymphoid cell proliferation. The liquid emulsion technique was employed following the general recommendations of Rogers (1967). The fish were injected with tritium-labelled thymidine 18 hours before sacrifice, i.p. at the rate of 1 µCi/g body weight.

Experimental design

Fish in the groups primed by injection received one injection of antigen delivered in saline at 4 weeks old. One group (A) was then challenged at 9-10 weeks old, other groups (B and C) received a second injection in saline at 9-10 weeks old, followed by challenge with antigen in adjuvant at the age of 13-14 weeks. Fish primed by direct immersion received either 5 (group F) or 10 (groups G and H) immersions at weekly intervals commencing when the fish were 4 weeks old. Group F was challenged using an i.p. injection of antigen in adjuvant when the fish were aged 10 weeks, while in groups G and H the fish were similarly challenged when 15 weeks old.

Serum antibody levels were tested 5-6 weeks after challenge for fish in groups A and B, F and G or were postponed to 13-14 weeks after challenge for groups C and H. This later timing was used to ascertain that any possible tolerogenic effect represented a failure, rather than a delay, of antibody production. Fish to be examined by autoradiography were killed before those whose antibody responses were to be studied, at 3-4 weeks after challenge, because previous experience in our laboratory has shown that the peak of the proliferative response preceeds that of antibody formation.

RESULTS

Priming by injection

Fig. 1 summarizes the results of experiments A, B and C in which the initial exposure of 4 -week old carp to antigen was made by intraperitoneal injection; for details see Mughal (1984). Injection of the thymus dependent antigen HGG into 4 week old carp resulted in immunological tolerance. This was manifested by a failure to produce anti-HGG antibody when the fish were challenged at an age when normal fish are capable of yielding a positive anti-HGG humoral antibody response. (Previous results from our laboratory (see Mughal, 1984) have shown that by the age of 9-10 weeks, HGG no longer induces tolerance; on the contrary, 9-10 week old carp can react positively to the antigen and a second encounter with HGG produces some enhancement of antibody levels). From Fig. 1 it can be seen that the tolerance effect of exposure at the younger age of 4 weeks is similar whether HGG is injected in solution or bound to latex particles.

The results from injecting a thymus independent antigen, formalin-killed *A. salmonicida* bacteria, were strikingly different from those using HGG (Fig. 1). 4 week old carp were able to give a primary antibody response to this antigen (Mughal, 1984; Manning and Mughal, 1985) and priming led to good enhanced antibody responses on secondary exposure (Fig. 1).

The autoradiographic studies showed that when *A. salmonicida* vaccine was used as the antigen, lymphoid tissue in both the spleen and the kidney gave a proliferative reaction to the primary injection, followed by an antigen-related enhancement of proliferation in response to the challenge injection. This enhancement indicates a positive memory component and correlates well with the findings for antibody production; for details see Mughal (1984).

The results where HGG was used as the antigen, injected either on latex particles or in solution, were perhaps more surprising. A secondary enhancement of proliferation following challenge after priming with HGG by injection at 4 weeks old was again obtained despite the fact that HGG priming of young fish had an opposite (tolerogenic) effect on antibody production. Thus the enhancement of proliferation following priming was found for all three forms of antigen used and was not related to their thymic dependency.

Priming by direct immersion

Fig. 2 summarizes the levels of antibody produced by fish in groups F, G and H which received their primary exposure to antigen by the direct

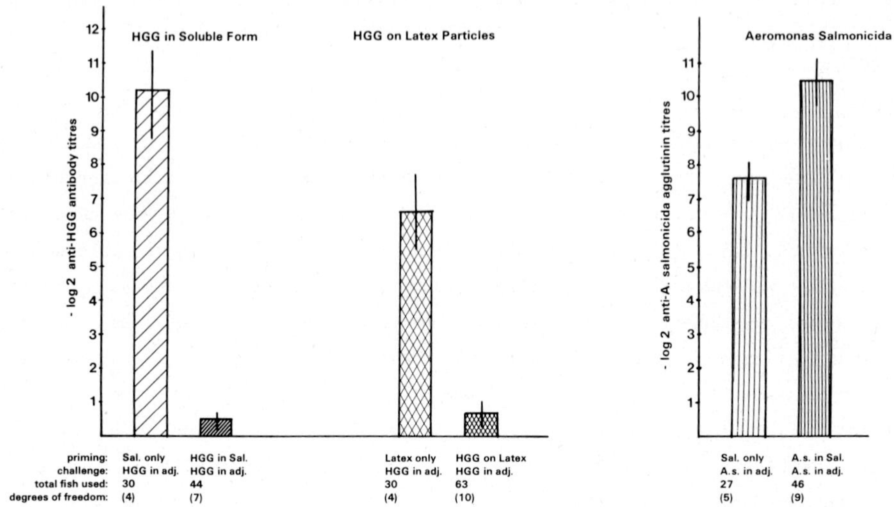

Fig. 1. Humoral antibody production in young carp, Cyprinus carpio, primed and challenged by intraperitoneal injection using soluble or particulate antigens. The diagram shows pooled data for groups A, B and C. *

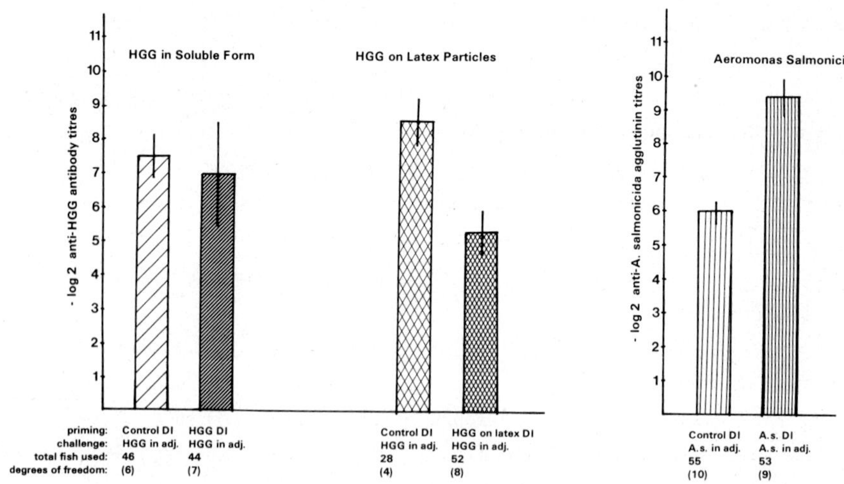

Fig. 2. Humoral antibody production in young carp, Cyprinus carpio, primed by direct immersion (D.I.) and challenged by intraperitoneal injection using soluble or particulate antigens. The diagram shows pooled data for groups F, G and H. *

* All fish were 4 weeks old at the beginning of the experiment. Vertical bar indicates standard error; (d.f.), degrees of freedom.

Tables 1 and 2 Mean autoradiography counts mm^{-2} (± standard error) in young carp immunized with HGG (human gamma globulin) by direct immersion ($5mg\ HGG\ dm^{-3}$), kept at room temperature (20 ± 2°C). All fish were 4 weeks old at the time of primary treatment.

Table 1 HGG in soluble form

Primary treatment by immersion	Challenge by injection in adjuvant	Mean autorad. counts mm^{-2} (± standard error)				Mean autorad. counts mm^{-2} (± S.E., n as for spleen)	
		Group F		Group G		Group F	Group G
		Count	No. fish	Count	No. fish	Count	Count
		SPLEEN				KIDNEY	
None	None	5 ± 3	(6)	10 ± 5	(5)	13 ± 4	13 ± 6
Control	Saline	33 ± 6	(6)	33 ± 13	(6)	118 ± 26	64 ± 22
HGG	Saline	7 ± 3	(6)	13 ± 5	(6)	13 ± 7	62 ± 30
HGG	None	6 ± 3	(5)	14 ± 5	(6)	7 ± 3	26 ± 11
Control	HGG	66 ± 20	(6)	233 ± 66	(6)	190 ± 50	288 ± 48
HGG	HGG	100 ± 39	(6)	211 ± 31	(6)	167 ± 32	286 ± 30

Figures in parentheses represent number of fish used (n).

Table 2 HGG on latex particles

Primary treatment by immersion	Challenge by injection in adjuvant	Mean autorad. counts mm^{-2} (± standard error)				Mean autorad. counts mm^{-2} (S.E., n as for spleen)	
		Group F		Group G		Group F	Group G
		Count	No. fish	Count	No. fish	Count	Count
		SPLEEN				KIDNEY	
None	None	10 ± 6	(6)	11 ± 5	(5)	20 ± 6	20 ± 6
Latex particles	Saline	85 ± 31	(6)	19 ± 12	(6)	210 ± 49	133 ± 40
HGG on latex particles	Saline	12 ± 10	(5)	93 ± 33	(10)	92 ± 19	197 ± 39
HGG on latex particles	None	52 ± 29	(5)	100 ± 39	(5)	105 ± 26	126 ± 45
Latex particles	HGG	299 ± 43	(5)	205 ± 46	(6)	355 ± 55	332 ± 26
HGG on latex particles	HGG	437 ± 53	(10)	461 ± 53	(11)	1047 ± 119	795 ± 70

Table 3 Mean autoradiography counts mm $^{-2}$ ($\pm$ standard error) in young carp immunized with *Aeromonas salmonicida* vaccine by direct immersions (DI)(10^9 formalin killed cells dm^{-3}), kept at room temperature (20 $\pm$ 2°C). All fish were 4 weeks old at the time of primary treatment.

Primary treatment by immersion	Challenge by injection in adjuvant	Mean autorad. counts mm^{-2} ($\pm$ standard error)				Mean autorad. counts mm^{-2} ($\pm$S.E., n as for spleen)	
		Group F		Group G		Group F	Group G
		Count	No. fish	Count	No. fish	Count	Count
		SPLEEN				KIDNEY	
None	None	N.T.		N.T.			
Latex particles	Saline	12 $\pm$ 5	(6)	12 $\pm$ 4	(5)	95 $\pm$ 15	126 $\pm$ 26
Control	Saline	34 $\pm$ 13	(6)	30 $\pm$ 13	(6)	121 $\pm$ 43	57 $\pm$ 22
Aeromonas salmonicida	Saline	59 $\pm$ 24	(6)	94 $\pm$ 26	(5)	167 $\pm$ 39	117 $\pm$ 23
Aeromonas salmonicida	None	N.T.		47 $\pm$ 16	(5)	N.T.	89 $\pm$ 19
Latex particles	*Aeromonas salmonicida*	N.T.		179 $\pm$ 29	(7)	N.T.	292 $\pm$ 29
Control	*Aeromonas salmonicida*	86 $\pm$ 26	(6)	192 $\pm$ 34	(6)	140 $\pm$ 24	271 $\pm$ 36
Aeromonas salmonicida	*Aeromonas salmonicida*	249 $\pm$ 43	(5)	339 $\pm$ 35	(6)	381 $\pm$ 59	440 $\pm$ 39

N.T. = Not tested

immersion method; for details see Mughal (1984). When young carp were immersed in HGG in soluble form, the procedure was ineffective. The young fish showed no significant antibody production following direct immersions in the primary series, nor did priming by direct immersion yield any enhancement of antibody production on challenge. Certainly, unlike the administration of soluble HGG by injection, there was no ensuing tolerance as a result of direct immersion in soluble HGG. When the HGG was attached to latex particles, on the other hand, direct immersion of the young carp led to a slight suppression of antibody levels following challenge. In contrast, when the bacterial antigen, *A. salmonicida* vaccine, was employed by direct immersion, there was no hint of tolerance induction. Primary antibody levels in response to direct immersion alone were poor, but the direct immersion vaccination considerably enhanced the antibody responses after challenge. This indicates that a positive memory response can be induced to the bacterial antigen by the direct immersion technique in these young fish.

The results of the autoradiographic studies are shown in Tables 1, 2 and 3. When direct immersion was employed as the method of antigen administration, the use of tritium labelled thymidine again demonstrated a proliferative effect in the lymphoid tissue of the spleen and kidney which had an antigen-related positive memory component after challenge. This occurred in fish primed with A. salmonicida vaccine (again in consonance with the antibody results); see Table 3, line 8 cf. line 7. It also occurred in fish primed by direct immersion in latex particle-borne HGG (again, as for the injected groups A and B, despite the suppression of antibody production); see Table 2, line 6 cf. line 5. In the case of fish directly immersed in HGG in soluble form, both the results of autoradiography (Table 1) and the results of the antibody studies point in the same direction. Both suggest that the procedure had been ineffective and had had no influence on subsequent immunological memory.

DISCUSSION

The fact that positive immunological memory, demonstrated after challenge, could be elicited following priming by direct immersion (as well as by injection) in young fish using the A. salmonicida antigen is consonant with the findings of other workers that direct immersion in bacterial vaccines can bestow protective immunity. However, no antibody was detected in the primary series alone, following 5 or 10 antigen immersions, in the young carp. We have shown in our laboratory that by the time they are 3 months old (at 20 $\pm$ 2°C), carp can produce antibodies to A. salmonicida when these are administered by direct immersion (Watson, 1984). The levels are relatively low compared with those obtained by injection but nevertheless reveal a capability which was not yet present in the 4 week old fish. Unlike the 4 week old fish, 3 month old carp can also produce antibody in response to direct immersion in HGG administered in solution (Watson, 1984). Possibly young fish are more refractory than adults to the uptake of antigen, as was suggested by Tatner and Horne (1983a) for Vibrio anguillarum uptake in young rainbow trout fry.

The comparison between particle-borne HGG and soluble HGG was initiated in the present work following the report of Smith (1982) that the particulate form of this type of antigen was taken up more rapidly across the gills of rainbow trout fry after direct immersion than was the soluble form of antigen. Farley-Ewens (1983) obtained similar results in 9 month old carp, Cyprinus carpio. The more rapid uptake and clearance from the gills of the latex-borne antigen did not, however, result in better memory induction. Thus when primed by direct immersion and challenged by intraperitoneal injection in adjuvant, the overall anti-HGG antibody titres expressed as -log 2 were respectively 19.4 $\pm$ 2.3 (SD), n = 12 for fish primed in HGG in solution and 14.6 $\pm$ 2.7, n = 12 for those primed in latex-bound HGG ($P<0.05$).

These secondary levels were not higher than the primary response to an injection of HGG in adjuvant (see also the results of Lamers et al., 1985). Indeed there may even have been a slight immunosuppressive effect, although this has still to be confirmed (Farley-Ewens, 1983).

It has yet to be demonstrated whether the tolerogenic effect on antibody production which results from exposing young carp to a thymus dependent antigen is antigen specific. The mechanisms are as yet unknown. The treatment did not adversely affect the proliferative reaction to HGG, since injection of the antigen into young carp, or administration in latex-borne form by direct immersion, induced enhanced secondary proliferative responses. However, the method of tritium labelled thymidine autoradiography did not reveal the nature of the proliferating cells. A possible explanation of the results is that administration of the thymus dependent antigen, HGG, induced tolerance in the B cell and/or T helper cell populations when administered to 4 week old carp while at the same time, positively sensitizing the cells which are concerned with cell-mediated immunity, the latter perhaps being the cells which responded by proliferating. It is known that both specific and non-specific cell mediated responses develop early in fish (see Manning et al., 1982). Nevertheless, the possibility remains that the proliferation revealed by autoradiography may be partly a B-cell response which, in the case of the antibody tolerant animals, did not proceed to antibody secretion, or it may have been due to some non-immune component. In the case of the HGG-treated fish, it is even conceivable that one may have been observing the generation of suppressor cells responsible for the antibody tolerance.

It should be noted that fish vaccination programmes to date have concentrated mainly on the use of bacterial vaccines and this type of antigen is shown in this report to carry no risk of tolerance induction. We have, however, demonstrated tolerance using a thymus dependent antigen. This is a possibility which must therefore be considered in new vaccine development and any conditions which may influence tolerance versus immunity require careful study (for example, physical presentation, such as particle size in direct immersion vaccination). The immune status of our humoral antibody-tolerant fish which were still showing enhanced secondary proliferative responses is far from clear. This highlights the need for further investigation of the role of cell-mediated reactions and local immunity, both specific and non-specific, in the immune responses of fish.

ACKNOWLEDGEMENTS

The work of our laboratory is supported by a research grant (GR3/4431) from the Natural Environment Research Council.

REFERENCES

Anderson, D.F., Van Muiswinkel, W.B. and Roberson, B.S., 1984. Effects of chemically induced immune modulation on infectious diseases of fish. In: M. Kende, J. Gainer and M. Chirigos (Editors), Chemical Regulation of Immunity in Veterinary Medicine, A.L. Liss, Inc., New York, pp. 187-211.

Bowers, A. and Alexander, J.B., 1981. Hyperosmotic infiltration: Immunological demonstration of infiltrating bacteria in brown trout *Salmo trutta* (L.). Journal of Fish Biology, 18: 9-13.

Egidius, E.C. and Anderson, K., 1979. Bath immunization - a practical and non-stressing method of vaccinating sea farmed rainbow trout *Salmo gairdneri* Richardson against vibriosis. Journal of Fish Diseases, 2: 405-410.

Farley-Ewens, E.K., 1983. Immunization of carp, *Cyprinus carpio* (L.), by bath immersion: Antigen uptake and subsequent antibody production. M.Sc. Thesis, C.N.A.A., Plymouth Polytechnic, U.K. (unpubl.) 44pp.

Hudson, L. and Hay, F.C., 1980. Practical Immunology, Blackwell Scientific Publications, Oxford.

Johnson, K.A., Flynn, J.K. and Amend, D.F., 1982a. Duration of immunity in salmonids vaccinated by direct immersion in *Vibrio anguillarum* and *Yersinia ruckeri* bacterins. Journal of Fish Diseases, 5: 197-205.

Johnson, K.A., Flynn, J.K. and Amend, D.F., 1982b. Duration of immunity in salmonids vaccinated by direct immersion with *Yersinia ruckeri* and *Vibrio anguillarum* bacterins. Journal of Fish Diseases, 5: 207-213.

Lamers, C.H.J., de Haas, M.J.H. and Van Muiswinkel, W.B., 1985. The reaction of the immune system of fish to vaccination. Development of immunological memory in carp (*Cyprinus carpio*) following direct immersion in *Aeromonas hydrophila* bacterin. Journal of Fish Diseases, 8: (in press).

Manning, M.J. and Mughal, M.S., 1985. Factors affecting the immune responses of immature fish. In: A.E. Ellis (Editor), Fish and Shellfish Pathology, Academic Press, London/Orlando/San Diego, pp. 27-40.

Manning, M.J., Grace, M.F. and Secombes, C.J., 1982. Developmental aspects of immunity and tolerance in fish. In: R.J. Roberts (Editor), Microbial Diseases of Fish, Academic Press, London, pp. 31-46.

Mughal, M.S., 1984. Immunological Memory in Young Fish and Amphibians: Studies on *Cyprinus carpio*, *Chelon labrosus* and *Xenopus laevis*. Ph.D. Thesis, C.N.A.A., Plymouth Polytechnic, U.K.

Mughal, M.S. and Manning, M.J., 1985. Antibody responses of young carp, *Cyprinus carpio*, and grey mullet, *Chelon labrosus*, immunized with soluble antigen by various routes. In: M.J. Manning and M.F. Tatner (Editors), Fish Immunology, Academic Press, London/Orlando/San Diego, pp. 313-325.

Newman, S.G. and Majnarich, J.J., 1982. Direct immersion vaccination of juvenile rainbow trout, *Salmo gairdneri* Richardson, and juvenile coho salmon, *Oncorhynchus kisutch* (Walbiaum) with a *Yersinia ruckeri* bacterin. Journal of Fish Diseases, 5: 339-341.

Rogers, A.W., 1967. Techniques of Autoradiography, Elsevier Publishing Company, Amsterdam.

Secombes, C.J., 1981. Comparative Studies on the Structure and Function of Teleost Lymphoid Organs. Ph.D. Thesis, University of Hull, U.K.

Smith, P.D., 1982. Analysis of the hyperosmotic and bath methods for fish vaccination - comparison of uptake of particulate and non-particulate antigens. Developmental and Comparative Immunology, suppl. 2: 181-186.

Stavitsky, A.B., 1954. Micromethods for the study of proteins and antibodies. I. Procedure and general applications of haemagglutination and haemagglutination-inhibition reactions with tannic acid and protein-treated red blood cells. Journal of Immunology, 72: 360-375.

Tatner, M.F. and Horne, M.T., 1983a. Susceptibility and immunity to *Vibrio anguillarum* in post-hatching rainbow trout fry *Salmo gairdneri* Richardson 1836. Developmental and Comparative Immunology, 7: 465-472.

Tatner, M.F. and Horne, M.T., 1983b. Factors influencing the uptake of C^{14} -labelled Vibrio anguillarum vaccine in direct immersion experiments with rainbow trout Salmo gairdneri Richardson. Journal of Fish Biology, 22: 585-592.

Van Loon, J.J.A., Van Oosterom, R. and Van Muiswinkel, W.B., 1981. Development of the immune system in carp, Cyprinus carpio. In: J.B. Solomon (Editor), Aspects of Developmental and Comparative Immunology I, Pergamon Press, Oxford, pp. 469-470.

Watson, I.D., 1984. The Responses of Mullet, Chelon labrosus, and Carp, Cyprinus carpio, to Antigen Administered by Injection or Direct Immersion. M.Phil. Thesis, C.N.A.A., Plymouth Polytechnic, U.K.

Wolf, K. and Markiw, M.E., 1982. Ichthyophthiriasis: Immersion immunization of rainbow trout, Salmo gairdneri using Tetrahymena thermophilia as a protective immunogen. Canadian Journal of Fisheries and Aquatic Sciences, 39: 1722-1725.

Veterinary Immunology and Immunopathology, 12 (1986) 193—201
Elsevier Science Publishers B.V., Amsterdam — Printed in The Netherlands

IMMUNOLOGICAL ACTIVATION OF RAINBOW TROUT MACROPHAGES INDUCED IN VITRO BY SPERM AUTOANTIBODIES AND FACTORS DERIVED FROM TESTIS SENSITISED LEUCOCYTES

C.J. SECOMBES, Department of Zoology, University of Aberdeen, Tillydrone Avenue, Aberdeen, AB9 2TN, Scotland

ABSTRACT

Secombes, C.J., 1986. Immunological activation of rainbow trout macrophages induced in vitro by sperm autoantibodies and factors derived from testis sensitised leucocytes. Vet. Immunol. Immunopathol., 12: 193-201.

Young cultures of rainbow trout macrophages were found to significantly increase in diameter following addition of muramyl dipeptide or of supernatants from testis/FCA sensitised leucocytes incubated with spermatozoa, or a testis extract. However, such supernatants caused little migration inhibition or increase in phagocytosis of spermatozoa by macrophages, whereas opsonization of spermatozoa with anti-sperm serum caused an almost six-fold increase in phagocytosis. These results suggest an interplay between humoral and cell-mediated immune reactions upon macrophages during experimental autoimmunity to the testis in trout.

INTRODUCTION

Recent studies have shown that immunisation of mature male rainbow trout *Salmo gairdneri* with an allogeneic testis solution emulsified in Freund's complete adjuvant elicits an autoimmune response to the testis (Secombes *et al.*, 1984, 1985). This response is characterised by the appearance of sperm agglutinating autoantibodies in the serum and focal macrophage invasion into the seminiferous tubules. Subsequent ingestion and destruction of spermatozoa by the macrophages gives rise to severe lesions. In mammalian experimental allergic orchitis such immunopathological reactions are the result of a complex interplay between humoral and cell-mediated immunity. Whether the same is true for the fish autoimmune response is not known. Some possible actions that antibodies and lymphokines may have upon macrophages during these responses were investigated *in vitro* in the present study, using cultures of macrophages from unimmunised fish.

MATERIALS AND METHODS

Macrophages cultures

Monolayers of macrophages were prepared from a suspension of pronephros cells following the method of Braun-Nesje *et al.* (1981), with modifications of the Percoll densities as described by Secombes (1985). Cells were seeded onto flying coverslips in Leighton tubes containing L-15 medium (Gibco, Paisley), 10%

0165-2427/86/$03.50 © 1986 Elsevier Science Publishers B.V.

(Gibco, Paisley) per ml. After 2 hours at 14°C the cells were washed to remove non-adherent cells and were either used immediately (for cell spreading) or were cultured for 3 days before use. By day 3 a homogenous population of well spread adherent cells was present. These cells were phagocytic for sheep erythrocytes (>90%) and positive for non-specific esterase (>95%), confirming them to be macrophages.

Macrophage spreading

Increased spreading of macrophages *in vitro* is one of the earliest expressions of the activated phenotype (Cohn, 1978) and provides a simple and effective measure of macrophage activation. A quantitative spreading assay of macrophage activation has recently been described (Donaldson *et al*., 1984) and was adopted in the present investigation. Immediately after rinsing to remove non-adherent cells the macrophages were incubated with the well known activating agent muramyl dipeptide (MDP) (Sigma, St. Louis) at 10 or 20 μg/ml L-15 for 5, 10 or 20 h at 14°C. Subsequently the cultures were fixed and stained and the maximum diameters of 200 macrophages were measured. This was then repeated using supernatants from testis/adjuvant sensitised leucocytes incubated with spermatozoa or a testis extract. Pronephros leucocytes from rainbow trout kept at 14°C that had been immunised 8 weeks earlier with a testis homogenate (as described by Secombes *et al*., 1984, 1985) were washed and resuspended to 2.5 x 10^{6} cells/ml L-15 medium, supplemented with 10% FCS, 2.1 mg $NaHCO_3$ and 200 i.u. penicillin/streptomycin. A 10 ml suspension of these cells was then cultured in the presence of 10^{6}, 10^{7} or 10^{8} spermatozoa per ml at 20°C in 25 cm^{2} tissue culture flasks (Nunc, Gibco, Paisley). In addition the leucocytes were cultured in the presence of 100 or 200 μg/ml of the ammonium sulphate precipitable material (ASPM) from an acetic acid (0.1 N) extract of testis, prepared according to the method of Freund *et al*. (1955). After 24 or 48 h the supernatants were collected following centrifugation and were stored at -20°C. Controls consisted of pronephros leucocytes from the same fish incubated without antigen, followed by removal of the leucocytes and addition of antigen to the supernatants. The control supernatants for leucocytes incubated with whole spermatozoa were subsequently recentrifuged to remove the sperm, because they were removed from the active supernatants along with the leucocytes. These supernatants were diluted 50% with tissue culture medium prior to their addition to macrophage cultures. After 20 h the macrophages were stained and measured as described above.

Macrophage migration inhibition

Macrophage enriched Percoll fractions were washed and adjusted to 5 x 10^{7} cells/ml. Fifty ul capillary tubes were then filled with the cell suspension, sealed with cristaseal (Hawksley, Lancing) and centrifuged at 300 g for 5 min. After centrifugation the tubes were cut at the cell/fluid interface and the portions containing the cell pellet were attached to the bottom of wells in migration inhibition plates (Sterilin, Teddington) with silicone grease. The supernatants employed in the spreading assay, again diluted 50%, were used to fill the wells before sealing with a coverslip. At least four replicates were performed for each different supernatant. After 24 and 48 h the perimeter of the cells migrating out of the capillary tubes was drawn around using a camera lucida, and the area was calculated by planimetry. The perimeters were redrawn following inversion of the plates for 2 h to confirm that the macrophages (adherent cells) were indeed at the periphery.

Macrophage phagocytosis

Phagocytosis was assessed using 3 day old macrophage cultures. Prior to incubation with macrophages autologous spermatozoa (10^8/ml) were incubated with pooled sperm agglutinating antiserum (SAC) or normal trout serum (SC), with heat inactivated antiserum (SA), or with heat inactivated antiserum plus normal serum (SA+C), for half an hour at 14°C. In addition spermatozoa were incubated without trout serum (S) as a non-opsonized control. After this treatment the spermatozoa were washed and added to the macrophages. Two hours later non-phagocytosed spermatozoa were washed off the flying coverslips and the macrophages were fixed in methanol and stained with methyl green-pyronin. Counts were made of the number of sperm phagocytosed by 200 macrophages, the number of macrophages phagocytosing spermatozoa and the number of spermatozoa phagocytosed by 100 phagocytosing macrophages.

In a similar manner macrophages were incubated with SA or SAC opsonized and non-opsonized spermatozoa following exposure of 3 day old cultures to supernatants (obtained as described above) for 1, 2 or 3 days.

RESULTS

Macrophage spreading

Incubation of macrophages with MDP for 5 h caused no significant increase in cell diameter (Fig. 1). However, a longer incubation for either 10 or 20 h did cause a significant increase ($p < 0.01$); particularly after 20 h when cells incubated with 20 µg MDP/ml were significantly larger ($p < 0.01$) than cells incubated with 10 µg MDP/ml. Longer incubations than this were not used because after this time control cultures began to spread. An incubation of 20 h was therefore used for routine assessment of macrophage spreading.

Macrophages incubated with active supernatants for 20 h similarly showed significant increases ($p < 0.05$) in maximum cell diameter. In Fig. 2 the results using supernatants from leucocytes incubated with antigen for 24 h can be seen. With both whole spermatozoa and ASPM the larger the antigen dose used to stimulate the leucocytes the larger the increase in cell spreading. The results using supernatants from leucocytes incubated with antigen for 48 h were essentially the same. If the supernatants were incubated with the macrophages for only 2 h, followed by an 18 h incubation in culture medium, only minor increases in cell diameter were seen. On the basis of these results supernatants from leucocytes incubated with 10^8 spermatozoa per ml or 200 µg ASPM per ml for 24 h were used further for macrophage migration inhibition and phagocytosis experiments.

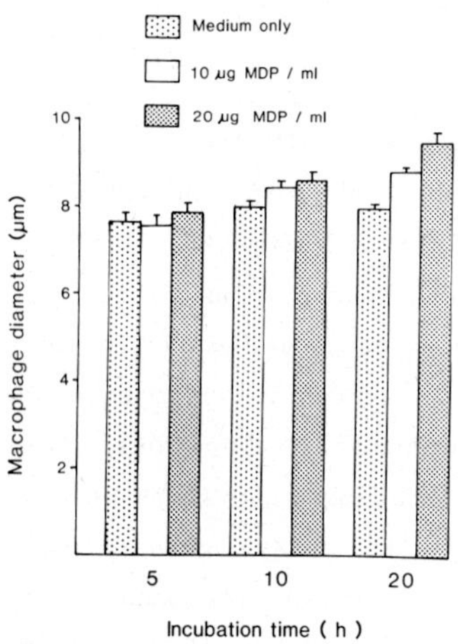

Fig. 1. Mean macrophage diameters following incubation with muramyl dipeptide. Vertical bars represent the standard errors of the means.

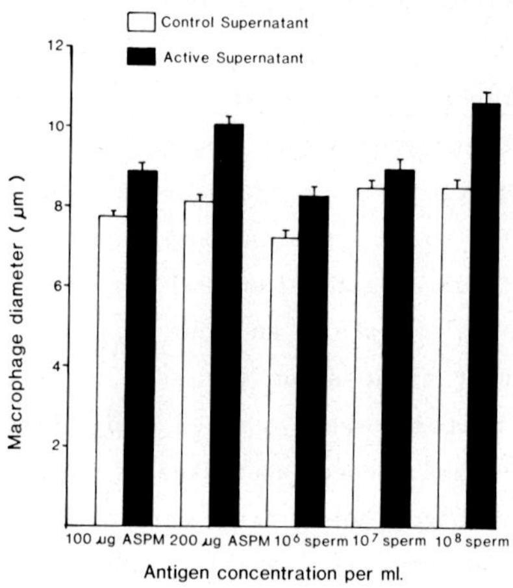

Fig. 2. Mean macrophage diameters following incubation for 20h with supernatants from testis sensitised leucocytes cultured with ASPM or sperm for 24h. Vertical bars represent the standard errors of the means.

Macrophage migration inhibition

As can be seen in Fig. 3, clear reductions in mean migration areas were seen after 24 h incubation with active supernatants. However, these differences were not statistically significant using active supernatants from leucocytes incubated with 200 µg ASPM per ml and were only just at the level of statistical significance using active supernatants from leucocytes incubated with 10^8 spermatozoa per ml. By 48 h the migration inhibition was even more marked, but was still only just bordering significance. Inversion of the plates for 2 h caused no significant differences in migration areas, confirming that the migrating cells being measured and inhibited were macrophages.

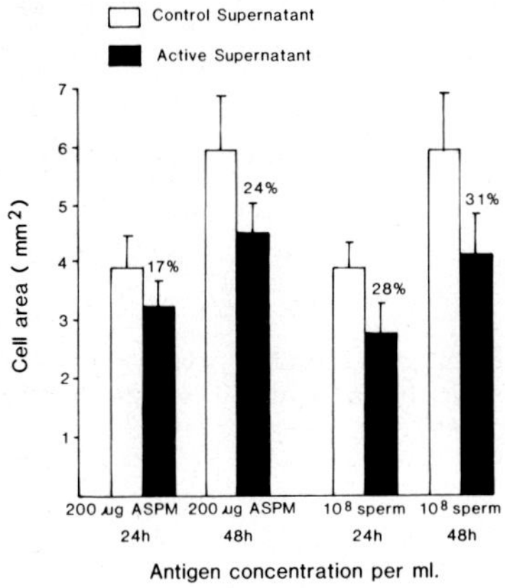

Fig. 3. Mean macrophage migration areas following 24h or 48h incubation with supernatants from testis sensitised leucocytes cultured with 200µg ASPM or 10^8 sperm for 24h. The percentage inhibition is given for each pair. Vertical bars represent the standard errors of the means.

Macrophage phagocytosis

As can be seen in Fig. 4 (data from 2 fish), incubation of spermatozoa with SAC showed a marked opsonic effect which involved both an increase in the number of cells phagocytosing spermatozoa and an increase in the number of spermatozoa phagocytosed per macrophage. Data averaged from 6 fish showed the overall increase to be almost six times the value of non-opsonized sperm. This effect was removed by heat inactivation of the antiserum (SA) and restored, at least in part, by the addition of fresh normal serum (SA+C). Incubation of spermatozoa with SC sometimes had an opsonic effect, but overall this was not significantly higher than the non-opsonized values.

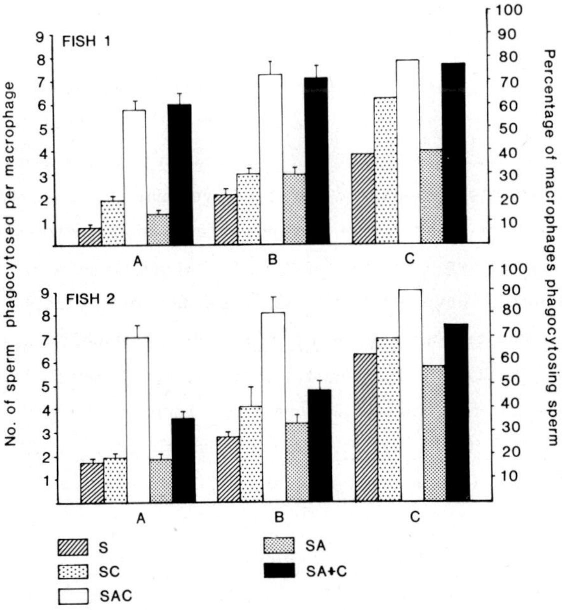

Fig. 4. Macrophage phagocytosis of opsonized autologous spermatozoa. A, mean number of sperm phagocytosed per macrophage by 200 macrophages. B, mean number of sperm phagocytosed per macrophage by 100 phagocytosing macrophages. C, percentage of macrophages phagocytosing sperm out of 200 macrophages. Vertical bars represent the standard errors of the means.

Macrophages incubated with active supernatants for 1, 2 or 3 days showed only small increases (if any) in phagocytosis relative to macrophages incubated with control supernatants (Table 1), especially when compared with the above increases for SAC opsonized sperm. Using SA or SAC opsonized spermatozoa (data not shown) did not cause any further increase relative to the controls.

TABLE 1

Increase in phagocytosis of spermatozoa following incubation with active supernatants from testis/adjuvant sensitised leucocytes incubated for 24 h with 10^8 spermatozoa per ml (Sp) or 200 μg ASPM per ml (As).

Incubation time		1 day		2 days		3 days	
		Sp	As	Sp	As	Sp	As
Percentage increase in phagocytosis	A	6.0	13.5	6.5	20.5	18	-3
	B	3.5	17	9	11.5	19	17

A, number of sperm phagocytosed per 200 macrophages.
B, number of sperm phagocytosed per 100 phagocytosing macrophages.

DISCUSSION

It is well known that macrophages may be activated by a variety of soluble factors produced by lymphocytes called lymphokines, resulting in both functional and morphological changes. For example, lymphokine-stimulated macrophages may exhibit increased metabolic activity and cytotoxicity (Gemsa *et al.*, 1984), increased phagocytosis (Nathan *et al.*, 1971; Dunn *et al.*, 1983), increased spreading and adherence (Adams *et al.*, 1973) and migration inhibition (Bloom and Bennett, 1966; David, 1966). In the present study investigating macrophage-lymphocyte interactions during autoimmune responses in rainbow trout, leucocytes from testis sensitized fish incubated in the presence of specific antigen were shown to release factors that had a marked effect upon macrophage spreading *in vitro*. Spreading provides a potentially reliable measure of cell function and many mammalian studies have used it as a marker of macrophage activation (Rabinovitch, 1975; Phaire-Washington *et al.*, 1980; Donaldson *et al.*, 1984). Although it has still to be formally proven that macrophage spreading in fish correlates with functional activation, incubation with a potent activator of macrophages, MDP (Wahl *et al.*, 1979; Tanaka *et al.*, 1980; Iribe *et al.*, 1981), was shown to induce the same effect and supports this concept.

Functional assays for lymphokine-stimulated macrophages were also carried out, using the active supernatants that gave the largest increase in cell spreading. However, both phagocytosis of spermatozoa and migration inhibition were found to be only marginally positive. This may indicate that the measurement of cell spreading was a more sensitive assay, and was able to detect concentrations of lymphokines too low to induce substantial phagocytosis or migration inhibition, or that the lymphokine(s) present did not affect these particular functions. An example of the latter in mammals is γ-interferon, which has many of the properties associated with a macrophage activating factor (Roberts and Vasil, 1982; Fukazawa et al., 1984), including being able to induce morphological changes in macrophages, but does not cause an increase in non-specific (non-receptor mediated) phagocytosis (Vogel and Friedman, 1984). For these reasons further functional tests and ways to increase lymphokine levels are currently being investigated.

Immune-mediated phagocytosis of spermatozoa was also investigated, following incubation with anti-sperm sera. Such treatment caused the number of spermatozoa phagocytosed per macrophage to increase almost six-fold. This effect appeared to be mediated via receptors for complement, as heat inactivation of the antiserum completely removed the opsonic effect and addition of complement (fresh normal serum) to such sera restored it. Several other studies on phagocytosis in fish have also shown that complement may play an important role in opsonization and phagocytosis (Sakai, 1984; Johnson & Smith, 1984; Scott et al., 1985). This is interesting when one considers that in anuran amphibians and mammals complement receptors promote only binding of particles to macrophages and not phagocytosis (Sekizawa et al., 1984), although they can be induced to do so in certain circumstances (Bianco et al., 1975; Griffin et al., 1984).

Specific antibody, although perhaps indirectly responsible, clearly has an important role in increasing phagocytosis of sperm. If macrophages that exhibit increased spreading are indeed more active they may be more able to kill and degrade these larger quantities of phagocytosed sperm in vivo, and the ability of lymphokines to increase phagocytosis further may be of only secondary importance in this model. Such immunologically-mediated effects upon macrophage function and morphology suggest that in fish, as in mammals, there is an interplay between humoral and cell-mediated immune reactions during the experimental autoimmune response to the testis.

ACKNOWLEDGEMENTS

This work was supported by grant No. GR/B/743 68 from the Science and Engineering Research Council, awarded to Dr. I.G. Priede.

REFERENCES

Adams, D.O., Biesecker, J.L. and Koss, L.G., 1973. The activation of mononuclear phagocytes in vitro: immunologically mediated enhancement. J. Reticuloendothel. Soc., 14: 550-570.

Bianco, C., Griffin, F.M.Jr. and Silverstein, S.C., 1975. Studies of the macrophage complement receptor. Alteration of receptor function upon macrophage activation.

Bloom, B.R. and Bennett, B., 1966. Mechanism of a reaction in vitro associated with delayed-type hypersensitivity. Science, 153: 80-82.

Braun-Nesje, R., Bertheussen, K., Kaplan, G. and Seljelid, R., 1981. Salmonid macrophages: separation in vitro culture and characterization. J. Fish Dis., 4: 141-151.

Cohn, Z.A., 1978. The activation of mononuclear phagocytes. Fact, fancy and future. J. Immunol., 121: 813-816.

David, J.R., 1966. Delayed hypersensitivity in vitro: its mediation by cell-free substances formed by lymphoid cell-antigen interaction. Proc. Natl. Acad. Sci., 56: 72-77.

Donaldson, K., Bolton, R.E., Brown, D. and Douglas, A., 1984. An improved macrophage spreading assay - a simple and effective measure of activation. Immun. Comm., 13: 229-244.

Dunn, P.A., Eaton, W.R., Lopatin, E.D., McEntire, J.E. and Papermaster, B.W., 1983. Lymphokine-stimulated macrophage phagocytosis of fluorescent microspheres: a rapid new assay. J. Immunol. Methods, 64: 71-83.

Freund, J., Thompson, G.E. and Lipton, M.M., 1955. Aspermatogenesis, anaphylaxis, and cutaneous sensitization induced in the guinea pig by homologous testicular extract. J. Exp. Med., 101: 591-604.

Fukazawa, Y., Kagaya, K., Miura, H., Shinoda, T., Natori, K. and Yamazaki, S., 1984. Biological and biochemical characterization of macrophage activating factor (MAF) in murine lymphocytes: physicochemical similarity of MAF to gamma interferon (IFN-γ). Microbiol. Immunol., 28: 691-702.

Gemsa, D., Kubelka, C., Debatin, K.-M. and Krammer, P.H., 1984. Activation of macrophages by lymphokines from T-cell clones: evidence for different macrophage-activating factors. Molec. Immunol., 21: 1267-1276.

Griffin, F.M.Jr., Luben, R.A. and Golde, D.W., 1984. A human lymphokine activates macrophage C_3 receptors for phagocytosis: studies using monoclonal anti-lymphokine antibodies. J. Leuk. Biol., 36: 95-109.

Iribe, H., Koga, T., Onone, K., Kotani, S., Kusumoto, S. and Shiba, T., 1981. Macrophage-stimulating effect of a synthetic muramyl dipeptide and its adjuvant-active and inactive analogs for the production of a T-cell activating monokine cell. Immunol., 64: 73-83.

Johnson, E. and Smith, P.D., 1984. Attachment and phagocytosis by salmon macrophages of agarose beads coated with human C_3b and C_3bi. Dev. Comp. Immunol., 8: 623-630.

Nathan, C.F., Karnovsky, M.L. and David, J.R., 1971. Alterations of macrophage functions by mediators from lymphocytes. J. Exp. Med., 133: 1356-1376.

Phaire-Washington, L., Wang, E. and Silverstein, S., 1980. Phorbol myristate acetate stimulate pinocytosis and membrane spreading in mouse peritoneal macrophages. J. Cell Biol., 86: 634- .

Rabinovitch, M., 1975. Macrophage spreading in vitro. In: R. van Furth (Editor), Mononuclear phagocytes in immunity, infection, and pathology. Blackwell Scientific Publications, Oxford, pp.369-383.

Roberts, W.K. and Vasil, A., 1982. Evidence for the identity of murine gamma interferon and macrophage activating factor. J. Interferon Res., 2: 519-532.

Sakai, D.K., 1984. Opsonization by fish antibody and complement in the immune phagocytosis by peritoneal exudate cells isolated from salmonid fishes. J. Fish Dis., 7: 29-38.

Scott, A.L., Rogers, W.A. and Klesius, P.H., 1985. Chemiluminescence by peripheral blood phagocytes from channel catfish: function of opsonin and temperature. Dev. Comp. Immunol., 9: 241-250.

Secombes, C.J., 1985. The in vitro formation of teleost multinucleate giant cells. J. Fish Dis., 8: 461-464.

Secombes, C.J., Lewis, A.E., Laird, L.M., Needham, E.A. and Priede, I.G., 1984. Agglutination of spermatozoa by autoantibodies in the rainbow trout, Salmo gairdneri. J. Fish Biol., 25: 691-696.

Secombes, C.J., Lewis, A.E., Laird, L.M., Needham, E.A. and Priede, I.G., 1985. Experimentally induced immune reactions to gonad in rainbow trout (*Salmo gairdneri*). In: M.J. Manning and M.F. Tatner (Editors), Fish Immunology. Academic Press, Orlando, pp.343-355.

Sekizawa, A., Fujii, T. and Tochinai, S., 1984. Membrane receptors on *Xenopus* macrophages for two classes of immunoglobulins (IgM and IgY) and the third complement component (C3). J. Immunol., 133: 1431-1435.

Tanaka, A., Nagao, S., Imai, K. and Mori, R., 1980. Macrophage activation by muramyl dipeptide as measured by macrophage spreading and attachment. Microbiol. Immunol., 24: 547-557.

Vogel, S.N. and Friedman, R.M., 1984. Interferon and macrophages: activation and cell surface changes. In: J. Vilcek and E. De Maeyer (Editors), Interferon, volume 2: Interferons and the immune system. Elsevier Science Publishers B.V., Amsterdam, pp. 33-59.

Wahl, S.M., Wahl, L.M., McCarthy, J.B., Chedid, L. and Mergenhagen, S.E., 1979. Macrophage activation by mycobacterial water soluble compounds and synthetic muramyl dipeptide. J. Immunol., 122: 2226-2231.

Veterinary Immunology and Immunopathology, 12 (1986) 203—211
Elsevier Science Publishers B.V., Amsterdam — Printed in The Netherlands

IMMUNIZATION AND CULTURE OF RAINBOW TROUT ORGAN SECTIONS IN VITRO

D. P. Anderson[1], O. W. Dixon[1] and E. F. Lizzio[2]

[1]U.S. Fish and Wildlife Service, National Fish Health Research Laboratory, Box 700, Kearneysville, West Virginia 25430, USA

[2]Immunohematology Branch, Division of Blood and Blood Products, Office of Biologics, Food and Drug Administration, Bethesda, Maryland 20892, USA

ABSTRACT

Anderson, D. P., Dixon, O. W. and Lizzio, E. F., 1986. Immunization and culture of rainbow trout organ sections in vitro. Vet. Immunol. Immunopathol., 12: 203-211.

Splenic and anterior kidney sections or whole organs were excised from large (1 kg) or small (200 g) rainbow trout (Salmo gairdneri) and placed in sterile 60 mm plastic plates containing 10 ml of Eagle's minimal essential medium (EMEM) supplemented with normal or fetal calf serum for in vitro culture. The organ samples were immunized in vitro by direct injection or by mixing in the medium Yersinia ruckeri O-antigen or dinitrophenyl-Ficoll. The medium was changed once during the 10-day incubation at 15 C. The passive hemolytic plaque assay demonstrated antibody production from the plaque-forming cells (PFC); passive hemagglutination was used to measure antibody titers in the media. High numbers of PFC occurred in cultures of either kidney or spleen, demonstrating that these organs can function independently for antibody production. Splenic sections from large fish produced more PFC than comparable whole organs from small fish. EMEM supplemented with 2% normal calf serum was a satisfactory culture medium. 2-hydroxyethyl-mercaptan an ingredient used in mammalian cell culture, inhibited antibody production in trout cells. These techniques are being used in the culture of organs and cells to elucidate pathways and sequences of antigen uptake and delivery of the immunopoietic tissues in trout.

INTRODUCTION

For the past several years we have been studying the kinetics of the immune response in salmonids, particularly rainbow trout (Salmo gairdneri). The constant flow, constant temperature springwater available for holding fish at the National Fish Health Research Laboratory offers unique opportunities to conduct experiments year-around with minimum external environmental influences for these poikilothermic animals; thus, the potency and efficacy of bacterins can be standardized and parameters of the immune response easily predicted. By holding the environment constant, one can study separately the effects of temperature, age of fish, pollutants in water, and the administration of drugs and antibiotics on the immune response.

0165-2427/86/$03.50 © 1986 Elsevier Science Publishers B.V.

Problems arise, however, in accounting for the wide variation of the immune response among individuals in the heterologous populations of hatchery trout used for these studies. There is also a need to further control and standardize laboratory environmental conditions so that immunological organs and cells can be sampled at field locations and transported to central laboratories for further immune assays. Therefore, we began experiments to test in vitro culture and immune stimulation of the immunopoietic organs of rainbow trout--primarily the anterior kidney and the spleen.

Cell culture of lines derived from fish tissues have been available for some time (Wolf and Mann, 1980). The culture media used with fish lines are similar to those used with mammalian tissues; however, the culture incubation temperature may be lower for fish and it is not necessary to lower oxygen potentials by CO_2 incubation. These fish cell lines have been used in toxicology studies. Bols et al. (1985) used a rainbow trout cell line (Wolf and Quimby, 1962) to demonstrate that the addition of phenol and related analogs to the medium reduced the ability of the cells to adhere in vitro to their substrate. They believed that their assays gave clues to the effects of pollutants on fish in the environment.

In vitro organ culture and immunostimulation have been done with mice spleens (Globerson and Auerbach, 1966) by excising the organ and exposing it to sheep red blood cells. Antibody in the medium was measured by agglutination tests. This assay was further refined by Mishell and Dutton (1967) who used the same antigens, exposed spleen cell suspensions, and tested the immune response by using the Jerne (direct hemolytic plaque) assay 4 days after immunization. The Mishell-Dutton tests have been used for analyzing the in vitro primary and secondary response of channel catfish (*Ictalurus punctatus*) immunized with hapten carrier conjugates (Miller and Clem, 1984).

In the present experiments, we adapted the above protocols, using standardized antigens, *Yersinia ruckeri* O-antigen, and dinitrophenyl (DNP)-Ficoll, for immunostimulation in rainbow trout organs held in vitro. The immune response was assayed 10 days after immunization by the passive hemolytic plaque assay to demonstrate individual antibody-producing cells and by passive hemagglutination to monitor antibody titers in the media.

MATERIALS AND METHODS

Experimental animals

Large and small rainbow trout (1.0-1.5 kg and 0.2-0.4 kg) were transferred from the White Sulphur Springs (West Virginia) National Fish Hatchery to the Aquaculture Production/Demonstration Station then to the National Fish Health Research Laboratory (Kearneysville, West Virginia) holding facilities. Fish were placed in 340 liter fiberglass tanks fed with 12 C springwater at the rate of 5 liters/min. All trout were fed a commercial pelletized dry feed (#PR 11-30, Zeigler Brothers, Inc., Gardners, Pennsylvania*).

Antigens for immunization

Antigens previously used for in vivo immunization were optimized and standardized for in vitro immunization (Anderson et al., 1979). The *Yersinia ruckeri* O-antigen is derived from the etiological agent causing enteric redmouth disease of salmonid fishes. The bacteria were cultured in a 20 liter fermenter in tryptic soy broth for 48 h at 17 C, harvested and prepared according to Edwards and Ewing (1972). The DNP-Ficoll was prepared according to Inman et al. (1973) and used as described by Anderson et al. (1983).

Preparation and incubation of the organ section

After the trout were anesthetized in 1:20,000 dilution of MS-222 for 3 min, they were killed by a sharp blow to the head. The area where the incision was to be made was rubbed with alcohol, and the organ was excised with sterilized tools. The organ was placed in an individual, sterile, 60 mm plastic petri dish containing 10 ml phosphate buffered saline (PBS), pH 7.2. When large fish were used sections of organs (5 mm cubes, weighing about 0.2 g) were placed in incubation petri dishes containing 10 ml medium; when smaller sized fish were used, organs were left whole. After injection of immunogen, the organs or sections were incubated for 10 days at 15 C before sampling for immune response. The medium was changed on day 5 by taking off 5 ml of the original medium and adding 5 ml of medium of the same formula, excluding antigen (Fig. 1).

*Reference to a trade name or supplier does not imply Government endorsement of a commercial product.

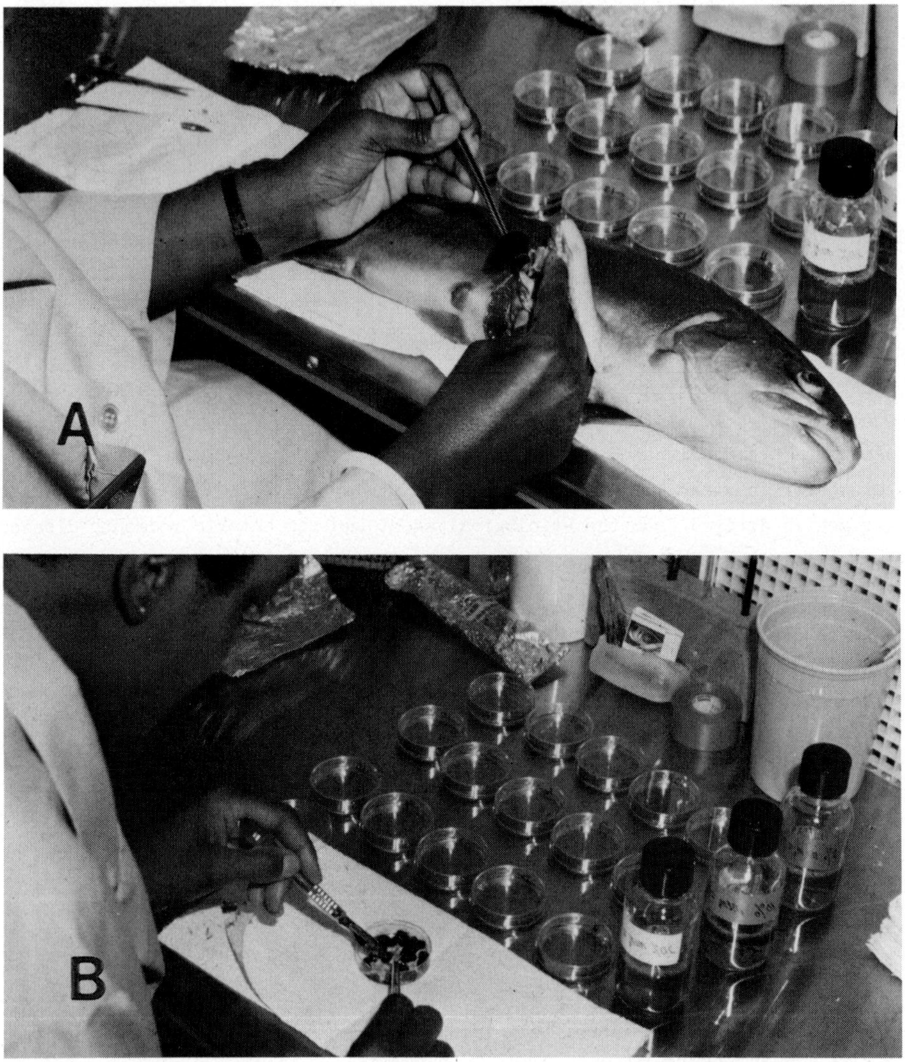

Fig. 1. The spleen, excised from a large Rainbow trout (A), is divided (B) and each section is immunized and cultured for 10 days before analysis of the in vitro immune response.

Immunization of the organ section

Direct injection--0.1 ml of immunogen suspended in 0.1 ml of sterile PBS using a 25 gauge needle--of the organ section was done after the section was placed in the dish. In other experiments the inoculum was mixed with just the EMEM. The *Yersinia ruckeri* O-antigen dosage was 100 µg, the DNP-Ficoll, 100 µg.

Culture media tests

Experiments were conducted to determine the effects of various medium components on optimization of immunization and the development of numbers of antibody-producing cells. In the first experiment we tested the effects of 2, 10, or 20% normal calf serum (Armour Pharmaceuticals, Terrytown, New York) as a supplement in EMEM. In the second test we compared the addition of 2-hydroxyethyl-mercaptan (2-ME) Type 1 (Sigma Chemical Co., St. Louis, Missouri) to the EMEM supplemented with 2% normal calf serum. In the third experiment we contrasted the use of normal calf serum or the use of fetal calf serum. In each test the EMEM contained 100 IU/ml penicillin and 100 µg/ml streptomycin.

Assays for the immune response

The passive hemolytic plaque assay (Jerne assay) was used to determine the numbers of plaque forming cells (PFC) producing antibody. At sampling time, the organs or sections were vigorously scraped on a metal screen to separate individual cells. The suspension was centrifuged (800 g) for 10 min, the cell pellet was then resuspended and filtered through glass wool. Cells were mixed with appropriate antigen-labeled sheep red blood cell liquid media and warm agar, the mixture was then poured on glass slides. After overnight incubation over ice, homologous complement--diluted 1:20 in PBS, pH 7.2--was overlaid and slides were incubated for another 3 h before PFCs were counted. Two slides were poured for each sample.

Supernatant media from the first centrifugation were sometimes sampled for the presence of antibody. Titers were determined by using the same labeled sheep red blood cells in the cellular assay.

RESULTS AND DISCUSSION

The development of in vitro culture and immunization of fish immunopoietic tissues makes available new methods for analyzing organs and cells of the immune system for such experiments as demonstrating effectors that induced immunosuppression or stimulation. Also, these methods might be used for taking samples of fish organs in the field and transporting them to the laboratory where immunological assays can be done less expensively and more reliably. In facilities where fish immunological experiments are done, it is difficult to hold large numbers of fish by the in vitro techniques presented here. In addition, the number of fish used can be reduced by dividing large organs into sections. These techniques will help us with one of the continuing problems--the wide variation among individuals--of assaying the immune response in fish. Using in vitro methods, the investigator can cut one spleen or anterior kidney into multiple sections; single fish organ cultures result in a more consistent immune analysis independent of individual variation (Table 1). Thus, there is the dampening of the variation of results among sample groups when effectors are tested in vitro.

TABLE 1

Column A shows numbers of splenic plaque forming cells from fish individually injected and held in aquaria before sampling whole organ. Columns B, C, and D each represent numbers from a single fish spleen divided into sections and held in vitro before sampling. Each fish or organ section was injected with 100 μg of *Yersinia ruckeri* and sampled 10 days later.

	A	B	C	D
	38	51	47	15
	64	42	29	5
	30	52	35	9
	17	44	36	11
	0		19	16
	67			
	120			
	72			
	11			
	32			
	24			
	1			
	104			
	2			
Mean:	39.6	47.3	33.2	11.2
S.D.	39.2	5.0	10.3	4.5

Many of the parameters for maximizing the in vitro immune response of trout immunopoietic cells have yet to be defined. The media and methods we used in these trials were selected on the basis of data obtained in previous experiments of in vitro immunization and in vivo analysis of the immune response by the passive hemolytic plaque assay. The selection of incubation temperatures was based on in vivo results that showed that the numbers of antibody-producing cells were highest between 14 and 21 days after immunization when fish were held at 12 C. We wanted to hold fish organ sections for as brief a time as possible to avoid contamination and cell death; therefore, the immune analysis tests were done 10 days after incubation of the sections at 15 C.

The different concentrations of 2, 10, or 20% normal calf serum added to EMEM seemed to have no affect on resultant numbers of PFC (Fig. 2). The more expensive fetal calf serum, used at concentrations of 2 and 10%, also showed no statistical differences in the numbers of PFCs found when compared with the 2% normal calf serum. It therefore seems that the least expensive supplement is adequate.

A concentration of 5 X 10^{-5} M of 2-ME is recommended in many formulae for mammalian in vitro immunization tests (Rijkers and Mosier, 1985). However, this chemical abrogated the immune response for trout cells in vitro, in direct contrast to reports of mouse in vitro immunization (Figs. 3, 4). Possible immuno-

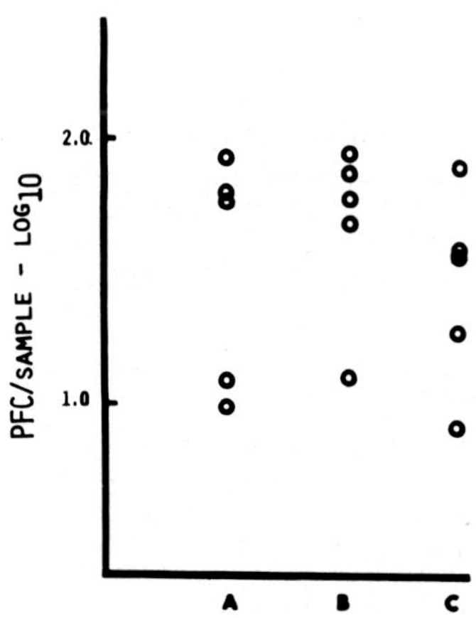

Fig. 2. Numbers of plaque-forming cells per sample from a single large trout spleen sectioned, injected with Yersinia ruckeri and cultured in (A) 2%, (B) 10%, or (C) 20% normal calf serum supplement in EMEM.

globulin, being a large tetrameric 17S molecule held together by a joining chain, was disrupted and inactivated by the 2-ME that is known to break disulfide bonds. In contrast, the mammalian 7S, IgG immunoglobulin is 2-ME resistant. These results are in contrast to those reported by Miller and Clem (1984) who showed that the addition of 2-ME into in vitro experiments caused no marked changes in numbers of PFC in channel catfish when the Mishell-Dutton tests were used.

Both the spleen and anterior kidney of young fish had full immunocompetence for antibody-producing cells in vitro, demonstrating that the organs can act independently. The trout anterior kidney is a diffuse hemopoietic organ, somewhat analogous to the bone marrow of mammals, whereas the trout spleen resembles a mature lymph node. The in vitro tests will be important in studying the residences and migrations of subpopulations of lymphocytes in the organs of fishes. Indeed, the point of action of a suppressant or a stimulant on the immune response might be demonstrated in vitro by adding the effectors at different times in an immunization regimen--perhaps giving information on how to make bacterins and vaccines more effective and potent. The in vitro culture and immunization of organs and cells offers many additional opportunities for analyzing the immune response in fish.

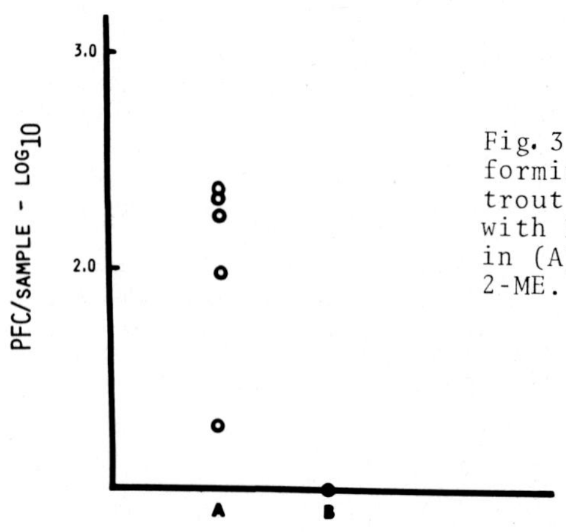

Fig. 3. Numbers of plaque-forming cells per sample from trout whole spleens injected with DNP-Ficoll and cultured in (A) without or (B) with 2-ME.

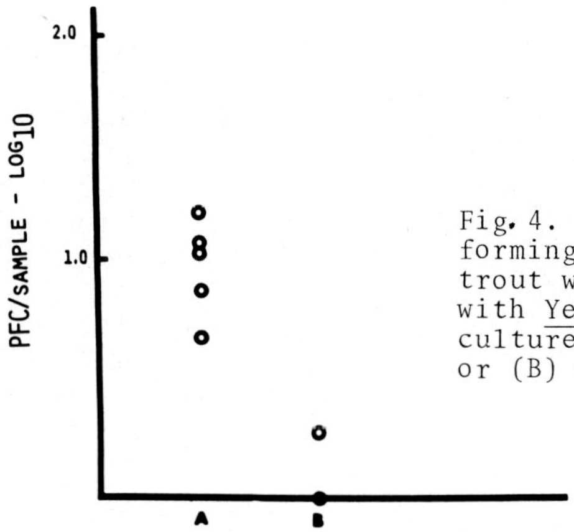

Fig. 4. Numbers of plaque-forming cells per sample from trout whole spleens injected with Yersinia ruckeri and cultured in media (A) without or (B) with 2-ME.

REFERENCES

Anderson, D. P., Dixon, O. W. and Roberson, B. S., 1979. Kinetics of the primary immune response in rainbow trout administered Yersinia ruckeri O-antigen by flush exposure. Dev. Comp. Immunol., 3: 739-744.

Anderson, D. P., Merchant, B., Dixon, O. W., Schott, C. F. and Lizzio, E. F., 1983. Flush exposure and injection immunization of rainbow trout to selected DNP conjugates. Dev. Comp. Immunol., 7: 261-268.

Bols, N. C., Boliska, S. A., Dixon, D. G., Hodson, P. V. and Kaiser, K. L. E., 1985. The use of fish cell cultures as an indication of contaminant toxicity to fish. Aquat. Toxicol., 6: 147-155.

Edwards, P. R. and Ewing, W. H., 1972. Identification of Enterobacteriaceae. Burgess Publishing Company, Minneapolis, Minnesota, 258 pp.

Globerson, A. and Auerbach, R., 1966. Primary antibody response in organ cultures. J. Exp. Med., 124: 1001-1016.

Inman, J. K., Merchant, B., Claflin, L. and Tacey, S. E., 1973. Coupling of large haptens to proteins and cell surfaces: preparation of stable, optimally sensitized erythrocytes for hapten-specific, hemolytic plaque assays. Immunochemistry, 10: 165-174.

Miller, N. W. and Clem L. W., 1984. Microsystem for in vitro primary and secondary immunization of channel catfish (Ictalurus punctatus) leukocytes with hapten-carrier conjugates. J. Immunol. Methods, 72: 367-379.

Mishell, R. I. and Dutton, R. W., 1967. Immunization of dissociated spleen cell cultures from normal mice. J. Exp. Med., 126: 423-442.

Rijkers, G. T. and Mosier, D. E. 1985. Pneumococcal polysaccharides induce antibody formation by human B lymphocytes in vitro. J. Immunol., 135: 1-4.

Wolf, K. and Mann, J. A., 1980. Poikilotherm vertebrate cell lines and viruses: a current listing for fishes. In Vitro, 16: 168-179.

Wolf, K. and Quimby, M. C., 1962. Established eurythermic line of fish cells in vitro. Science 135: 1065-1066.

Veterinary Immunology and Immunopathology, 12 (1986) 213—221
Elsevier Science Publishers B.V., Amsterdam — Printed in The Netherlands

SEASONAL CHANGES IN THE HUMORAL IMMUNE RESPONSE AND THE LYMPHOID TISSUES OF THE MARINE TELEOST, SEBASTISCUS MARMORATUS

T. Nakanishi

National Research Institute of Aquaculture, Tamaki, Mie 519-04 (Japan)

ABSTRACT

Nakanishi, T., 1986. Seasonal changes in the humoral immune response and the lymphoid tissues of the marine teleost, Sebastiscus marmoratus. Vet. Immunol. Immunopathol., 12: 213-221.

Seasonal modulation in antibody production in relation to the state of lymphoid tissue development was studied in the ovoviviparous fish, S. marmoratus. Animals were kept in tanks with running seawater at 23$\pm$1°C for a minimum 2 week acclimatization period and then immunized three times at 2 day intervals with 20% SRBC (5μl/g body weight) intraperitoneally. Immunized fish were bled 2 weeks after the first injection at the time of peak response and plasma were analyzed for titration. The thymus and pronephros were weighed and the number of leukocytes counted in the cell suspension. Antibody levels in fish immunized in summer were higher than those in fish immunized in winter, even if the environmental temperature was held constant. Furthermore, the reactivity of mature females to SRBC was lower than that of males or immature females in the spawning season(winter). The antibody titre was inversely related to the weight of the thymus with the exception of females during the spawning season, while the weight of the pronephros did not show any significant change throughout the year. In addition, the thymus of pregnant, and especially post-spawning females, was entirely involuted, showing a marked decrease in the number of lymphocytes in both the cortex and medulla. Preliminary experiments to examine the effect of photoperiod on antibody production indicated a slight increase in titre among adult fish under a long photoperiod regimen. The present data show that both the season and stage of sexual maturity affect the humoral immune response and lymphoid tissues, and suggest that the thymus might have a function other than that concerned with immunity.

INTRODUCTION

Seasonal variation in immune responsiveness has been reported in rainbow trout, Salmo gairdneri(Yamaguchi et al., 1980) and in perch, Perca fluviatilis(Pontius and Ambrosius, 1972). Seasonal changes in thymic activity and other lymphoid organs have been studied in a number of fish species (Tamura and Honma, 1973, 1974, 1975, 1977, Tamura, 1978, Tamura et al., 1981), however, no attempt was made to correlate the seasonal changes of the immune response to that of the lymphoid tissues. In the present study, suppression of antibody production was found in pregnant, especially post-spawning females, accompanied by an extreme involution of the thymus. This finding is of interest with respect to the post-spawning death which occurs in many species of fish. This paper describes the seasonal changes, and sexual differences in relation to

0165-2427/86/$03.50 © 1986 Elsevier Science Publishers B.V.

sexual maturity, found in both the humoral immune response and the lymphoid tissues of the ovoviviparous fish, S. marmoratus.

MATERIALS AND METHODS

Animals

Sebastiscus marmoratus were collected in Gokasho Bay in the vicinity of our Institute at monthly intervals from May 1981 to April 1983. Prior to immunization, animals were acclimated in tanks with running seawater at 23±1°C for at least 2 weeks and were fed krill. Lymphoid tissues were examined from animals sacrificed shortly after capture. The fish used in these studies consisted of 282 adults weighing 70-200 g and 44 immature fish weighing 25-55 g.

Immunization

Sheep red blood cells(SRBC) in Alsever's solution were washed three times with phosphate-buffered saline(PBS) and adjusted to a 20% suspension. Animals were given three intraperitoneal injections of SRBC(5µl/g body weight) at 2 day intervals. The fish were anesthetized with ethyl p-amino benzoate (100mg/l) prior to manipulation. Immunized fish were bled with heparinized syringe 2 weeks after the first injection at the time of peak response, and the plasma samples analyzed for haemagglutination titres.

Lymphoid tissues

One side of the thymus and the pronephros were dissected free of other tissues and fixed in Bouin's fluid for weighing and histological examination. Serial sections of 7 µm were prepared and stained with haematoxylin and eosin. The other side of the thymus was put on a steelmesh filter (100µm) with a small amount of saline suitable for marine fish(0.2M NaCl) and squeezed to give a single cell suspension. The number of thymocytes was counted in a haemocytometer.

Long photoperiod regimen

Three to eight immature fish of each sex were exposed to a photoperiod of 18 h light : 6 h dark for two months at 23±1°C during the period from January to March, after which their lymphoid tissues and immune responses were examined. Six adults of each sex were also subjected to the same regimen for 2.5 months during the period from February to April and then immunized.

RESULTS

Seasonal changes in humoral immune response

Fig. 1 shows the humoral immune response of rock-fish to SRBC in each month. In August, the mean antibody titre of males and females reached a peak of

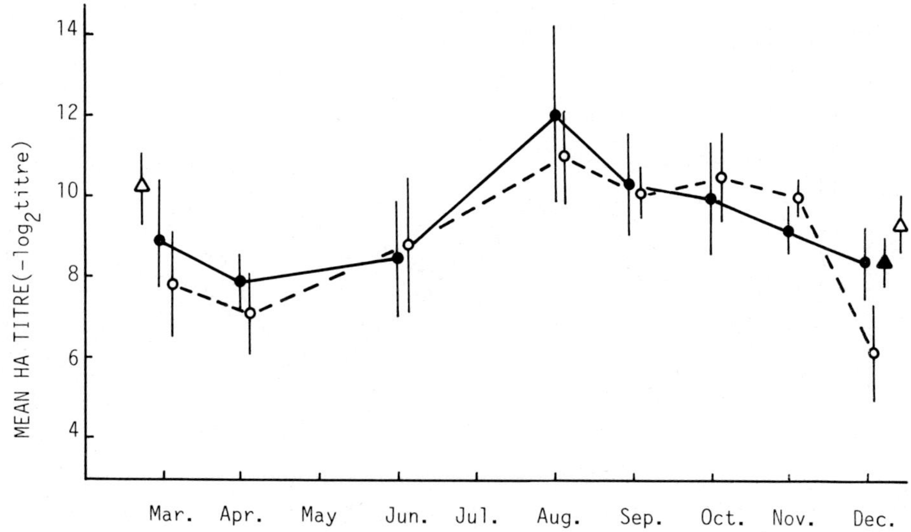

Fig. 1. Seasonal changes in the antibody response to SRBC in the rock fish. Each point represents the mean antibody titres for 6 fish. Vertical bars indicate standard deviations. ● ; adult male, ○ ; adult female, ▲ ; immature male, △ ; immature female.

($\log_2$) 12 and 11, respectively, at 2 weeks after the first injection. In contrast, administration of SRBC from winter to spring elicited a lower response than in summer. This cyclic pattern in immune reactivity was prominent in adults. Immunized mature females in winter exhibited the lowest level of antibody titre($\log_2$ 6), while males and immature females maintained higher responses.

Seasonal changes in lymphoid tissues

The weight of the thymus in both sexes was lowest in September(Fig. 2). The male thymus reached a peak weight in February, while the female thymus was extremely involuted at this time. Subsequently, enlargement was detected which reached a peak in April. These findings were confirmed in the number of thymocytes, that is, the thymus of pregnant or post-spawning females showed lower numbers than that of mature males or immature fish in late-winter(Fig. 3). Fig. 4 shows the remarkable contrast between the male and female thymus in late-winter. The thymus of the post-spawning female, caught in February, was entirely involuted, showing a marked decrease in the number of lymphocytes in both the cortex and medulla, while the male thymus was well developed and filled with a great number of lymphocytes. In contrast, the weight of the pronephros did not show any significant change throughout the year(Fig. 5).

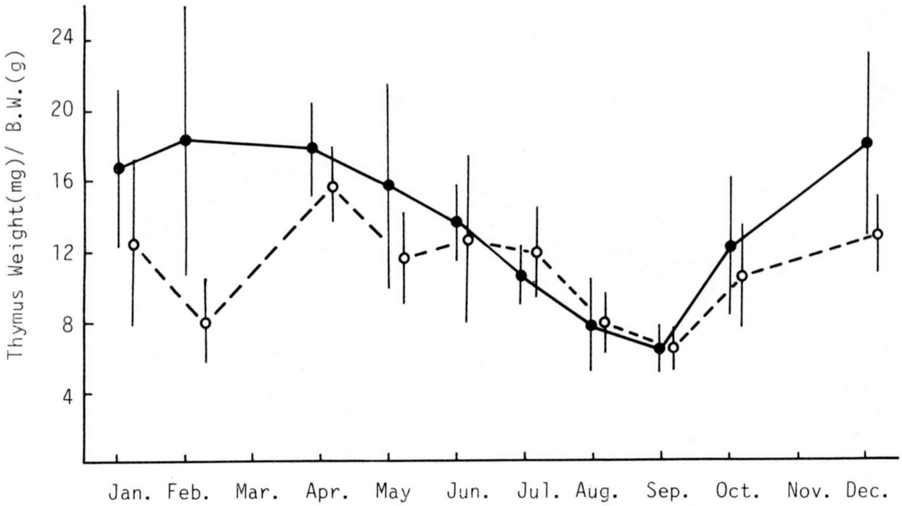

Fig. 2. Seasonal changes in thymus weight in the rock fish.
● ; male, ○ ; female. See footnotes of Figure 1 for each symbol.

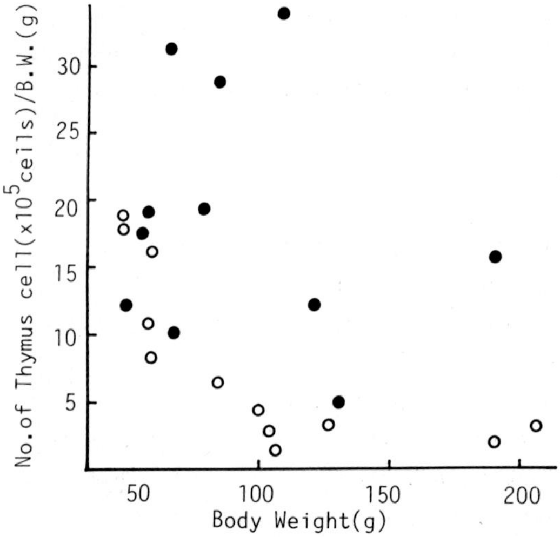

Fig. 3. Comparison of the number of thymus cells in male and female rock fish in late-winter. ● ; male, ○ ; female. See footnote of Figure 1 for each symbol.

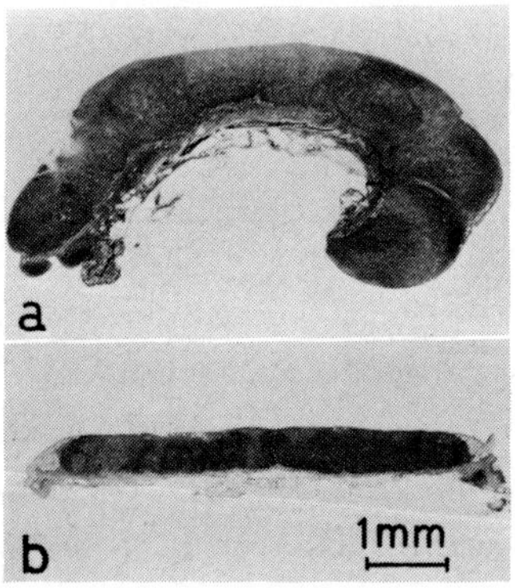

Fig. 4. Comparison of the thymus of an adult male and adult female in late-winter.
a ; male, b ; female. Note the extreme involution of the female thymus, to show a marked decrease in the number of lymphocytes in both the cortex and medulla.

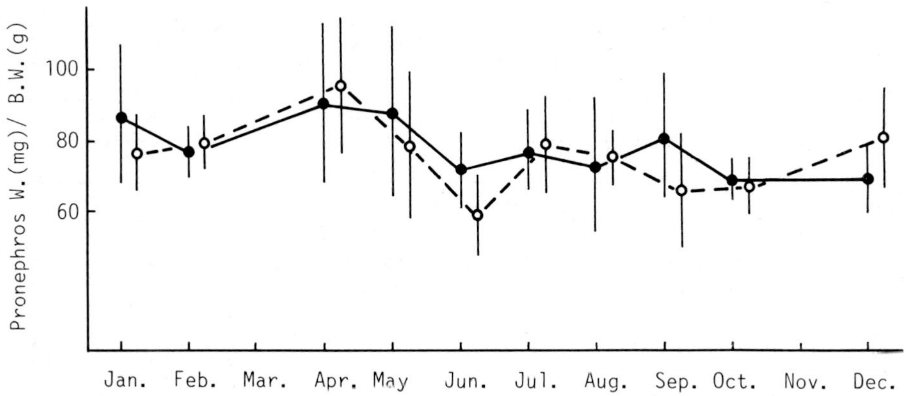

Fig. 5. Seasonal changes in pronephros weight in the rock fish. ● ; male, ○ ; female. See footnotes of Figure 1 for each symbol.

Effects of a long photoperiod regimen on the thymus and humoral immune response

Both sexes of immature fish were exposed to a long photoperiod in winter, and then sacrificed. The thymus was weighed and the number of thymocytes counted. There were no significant differences between experimental and control animals in the ratio of both thymus weight and number of thymocytes to body weight (Table 1). When immature females were immunized shortly after the long photoperiod regimen, peak titres were the same in both experimental and control animals. However, in adults, there was a significant difference in the titre level between experimental and control fish, except for one female fish($P<0.05$, Table 1).

DISCUSSION

Studies on the immune system of S. marmoratus indicate that seasonal variations affect both the level of immune response and the histological appearance of the lymphoid tissues. Similar season-dependent variations in both immune function and lymphoid tissues have also been reported in lizards(Hussein et al., 1979) and snakes(El Ridi et al., 1981), where the seasonal changes could be ascribed to the fluctuating environmental temperature(El Deeb et al., 1980). In rock-fish, temperature is also one of the most important factors affecting the humoral and cellular immune responses (Nakanishi, 1983b, 1985). However, a seasonal change was found even when the environmental temperature was held constant throughout the year. A similar phenomenon was reported in rainbow trout by Yamaguchi et al.(1980), who reported that when trout were immunized with Aeromonas salmonicida prior to spring, the antibody levels were much higher than those in fish immunized prior to winter, even when the animals were

TABLE 1
Effects of a long photoperiod regimen on thymus weight and antibody production to SRBC during the period from winter to spring.

		Thymus Weight(mg) / Body Weight(g)	No. of Thymus cells($x10^5$) /Body Weight(g)	HA titre ($-\log_2$)
(Immature)				
Experimental	Male	17.9 ± 4.0* (3)	13.4 ± 5.5 (3)	---
	Female	20.7 ± 6.0 (3)	18.6 ± 7.7 (3)	10.0 ± 1.5 (8)
Controls	Male	18.2 ± 6.6 (3)	14.8 ± 5.3 (3)	---
	Female	21.6 ± 3.7 (5)	14.4 ± 4.2 (5)	10.2 ± 0.9 (9)
(Adults)				
Experimental	Male	---	---	9.9 ± 1.9 (6)
	Female	---	---	8.7 ± 2.8 (6)
Controls	Male	---	---	7.9 ± 0.7 (7)
	Female	---	---	7.1 ± 1.0 (8)

* Standard deviation, number of animals used are given in parentheses

maintained at the same temperature of 18°C. Moreover, in perch P. fluviatilis, the number of plaque-forming cells in fish immunized in January was higher than that in fish immunized in September(Pontius and Ambrosius, 1972). These findings suggest the existence of seasonal factors other than temperature. In an attempt to understand the basis of this season-dependent variation on antibody production, the influence of a long photoperiod combined with a high water temperature(23°C) in winter was examined. The long photoperiod caused a slight elevation in the antibody level in adults of both sexes, however there was no effect in young adults. These results indicate that photoperiod is one of the factors which affect the humoral immune response in this species.

Seasonal changes were also found in the lymphoid tissues of rock fish, especially in the thymus. The weight of the thymus of both sexes was lowest in September, and the male and female thymus reached a peak in February and April respectively. These observations do not coincide with those reported for other fish species by Honma and Tamura(1984). They described that peak enlargement of the thymus in adults of both sexes occurs in June and is concomittant with the annual pattern of photoperiod in many species. In rock fish, it seems that photoperiod is not the factor affecting thymic change, since the annual fluctuation of day length in this district is not much different from that reported by Honma and Tamura(1984), and a long photoperiod regimen resulted in no alteration of thymic tissue in immatures. Furthermore, other than the results obtained in snakes(El Ridi et al., 1981) and lizards (Hussein et al., 1979), the magnitude of the humoral response to SRBC has not correlated with the state of lymphoid tissue development.

There are two possible explanations concerning the relationship between the immune response and thymic change in the rock fish. First, seasonal changes in immune reactivity or thymic tissue might be attributed not to the whole cell population but to lymphocyte subpopulations such as helper or suppressor T cells in the thymus, providing that thymus cells are responsible for the humoral reactivity of the rock-fish to SRBC. Alternatively, the thymic change might be a secondary effect, with the thymus being a target organ for endocrinological factors affecting the humoral immune response.

It is of interest to note that a sexual difference exists in antibody production of adult fish immunized in winter. This difference was also related to sexual maturation. Namely, reactivity of mature females to SRBC was lower than that of males or immature females in the spawning season. These findings are suggestive of hormonal regulation in the humoral immune system. Recent studies with rock fish in our laboratory show no correlation in the seasonal change between immune reactivity and hormones such as estradiol-17β, methyl testosterone and progesterone. Moreover, no effects on antibody production were observed following hormonal administration(estradiol-17β) and removal of the ovary during the gestation period (unpublished data). Thus, the above mentioned hormones themselves seem to have little effect on antibody production, although more work is needed to determine the precise role of hormones in the immune system.

The present study with rock fish revealed that the female thymus is extremely atrophied shortly before and after spawning, while the male thymus is well developed. This dissimilarity between the sexes in this lymphoid tissues has also been reported in viviparous fish, the guppy and marine surfperch (Tamura and Honma, 1979, Tamura et al., 1981). These sexual differences might be attributed to different seasonal cycles of sexual maturity, although the seasonal pattern of the thymus in rock fish is independent of the seasonal cycle of sexual maturity, as found in every species studied by Tamura and Honma(1981). The cause of this seasonal and sexual variation in the thymus is still unknown.

A weak antibody responsiveness and death from general prostration were observed in the post-spawning females accompanied by an entire involution of the thymus, whereas the seasonal pattern of immune reactivity did not coincide with that of the thymus. It is well known that thymic involution occurs with sexual maturation and increasing age. In addition, loss of immunity in relation to thymic involution was found in senile fish such as the Pacific salmon, Ayu, three-spined stickleback and arctic lamprey(Honma and Tamura, 1972). It is possible that post-spawning death could be ascribed to the weak immune reactivity of post-spawning, aged females, irrespective of whether thymic involution is the cause or the result.

The data obtained show that both factors dependent on season and sexual maturation are involved in the changes of humoral reactivity and lymphoid tissues. External as well as internal factors affecting both immune function and lymphoid tissue are still unclear, although photoperiod was considered as one of the factors affecting the humoral immune response in the rock fish. The physiological status of an animal interacting with environmental factors in a complex manner has to be considered. The results indicate that the state of thymus development dose not always represent the state of immune reactivity, and the thymus may have a function other than in immunity, as suggested by Honma and Tamura(1984), although an important role of the thymus in the immune system has been demonstrated in this species(Nakanishi, 1983a).

ACKNOWLEDGEMENTS

The author would like to thank to Dr. M.F. Tatner, Institute of Aquaculture, Stirling University, Scotland for improving the manuscript.

REFERENCES

El Deeb, S., El Ridi, R and Badir, N., 1980. Effect of seasonal and temperature changes on humoral response of Eumeces schneideri(Reptilia, Sauria, Scincidae). Dev. Comp. Immunol., 4: 753-758.

El Ridi, R., Badir, N. and El Rouby, S., 1981. Effect of seasonal variations on the immune system of the snake, Psammophis schokari. J. Exp. Zool., 216: 357-365.

Honma, Y. and Tamura, E., 1984. Histological changes in the lymphoid system of fish with respect to age, seasonal and endocrine changes. Dev. Comp. Immunol. suppl. 3: 239-244.

Hussein, M. F., Badir, N., El Ridi, R. and El Deeb, S., 1979. Effect of seasonal variation on immune system of the lizard, Scincus scincus. J. Exp. Zool., 209: 91-96.

Nakanishi, T., 1983a. Studies on the role of the lymphoid organs in the immune response of the marine teleost, Sebastiscus marmoratus. PhD. Thesis, Hokkaido Univ., Hakodate.

Nakanishi, T., 1983b. The immune response of the rock fish, Sebastiscus marmoratus-II. Effects of temperature on the antibody production and plaque-forming cell response to SRBC. Bull. Natl. Res. Inst. Aquaculture, 4: 121-129.

Nakanishi, T., 1985. The immune response of the rock fish, Sebastiscus marmoratus-III. Eye transplantation immunity and effects of temperature on scale allograft rejection. Bull. Natl. Res. Inst. Aquaculture, 8: 43-50.

Pontius, H. and Ambrosius, H., 1972. Contribution to the immune biology of poikilothermic vertebrates. IX. Studies on the cellular mechanism of humoral immune reactions in perch(Perca fluviatilis L.). Acta Biol. Med. Germ., 29: 319-339.

Tamura, E., 1978. Studies on the morphology of the thymus in some Japanese fishes. Spec. Publ. Sado Mar. Biol. Stat., Niigata Univ., 1-75.

Tamura, E. and Honma, Y., 1973. Histological changes in the organs and tissues of gobiid fishes throughout the life-span-V. Seasonal changes in the branchial organs of the flat-head goby in relation to sexual maturity. Bull. Japan. Soc. Sci. Fish., 39: 1003-1011.

Tamura, E. and Honma, Y., 1974. Histological changes in the organs and tissues of the gobiid fishes throughout their life-span-VI. Seasonal changes in the lymphopoietic organs of the flat-head goby. Bull. Japan. Soc. Sci. Fish., 40: 447-455.

Tamura, E. and Honma, Y., 1975. Histological changes in the organs and tissues of the gobiid fishes throughout their life-span-VII. Seasonal changes in the hemopoietic organs of the fork-tongue goby. Bull. Japan. Soc. Sci. Fish., 41: 413-422.

Tamura, E. and Honma, Y., 1977. Histological changes in the organs and tissues of the gobiid fishes throughout their life-span-VIII. Seasonal changes in the thymus of four species of gobies. Bull. Japan. Soc. Sci. Fish., 43: 963-974.

Tamura, E. and Honma, Y., 1979. Seasonal changes in the thymus of young guppy. Abstract, Ann. Meet. Japan. Soc. Sci. Fish., April, 1979, p.101.

Tamura, E., Honma, Y. and Kitamura, Y., 1981. Seasonal changes in the thymus of the viviparous surfperch, *Ditrema temmincki*, with special reference to its maturity and gestation. Japan. J. Ichthyol., 28: 295-303.

Yamaguchi, N., Teshima, C., Kurashige, S., Saito, T. and Mitsuhashi, S., 1980. Seasonal modulation of antibody formation in rainbow trout(*Salmo gairdneri*). In: J.B. Solomon(Editor) Aspect of Developmental and Comparative Immunology-I, Pergamon Press, Oxford and New York, pp. 483-484.

Veterinary Immunology and Immunopathology, 12 (1986) 223—234
Elsevier Science Publishers B.V., Amsterdam — Printed in The Netherlands

INTERACTION BETWEEN *AEROMONAS SALMONICIDA* AND PERITONEAL MACROPHAGES OF BROOK TROUT (*SALVELINUS FONTINALIS*)

G. OLIVIER, C.A. EATON and N. CAMPBELL

Department of Fisheries and Oceans, Fisheries and Environmental Science Division, Fisheries Research Branch, Scotia-Fundy Region, Halifax Fisheries Research Laboratory, P.O. Box 550, Halifax, Nova Scotia, B3J 2S7, Canada

ABSTRACT

Olivier, G., Eaton, C.A. and Campbell, N., 1986. Interactions between *Aeromonas salmonicida* and peritoneal macrophages of brook trout (*Salvelinus fontinalis*). Vet. Immunol. Immunopathol., 12: 223-234.

The phagocytic and bactericidal properties of peritoneal macrophages obtained from brook trout (*Salvelinus fontinalis*), injected with either glycogen or a modified Freund's complete adjuvant (MFCA), were evaluated against an avirulent and a virulent strain of *Aeromonas salmonicida*. Avirulent bacteria were effectively phagocytized and killed by macrophages obtained from fish injected with both irritants. With glycogen-elicited macrophages, no enhancement of killing was observed following opsonization of avirulent bacteria with specific antibodies. A killing index (K.I.) of 38 was obtained, compared to a K.I. of 39 for unopsonized bacteria. When avirulent bacteria were opsonized with complement, the K.I. was increased to 67. Virulent bacteria were less susceptible to the phagocytic and the bactericidal activities of glycogen-elicited macrophages, even after opsonization with antibodies and/or complement, K.I. of 9 to 15. In contrast, MFCA-elicited macrophages showed increased phagocytic and bactericidal activities against both strains. The K.I. of unopsonized virulent bacteria was increased to 47 and 46 compared to K.I. of 4 and 7 obtained with glycogen-elicited macrophages.

INTRODUCTION

Furunculosis, caused by the bacterium *Aeromonas salmonicida*, continues to cause serious losses in cultured salmonids and has been the subject of several reviews (Paterson, 1981; Michel, 1982; Munroe, 1984). The nature of the immune response (cellular and/or humoral) that must be elicited to protect fish against furunculosis is still controversial. It was first believed that humoral agglutinins correlated well with and were responsible for enhanced protection (Krantz et al., 1963; Spence et al., 1965; Paterson and Fryer, 1974; Hara et al., 1976). Recent studies, however, suggest that the levels of anti-*A. salmonicida* aggulutinins are not necessarily indicative of protection (Cipriano, 1982; Michel and Faivre, 1982; Olivier et al.,

0165-2427/86/$03.50 © 1986 Elsevier Science Publishers B.V.

1985a). Smith et al. (1980) using a leukocyte migration inhibition test, provided the first evidence correlating increased levels of cellular immunity with protection against furunculosis. This view was subsequently supported by others (Munn et al., 1982; Munroe, 1984; Munn and Trust, 1984).

Using a different approach we have recently shown that a single injection of modified Freund's complete adjuvant (MFCA) could increase up to 450 fold, the LD_{50} of a virulent A. salmonicida strain (Olivier et al. 1985b) The protection conferred was strong, non-specific and mediated by macrophages. The hypothesis was raised that MFCA treated macrophages have an increased bactericidal activity against virulent A. salmonicida. In order to test this hypothesis peritoneal macrophages, obtained from glycogen or MFCA treated brook trout, were evaluated for their capacity to phagocytize and kill an avirulent and a virulent strain of A. salmonicida. The effect of antibody and complement on killing was also investigated.

MATERIALS AND METHODS

Experimental Animals

Adult brook trout (300-500 g) were obtained from the provincial hatchery at Fraser Mills, Nova Scotia. This hatchery has had no history of furunculosis. At the laboratory, the fish were held in dechlorinated city water at ambient temperature and fed daily on commercial pellets. Prior to the start of the experiment, the fish were acclimated at 15°C for at least three weeks.

Isolation and Culture of Peritoneal Exudate Cells

Peritoneal exudate cells (PEC) were obtained from fish previously treated with one intraperitoneal (i.p.) injection of either 1 ml of glycogen (2.5%, w/v) in saline or 1 ml of MFCA prepared as described previously (Olivier et al., 1985a). During handling, fish were anaesthesized with 2-phenoxyethanol. PEC were recovered from fish 4 to 12 days and 19 to 33 days post-treatment with glycogen or MFCA respectively. The fish were killed by stunning and bled through the caudal vessel. The ventral surface area was disinfected with 70% ethyl alcohol and the peritoneal cavity injected with 10 ml of ice-cold Ca^{2+} and Mg^{2+} free Hanks balanced salt solution (HBSS)(Flow Laboratories, McLean, VA) containing 10 I.U. heparin, 100 I.U. penicillin and 100 μg streptomycin per ml (HBSS-1). After ten minutes a small incision was made on the ventral mid-line and the cell-rich fluid extracted. The peritoneal cavity was further washed with 3 x 10 ml of HBSS. Cells were centrifuged at 1000 rpm for 10 min and resuspended in 2 ml of HBSS-1 containing Ca^{2+} and Mg^{2+} (HBSS-2). The cells were counted and viability determined by the trypan blue exclusion test. Over 85% of the cells were alive at this stage. Smears were prepared and stained with Diff-Quick (Dade Diagnostics Inc. Aguada, PR) for differential leukocyte counts. PEC were adjusted to a concentration of 2.5 x 10^6 cells per ml and 0.6 ml seeded in each well of an 8 well tissue culture slide (Lab-Tek, Miles Laboratories Inc., Naperville, IL). After 2 hours incubation at room temperature non-adherent cells were removed by washing with HBSS-2 (2 x 0.5 ml). Macrophages were cultured for 2 days at 15°C in 0.5 ml of minimal essential media (MEM, Flow) supplemented with; L-glutamine 2mM/ml (Flow); 10% heat inactivated newborn calf serum (Flow); antibiotics as for HBSS-1; Fungizone 0.25 μg/ml (Flow) and buffered to pH 7.2 with 10 mM Hepes (Flow)

Culture of Bacterial Strains

The virulent, autoaggregating *A. salmonicida* strain AS-76-30 and the avirulent strain AS-75-74 used in this study have been described previously (Olivier et al., 1985a). Bacteria were grown overnight at 15°C in static Brain Heart Infusion broth (Difco Laboratories, Detroit, MI). Bacterial cells were centrifuged (8,000 g, 15 min, 4°C) and resuspended in saline containing 0.1% peptone (P-S). Bacterial suspensions were adjusted to an optical density of 0.3 at 540 nm, at which point the virulent strain was passed several times through a syringe fitted with a 26 gauge needle to break bacterial clumps. Stock suspensions of bacteria routinely contained approximately 2.5 x 10^8 colony forming units (CFU) per ml determined by serial dilutions in P-S and plating on tryptic soy agar (TSA) (Difco).

Opsonization of Bacteria

Sera used in these experiments were obtained from untreated brook trout and from fish immunized with one i.p. injection of 1 mg wet weight of formalin-killed virulent cells emulsified in MFCA, as described previously (Olivier et al., 1985a). The anti-*A. salmonicida* titers were <1:10 for normal sera and 1:2560 for immune sera.

Stock suspension of bacteria were diluted 1:10 in HBSS containing Ca^{2+}, Mg^{2+} and 0.01% gelatin (HBSS-G) Bacteria were incubated for 30 min at room temperature in HBSS-G with or without 10% heat-inactivated (45°C, 30 min) normal serum. For the bactericidal assay the same bacterial suspensions were used. In addition, bacteria diluted 1:10 in HBSS-G were also opsonized for 30 min with 10% fresh normal serum (complement), 10% heat-inactivated (as above) immune serum (antibodies) or 5% each of the former sera (complement plus antibodies). A volume of 0.2 ml, estimated to contain approximately 5 x 10^6 CFU, of the various bacterial preparations was used to infect the wells. At the same time an aliquot of each preparation was diluted in P-S and plated on TSA. The resulting count established the number of CFU added per well at t-0.

Phagocytosis Assay

Duplicate wells containing macrophages were infected with 0.2 of the bacterial suspensions with and without 10% heat-inactivated normal serum. Phagocytosis was allowed to proceed for 1 h. Slides were rinsed in HBSS-G, air dried and stained with Diff-Quick. Two hundred macrophages per well were examined. Results are expressed as the percentage of macrophages exhibiting phagocytosis and the mean number of bacteria associated per macrophage.

Bactericidal Assay

During bacterial opsonization, cultured macrophages were carefully washed with several changes of HBSS-G. In each experiment duplicate wells containing macrophages (assay wells) and duplicate wells with no macrophages (control wells) were infected with 0.2 ml of the various bacterial suspensions. The assay was performed at room temperature. During the experiment, wells were washed with 0.4 ml of HBSS-G and all washings from each well, including the lysis step (see below), were pooled and kept on ice. After infection, (t-o), the wells were incubated for 1 hour, washed twice and incubated for an additional 1 hour in 0.4 ml of HBSS-G. At this time, (t-2), the HBSS-G was removed and added to the previous washings. Each well then received 0.4 ml of sterile distilled water containing 0.01% bovine serum albumin in order to lyse macrophages, followed, after 15 minutes, by a final wash. The total volume of washings recovered from each well was ≈ 2.2 ml. The washings were diluted in P-S and the total number of CFU/well at t_2 determined by plate count. Results are expressed as % Growth at t_2 and calculated for each well from the formula:

$$\% \text{ Growth at } t_2 = 100 \times \frac{\text{total CFU } t_2}{\text{toal CFU } t_2}$$

By comparing the % Growth t_2 in the contro and assay wells a Killing Index (K.I) was obtained.

$$\text{K.I.} = \frac{\% \text{ Growth } t_2 \text{ assay well}}{\% \text{ Growth } t_2 \text{ control well}}$$

The student's t test for independent means was used to determine the probabilities (P) for the bactericidal activity of macrophages.

Table 1: *In vitro* phagocytic activity of brook trout peritoneal macrophages against *A. salmonicida*.

Treatment of bacteria	Avirulent			Virulent		
	%Phagocytosis	No. of bacteria per macrophage	No. of wells	%Phagocytosis	No. of bacteria per macrophage	No. of wells
Glycogen-elicited macrophages						
No serum	62.1 ± 7.4	6.9 ± 1.8	6	31.4 ± 8.7	2.5 ± 0.8	6
10% heat inactivated normal serum	77.0 ± 5.7	10.1 ± 1.5	6	42.4 ± 9.4	3.4 ± 0.7	6
MFCA-elicited macrophages						
No serum	92.0 ± 3.1	8.6 ± 0.3	4	65.1 ± 6.3	7.8 ± 2.2	4
10% heat inactivated normal serum	91.0 ± 4.8	12.1 ± 2.5	3	75.2 ± 11.1	9.1 ± 2.3	4

RESULTS

Total counts of peritoneal exudate cells ranged from 2 to 7 x 10^7 cells for glycogen injected fish 4 to 12 days post-treatment and from 3 to 10x 10^7 cells for MFCA injected fish 19 to 33 days post treatment. Differential counts performed on stained smears revealed that exudates were mainly composed of mononuclear cells (70% or higher). After culture for 48 h at 15°C, cells were adherent, well spread and morphologically similar to salmonid kidney macrophages described by Braun-Nesje et al., (1981). Based on the morphology and their phagocytic activity (90% of the cells could phagocytize yeast particles, results not shown) these cells were considered macrophages.

With glycogen-elicited macrophages, the percentage phagocytosis and the mean number of associated avirulent bacteria per macrophage were approximately double that observed for the virulent strain (Table 1). The MFCA-elicited macrophages showed enhanced phagocytic activity and increased numbers of associated bacteria per macrophage compared to the glycogen-elicited macrophages. This was observed for the virulent as well as the avirulent strain. The pretreatment of the bacteria, with 10% heat inactivated normal serum, resulted in a slight increase in phagocytic activity and in the number of bacteria associated per macrophage.

Significant killing of the avirulent strain (K.I. 29 to 67) was obtained with glycogen elicited macrophages (Table 2). Opsonization of the bacteria with specific antibodies alone did not increase killing but opsonization with complement, with or without antibodies, resulted in enhanced killing (K.I. 58 and 67 respectively). The virulent strain was much less suceptible to the bactericidal activity of glycogen-elicited macrophages. The K.I. was statistically significant only when complement plus antibodies were used as opsonins, but even then, killing was minimal (K.I. 11). MFCA-elicited macrophages caused significant killing (indexes >40) of both the virulent and the avirulent strain.

Table II. *In vitro* bactericidal activity of brook trout peritoneal macrophages against *A. salmonicida*

Treatment of bacteria	Avirulent bacteria					Virulent bacteria				
	% Growth, t_2		No. of	P.	K.I.	% Growth, t_2		No. of	P.	K.I.
	Control	Assay	wells			Control	Assay	wells		
Glycogen-elicited macrophages										
No serum	134±28	95±38	14	<0.005	29	108±15	104±18	10	>0.5	4
10% heat inactivated normal serum	130±36	79±42	39	<0.001	39	153±33	143±22	22	>0.2	7
10% heat inactivated immune serum (antibodies)	115±44	71±33	20	<0.005	38	163±38	148±36	8	>0.4	9
10% fresh normal serum (complement)	114±15	31± 7	6	<0.001	67	100±15	85±25	7	>0.2	15
5% fresh normal serum plus 5% heat inactivated immune serum	116±42	49±13	10	<0.001	58	136±13	121±17	10	<0.05	11
MFCA-elicited macrophages										
no serum	121±45	71±44	12	<0.025	41	116±35	61±37	12	<0.005	47
10% heat inactivated normal serum	177±47	78±53	14	<0.001	56	107±17	58±44	13	<0.005	46

DISCUSSION

This study reveals that phagocytic and bactericidal activities of brook trout peritoneal macrophages varied depending on the irritant used to induce exudation and on the virulence of the *A. salmonicida* strain. Avtalion and Shahrabani (1975) and Griffin (1983) have reported that peripheral blood leukocytes possess antibacterial activity but the cell population (mononuclear or polymorphonuclear phagocytes) responsible for this activity could not be differentiated. Our experimental approach enabled us to demonstrate that macrophages were responsible for the bacterial killing observed. With glycogen-elicited macrophages, killing of avirulent bacteria was not increased following opsonization with specific antibodies. Similar results were obtained by Griffin (1983) using *Yersinia ruckeri*. Addition of complement, with or without antibodies, increased the killing activity of glycogen-elicited macrophages. These findings correlate well with other phagocytosis experiments, where it was found that the phagocytosis of avirulent bacteria only was substantially increased by opsonization with complement (Olivier et al., unpublished results).

By contrast other investigators have reported increased phagocytosis by fish leukocytes following opsonization of bacteria with specific antibodies alone (Song and Kow, 1981; Griffin, 1983) or with specific antibodies and complement (Sakai, 1984). Our results suggest that the principal opsonin in fish serum is complement. A similar conclusion was obtained by Scott et al., (1985). In addition, it was recently shown that salmonid macrophages possess receptors for the mammalian C3b molecule (Johnson and Smith, 1984). Nonaka et al., (1985) who isolated and purified rainbow trout C3 molecule stated that C3 was essential for immune phagocytosis of sheep red blood cells.

Virulent *A. salmonicida* possess an additional layer, the A layer, on the surface of the outer membrane which has been correlated with virulence, autoaggregation, and adherence to cultured fish cells including macrophages (Udey and Fryer, 1978; Ishiguro et al., 1981; Evenberg et al., 1982; Trust et al., 1983b; Sakai 1984). With the exception of the work of Munn et al., (1982) who demonstrated that the A layer was responsible for the resistance of virulent bacteria to the bactericidal effect of normal and immune fish sera, other roles of the A layer in host-pathogen interactions remain largely unknown. In view of the unimpaired growth of virulent bacteria once injected into fish, one hypothesis is that virulent bacteria must be able to survive within the macrophage (Trust et al., 1983a; Munn and Trust, 1984). Our results tend to support this hypothesis since virulent bacteria, which possess the A layer, were clearly more resistant to the bactericidal activity of glycogen-elicited macrophages than were avirulent bacteria. The A layer could also be responsible for the increased resistance of virulent bacteria to phagocytosis observed in this study and as recently reported by Sakai and Kimura (1985).

When it was demonstrated that MFCA could confer strong nonspecific protection against furunculosis (Olivier et al., 1985b), it was postulated that macrophages, stimulated by MFCA, would possess enhanced antimicrobial properties. The results reported here confirm this hypothesis, since only the MFCA-elicited macrophages caused significant killing of the virulent strain. These macrophages also possessed enhanced phagocytic activity. Our results indicate that in fish, as in mammals, adjuvant can enhance phagocytosis and bactericidal activity of macrophages.

As suggested by other investigators (Smith et al., 1980; Munn et al., 1982), and in view of our findings, we strongly feel that the role of cellular immunity in furunculosis needs to be reassessed as it appears to represent a major component of the fish immune system. This study also demonstrates that cultured macrophages are a valuable tool to investigate the host-pathogen relationships in fish, not only for *A. salmonicida* but for other pathogens as well.

ACKNOWLEDGEMENTS

The authors gratefully acknowledge the assistance of M. Hill, Department of Fisheries, Province of Nova Scotia for supplying the brook trout and of D. Casavechia and F. Rahey, Aquarium staff, Halifax Fisheries Research Laboratory.

REFERENCES

Avtalion, R.R. and Shahrabani, R., 1975. Studies on phagocytosis in fish 1. *In vitro* uptake and killing of living *Staphylococcus aureus* by peripheral leucocytes of carp (*Cyprinus carpio*). Immunology 29: 1181-1187

Braun-Nesje, R., Bertheussen, K., Kaplan, F. and Seljelid, R. 1981. Salmonid macrophages: separation, *in vitro* culture and characterization. J. Fish

Cipriano, R., 1982. Immunization of brook trout (*Salvelinus fontinalis*) against *Aeromonas salmonicida*: immunogenicity of virulent and avirulent isolates and protective ability of different antigens. Can. J. Fish. Aquat. Sci. 39: 218-221.

Evenberg, D., Van Boxtel, R., Lugtenberg B., Schurer, F., Blommaert, J. and Bootsma, R., 1982. Cell surface of fish pathogenic bacterium *Aeromonas salmonicida*. 1. Relationship between autoagglutination and the presence of major cell envelope protein. Biochem. Biophys. Acta. 684: 241-248

Griffin, B.R., 1983. Opsonic effect of rainbow trout (*Salmo gairdneri*) antibody on phagocytosis of *Yersinia ruckeri* by trout leukocytes. Dev. Comp. Immunol. 7: 253:255.

Hara, T., Inoue, K.,Morikawa, S. and Toshiro, F., 1976. Vaccination trials for control of furunculosis of salmonids in Japan. Fish Path. 10: 227:235

Ishiguro, E.E., Kay, W.W., Ainsworth, T., Chamberlain, J.B., Austen, R.A., Buckley, J.T. and Trust, T.J., 1981. Loss of virulence during culture of *Aeromonas salmonicida* at high temperature. J. Bacteriol. 148: 333-340.

Johnson, E. and Smith, P., 1984. Attachment and phagocytosis by salmon macrophages of agarose beads coated with human C3b and C3bi. Dev. Comp. Immunol. 8: 623-630.

Kranz, G.E., Reddecliff, J.M. and Heist, C.E., 1963. Development of antibodies against *Aeromonas salmonicida* in trout. J. Immunol. 91: 757-760.

Michel, C., 1982. Progress towards furunculosis vaccination. In: Microbial Diseases of Fish. R.J. Roberts (Ed.) Academic Press, London, p 151-169.

Michel, C. and Faivre B., 1982. Occurence and significance of agglutinating antibodies in experimental furunculosis of rainbow trout (*Salmo gairdneri* Richardson). J. Fish Dis. 5: 429-432. Munn, C.B., Ishiguro,

Munn, C.B., Ishiguro E.E., Kay, W.W. and Trust, T.J., 1982. Role of surface components in serum resistance of virulent *Aeromonas salmonicida*. Infect. and Immun. 36: 1069-1075.

Munn, C.B. and Trust, T.J., 1984. Role of additional protein layer in virulence of Aeromonas salmonicida. In: Fish Diseases, 4th COPRAQ-Session, Acuigrup (Eds.) Editora Att, Spain p 69-75

Munroe, A.L.S., 1984. A furunculosis vaccine. Illusion or achievable objective. In: Symposium on Fish Vaccination. P. de Kinkelin (Ed.) Office International des Epizooties, Paris, p. 97-120.

Nonaka, M. Iwaki, M. Nakai, C., Nozaki, M., Kaidoh, T., Nonaka, M. Natsuume, Sakai, S., and Takahashi, M., 1985. Purification of a major serum protein of rainbow trout (Salmo gairdneri) homologous to the third component of mammalian complement. J. Biol. Chem. 259: 6327-6333.

Olivier, G., Evelyn, T.P.T., and Lallier, R., 1985a. Immunogenicity of vaccines from virulent and an avirulent strain of Aeromonas salmonicida. J. Fish Dis. 8: 43-55.

Olivier, G., Evelyn, T.P.T., and Lallier, R., 1985b. Immunity to Aeromonas salmonicida in coho salmon (Oncorhynchus kisutch) induced by modified Freund's complete adjuvant: its nonspecific nature and the probable role of macrophages in the phenomenon. Dev. Comp. Immunol. 9: 419-432.

Paterson, W.D., 1981. Aeromonas salmonicida as an immunogen. In: International Symposium on Fish Biologies, Serodiagnostics and Vaccines. Developments in Biological Standardization 45: 375-385

Paterson, W.D. and Fryer, J.L., 1974. Immune responses of juvenile coho salmon (Oncorhynchus kisutch) to Aeromonas salmonicida cells administered intraperitoneally in Freund's complete adjuvant. J. Fish. Res. Board Can. 21: 1751-1755.

Sakai, D.K., 1984. Opsonization by fish antibody and complement in the immune phagocytosis by peritoneal exudate cells isolated from salmonid fishes. J. Fish Dis. 7: 29-38.

Sakai, D.K., 1985a. Loss of virulence in a protease-deficient mutant of Aeromonas salmonicida. Infect. Immun. 48: 146-152.

Sakai, D.K. and Kimura, T., 1985. Relationships between agglutinative properties of Aeromonas salmonicida strains isolated from fish in Japan and their resistance to mechanisms of host defense. Fish Pathol. 20: 9-21

Scott, A.L., Rogers, W.A., and Klesius, P., 1985. Chemiluminescence by peripheral blood phagocytes from channel catfish: Function of opsonin and temperature. Dev. Comp. Immunol. 3: 241-250.

Smith, P.D., McCarthy, D.H. and Paterson W.D., 1980. Further studies on furunculosis vaccination. In: Fish Disease, W. Ahne (Ed.) Springer Verlag, New York, p 113-119.

Song, K.L. and Kou, G.H. 1981. The immune response of eel (Anguilla japonica) against Edwardsiella angullimortifera as studied by the immersion method. Fish Pathol. 15: 249-255.

Spence, K.D., Fryer, J.L. and Pilcher, K.S., 1965. Active and passive immunization of certain salmonid fishes against Aeromonas salmonicida. Can. J. Microbiol. 13: 397-405.

Trust, T.L, Ishiguro, E.E., Chart, H. and Kay, W.W., 1983a. Virulence properties of Aeromonas salmonicida. J. World Maricul. Soc. 14: 193-200.

Trust, T.J., Kay, W.W. and Ishiguro, E.E., 1983b. Cell surface hydrophobicity and macrophage association of Aeromonas salmonicida. Curr. Microbiol. 9: 315-318.

Udey, R.L. and Fryer, J.L., 1978. Immunization of fish with bacteria of Aeromonas salmonicida. Mar. Fish. Res. 40: 12-17.

Veterinary Immunology and Immunopathology, 12 (1986) 235—241
Elsevier Science Publishers B.V., Amsterdam — Printed in The Netherlands

MODULATION OF THE IMMUNE RESPONSE IN FISH

MAURICE ZEEMAN

Food and Drug Administration, Center for Veterinary Medicine (HFV-152),
5600 Fishers Lane, Rockville, MD 20857, USA

ABSTRACT

Zeeman, M., 1986, Modulation of the immune response in fish.
Vet. Immunol. Immunopathol., 12: 235-241.

This is a brief overview of the field of immune modulation in fish. Special attention is given to the effects of biological rhythms on the immune responses of animals. Biological rhythms in fish appear to be poorly studied and the effects of such rhythms on fish immune responses needs to be evaluated. Implications for research on the modulation of fish immune responses are discussed.

INTRODUCTION

In 1980, I finished a lengthy review of toxic agents that had been demonstrated to have effects upon the immune systems of fish (Zeeman and Brindley, 1981). I had been interested in fish and pesticides for a number of years. So naturally my review focused on pesticides, but it also dealt with the literature then available on drugs, radiation, and other environmental pollutants, such as heavy metals and PCB's.

There were several things that impressed themselves upon me as I tried to review the then nebulous field of research that is now called fish immunomodulation. First, it was quite apparent that the immune responses of fishes were very poorly understood in comparison to what was known about the immune responses of mammals and even birds.

Second, much of the research on fish immunomodulation appeared to have been conducted as a sidelight to some other research objective. Many of the results on fish immunosuppression were merely preliminary, or were footnotes to research projects in the really mature disciplines called Immunology, Toxicology or Ichthyology.

Third, the majority of researchers in immunology and toxicology were usually only interested in either extending their immunological techniques or testing for the toxic effects of their pet toxic agents.

0165-2427/86/$03.50 © 1986 Elsevier Science Publishers B.V.

Fish were just a different research animal to use, a little colder and wetter than the animals used in real research -- mammals!

This was evident by the number of individuals who did research on fish early in their careers, but soon after graduation went on to do their research using a mammalian model. Dr. Craig Lobb and I were graduate students together. I was impressed by the fact that he got to work with Dr. William Clem. This was because Dr. Clem had had a long sequence of students who had done some research in fish immunology. Dr. Clem admitted to me that he was surprised by Craig because this was the first student that he had had that was really interested in continuing to work with fish and their immune responses. I delighted in Dr. Lobb's resolve then and I note that he is still doing research and publishing on fish immunology right now.

It certainly seems that things have really started to change in the last five or so years. Not only are there semi-regular symposia that deal primarily with issues in fish immunology, now we even have an entire session that deals exclusively with the modulation of the immune response in fish. I am not being facetious when I say that I am impressed at the growth and maturity that this entire field of research appears to be gathering.

Fish immunology continues to be a field that is wide open to all sorts of new and innovative research opportunities. So much remains to be adapted from mammalian immunological techniques, so much remains to be tested for toxic or beneficial effects on fish, and so much remains to be learned about the similar and unique features of fish as animal models evolved to do their own immune business in the real world. In this regard, I would like to highlight an area of research that sorely needs to be explored in fish immunology.

IMMUNE MODULATION AND BIOLOGICAL RHYTHMS

Several fish immunologists are frustrated with the high variability seen in the individual responses of fish that were given the same treatment(s). Perhaps some of this variability can be accounted for by an experimental variable that, at this time, we are not paying sufficient attention to. Consider the following statements on and examples of how biological rhythms can influence research in mammalian immunology.

"Because the biological system is rhythmically changing, it follows that the organism is biochemically a different entity at different circadian phases." (Scheving, 1976)

"The basic principles of chronobiological experimentation need to be introduced immediately into immunological studies." (Pownall et al., 1978)

"It is no longer sufficient to consider the why and what of treatment; the when to treat, ... is a necessity." (Smolensky, 1981)

"It is now necessary in designing experimental protocols that careful consideration be given to the time of day at which medication is administered ..." (Hrushesky, 1984)

"Basic details such as lighting regimens, length of time the animals were stabilized on the regimen and the timing of procedures such as drug treatment should now become mandatory in all immunological publications. This could improve the reproducibility and decrease the variance of many immunological techniques." (Pownall and Knapp, 1980)

The immune systems of mammals are definitely influenced by their daily (circadian) biological rhythms (Haus et al., 1983). Circadian rhythms are found both in the proliferation and in the functioning of cells important in immune responses (Eskola et al., 1976; Kaplan et al., 1976; Szabo et al., 1978; Vallier and Donner, 1979; Laerum and Aardal, 1981). The light-dark cycle a mammal is exposed to can influence the resultant humoral and cell-mediated immune responses (Hayashi and Kikuchi, 1982). The time of day that an antigen is given to a mammal can significantly influence the magnitude of the resultant immune response (Pownall et al., 1979). The time of day that a foreign tissue is grafted to a host animal can influence its rate of rejection (Ratte et al., 1973). The time that chemotherapy is given during the day can significantly influence the side effects and therapeutic benefit of corticosteroids, anti-cancer drugs, and other medications (Smolensky, 1981; Hrushesky, 1984). The sensitivity of mammals to toxic agents, such as endotoxin, pesticides, etc., can vary with the time of day that the exposure(s) occur (Vea et al., 1977; Fatranska et al., 1978; Natalini, 1979). In addition to the circadian (daily) rhythms evident in mammalian immunology and toxicology, there are also longer term biological rhythms (e.g., weekly, seasonal, etc.) that are also being found to be of significance to these disciplines. (Laerum and Aardal, 1981; Shifrine et al., 1982; Haus et al., 1983).

It is likely that fish display similar circadian and seasonal rhythms in both their immune responses and in their sensitivity to agents (drugs, pesticides, etc.) which subsequently could modulate such fish immune responses. Biological rhythms, especially seasonal ones, have been demonstrated in fish (Schwassmann, 1971; Thorpe, 1978). However, the scientific literature dealing with daily or even seasonal rhythms in fish immunology appears to be quite scant, and there appears to be little literature that reports on rhythmic changes in the sensitivity of fish to drugs, pesticides, or other agents likely to modulate such fish immune responses. I am interested in these subjects, and a review of my files resulted in the following information on fish.

Over the period of a year, Lehmann et al., (1976) extensively recorded the seasonal changes seen in a variety of red and white blood cell parameters found in rainbow trout. Numbers of total leukocytes, as well as numbers of lymphocytes and granulocytes, were found to vary considerably during the year-long sampling period. Matty (1978) briefly reports that there are clear diurnal rhythms in fish plasma corticosteroids and Delahunty et al., (1978) demonstrates that goldfish show daily diurnal patterns in several plasma constituents, including total plasma corticosteroids. [Note that the mammalian literature illustrates that an inverse relationship exists between the serum corticosteroid levels and the numbers of leukocytes found in the circulation (Tavida et al., 1975; Eskola et al., 1976; Kawate et al., 1981)]. As relates to specific seasonal rhythms of interest in fish, White and Fletcher (1985) report some seasonal variations in the relative weights of two important hematopoietic organs (spleen and kidney) in plaice, while Nakanishi (1985) was able to demonstrate seasonal changes in the lymphoid tissues and immune response of a marine teleost. Chambers and Yarbrough (1979) report seasonal differences in the ability of mosquitofish to metabolize insecticides and Koivusaari et al (1981) found a seasonal variation in some xenobiotic metabolizing enzymes in the liver of rainbow trout.

The above information has several obvious implications for the initiation, conduct, and subsequent evaluation of research studies in fish immunology. The several items listed below will have special relevance for the sub-discipline of immune modulation as it attempts to deal with the changes in fish immune responses that are caused by physical agents (such as radiation) and chemical agents (such as drugs and environmental contaminants).

1. Where reasonable and feasible, fish used in immunology (and disease) studies need to be suitably stabilized to and maintained in a defined light:dark cycle.
2. The basic circadian (and seasonal, etc.) rhythms in fish hematology and immunology need to be determined in representative fish species (e.g., patterns of minimum and maximum sensitivity to immunizing agents and/or to immunomodulators, numbers of circulating leukocytes, etc.).
3. Fish immunology researchers using the *in vitro* techniques of cell, tissue, and organ culture need to be aware that biological rhythms are likely to persist in such living experimental materials.
4. In the design of an experiment, where the above *in vivo* and *in vitro* background immunology information is unavailable, then it becomes essential to consider whether or not each specific experimental procedure should be done at the same time every day [in actuality, at the same period(s) during the light and/or dark phase of the photoperiod]. The following experimental procedures would appear to need to be controlled: a) sampling of blood and other immunological tissues, b) immunization and exposure to other antigens, and c) the dosing of fish (or their cells or tissues) to compounds or agents that could modify their immune response.
5. Non-specific items, such as stress, can seriously affect fish immune systems. The time and duration of such occurrences need to be recorded. It is quite possible that the exact same stressor would have a different influence at different times of day.
6. The reporting of the results of experiments in fish immunology will now need to account for the biological rhythms inherent in fish.
7. Reviewers of research articles in fish immunology need to consider the significance of fish circadian and seasonal rhythms in the results being reviewed. Journals publishing fish immunology studies must be encouraged to acknowledge the importance of reporting such factors in the scientific articles that they publish.
8. Agencies, institutions, and companies funding research in fish immunology need to be made aware of the significance of fish biological rhythms and their probable influences on the research that they are supporting.

Whether we like it or not, it appears to be a fact that fish will exhibit dynamic biological rhythms and are in fact continually changing (cycling) right in front of our eyes. As researchers, we need to be aware of this and then be able to 1) determine what rhythms could have consequences for our studies, and/or 2) adjust how we conduct and report our studies in fish immunology.

REFERENCES -

Chambers, J.E. and Yarbrough, J.D. 1979. A seasonal study of microsomal mixed-function oxidase components in insecticide-resistant and susceptible mosquitofish, Gambusia affinis. Toxicol. Appl. Pharmacol. 48:497-507.

Delahunty, G., Olcese, J., Prack, M., Vodicnik, M.J., Schreck, C.B., and de Vlaming, V. 1978. Diurnal variations in the physiology of the goldfish, Carassius auratus. J. Interdiscipl. Cycle Res. 9:73-88.

Eskola, J., Frey, H., Molnar, G., and Sopi, E. 1976. Biological rhythm of cell-mediated immunity in man. Clin. Exp. Immunol. 26:253-257.

Fatranska, M., Vargova, M., Rosival, L., Batora, V., Nemeth, S., and Janekova, D. 1978. Circadian susceptibility rhythms to some organophosphate compounds in the rat. Chronobiologia. 5:39-44.

Haus, E., Lakatua, D.J., Swoyer, J., and Sackett-Lundeen, L. 1983. Chronobiology in hematology and immunology. Amer. J. Anat. 168:467-517.

Hayashi, O. and Kikuchi, M. 1982. The effects of the light-dark cycle on humoral and cell-mediated immune responses in mice. Chronobiologia. 9:291-300.

Hrushesky, W.J.M. 1984. Chemotherapy timing: an important variable in toxicity and response. In: M.C. Perty and J.W. Yarbro (Editors), Toxicity of Chemotherapy. Grune and Stratton, Inc., New York, pp. 449-477.

Kaplan, M.S., Byers, V.S., Levin, A.S., German, D.F., Fudenburg, H.H., and Lecam, L.N. 1976. Circadian rhythm of stimulated lymphocyte blastogenesis. J. Allergy Clin. Immunol. 58:180-189.

Kawate, T., Abo, T., Hinuma, S., and Kumagai, K. 1981. Studies on the bioperiodicity of the immune response. II. Co-variations of murine T and B cells and a role of corticosteroid. J. Immunol. 126:1364-1367.

Koivusaari, V., Harri, M., and Hanninen, O. 1981. Seasonal variation of hepatic biotransformation in female and male rainbow trout (Salmo gairdneri). Comp. Biochem. Physiol. 70C:149-157.

Laerum, O.D. and Aardel, N.P. 1981. Chronobiological aspects of bone marrow and blood cells. In: H.V. Mayersbach, L.E. Scheving, and J.E. Pauly (Editors), Eleventh International Congress of Anatomy: Biological Rhythms in Structure and Function. Alan R. Liss, Inc., New York, pp. 87-97.

Lehmann, J., Sturenburg, F.J., and Hesse,F. 1976. Haematologisch-serologische substratuntersuchungen an der regenbogenforelle (Salmo gairdneri). III. Normwerte des hemogramms unter berucksichtigung alters-und jahreszeitlich bedingter schwankungen. Gewasser Abwasser 59:1-32.

Matty, A.J. 1978. Pineal and some pituitary hormone rhythms in fish. In: J.E. Thorpe (Editor), Rhythmic Activity in Fishes. Academic Press, London, pp. 21-30.

Nakanishi, T. 1986. Seasonal changes in the humoral immune response and the lymphoid tissues of the marine teleost, Sebastiscus marmoratus. Vet. Immunol. Immunopathol. (this issue).

Natalini, J.J. 1979. Circadian rhythms: considerations in the laboratory. Amer. Lab. 11:97-102.

Pownall, R., Cove-Smith, J.R., Kabler, T.A., Kowanko, I., and Knapp, M.S. 1978. Circadian variation in immune response to oxazolone. Nature 275:346.

Pownall, R., Kabler, P.A., and Knapp, M.S. 1979. The time of day of antigen encounter influences the magnitude of the immune response. Clin. Exp. Immunol. 36:347-354.

Pownall, R. and Knapp, M.S. 1980. Immune responses have rhythms: are they important? Immunol. Today 1:vii-x.

Ratte, J., Halberg, F., Kuhl, J.F.W., and Najarian, J.S. 1973. Circadian variation in the rejection of rat kidney allografts. Surgery. 73:102-108.

Schwassmann, H.O. 1971. Biological rhythms. In: W.S. Hoar and D.J. Randall (Editors), Fish Physiology, Volume 6. Academic Press, New York, pp. 371-428.

Scheving, L.E. 1976. The discussion of time in biology and medicine - chronobiology. Endeavour. 35:66-72.

Shifrine, M., Garsd, A., and Rosenblatt, L.S. 1982. Seasonal variation in immunity of humans. J. Interdiscipl. Cycle Res. 13:157-165.

Smolensky, M.H. 1981. Chronotherapeutics: practical applications arising from chronopathology of disease processes and drug chronoavailability and chronotoxicity. In: C.A. Walker, K.F.A. Soliman and C.M. Winget (Editors), Chronopharmacology and Chronotherapeutics. Florida A and M University Foundation, Tallahassee, Florida, pp. 15-30.

Szabo, I., Kovats, T.G., and Halberg, F. 1978. Circadian rhythms in murine reticuloendothelial function. Chronobiologia. 5:137-143.

Tavida, H.B., Fleming, K.A., Hume, P.D., and Simpson, H.W. 1975. Circadian rhythmicity of human plasma cortisol and PHA-induced lymphocyte transformation. Clin. Exp. Immunol. 22:190-193.

Thorp, J.E. (Editor). 1978. Rhythmic Activity of Fishes. Academic Press, London, 312 pp.

Vailler, J. and Donner, M. 1979. Oscillatory nature of DNA, RNA, protein and lipid metabolisms in antigen-stimulated lymphocytes. Chronobiologia. 6:9-17.

Vea, E.V., Cutkomp, L.K., and Halberg, F. 1977. Interrelationships of oxygen consumption and insecticide sensitivity. Chronobiologia. 4:313-323.

White, A. and T.C. Fletcher. 1985. Seasonal changes in serum glucose and condition of the plaice, Pleuronectes platessa L. J. Fish Biol. 26:755-764.

Zeeman, M.G. and W.A. Brindley. 1981. Effects of toxic agents upon fish immune systems, In: R.P. Sharma (Editor), Immunologic Considerations in Toxicology, Volume II. CRC Press, Boca Raton, Florida, pp.1-60.

Veterinary Immunology and Immunopathology, 12 (1986) 243—250
Elsevier Science Publishers B.V., Amsterdam — Printed in The Netherlands

EFFECTS OF METALS ON THE CHEMILUMINESCENT RESPONSE OF RAINBOW TROUT (SALMO GAIRDNERI) PHAGOCYTES

M. S. ELSASSER, B. S. ROBERSON and F. M. HETRICK

Microbiology Dept., Univ. of Maryland, College Park, MD 20742. USA

ABSTRACT

Elsasser, M. S., Roberson, B. S., and Hetrick, F. M., 1986. Effects of Metals on the Chemiluminescent Response of Rainbow Trout (*Salmo gairdneri*) Phagocytes. Vet. Immunol. Immunopathol., 12: 243-250.

Quantification of an induced chemiluminescent (CL) response in phagocytes is currently being evaluated as an indicator system for determining those environmental pollutants that may predispose fish to disease. A CL assay was developed using phagocytes from the pronephros of rainbow trout (*Salmo gairdneri*). The CL response of phagocytes to phorbol myristate acetate, a chemical inducer of CL, was shown to be dose-dependent. The response to five species of bacteria was also evaluated. *Staphylococcus aureus* and *Aeromonas hydrophila* produced the most intense CL responses and the longest duration of response (100 min.) *Yersinia ruckeri* induced an immediate strong CL response of short duration (20 min.) whereas *Vibrio anguillarium* and *Aerococcus viridans* failed to stimulate CL under the test conditions employed.

The effect of sub-toxic levels of Cu, Al, and Cd on the CL response of phagocytes to *S. aureus* was examined using phagocytes exposed to the metals immediately before assay or after 1 hr or 24 hr exposure times. Copper caused a significant decrease in CL to the baseline level under all treatment conditions upon stimulation with *S. aureus*. Similar results were obtained with Al except that the decrease in CL, although significant, was not to the baseline level. In contrast, Cd caused a significant increase in CL when added 1 hr prior to or immediately before the assay; but, following a 24 hr exposure, the results were variable, in that either no change or a decrease was observed. The addition of Cu to phagocytes already exhibiting a strong CL response to *S. aureus* caused an immediate decrease in CL to that seen with the negative controls.

INTRODUCTION

Phagocytosis has been established as a major defense mechanism in fish (Finn and Nielson, 1971; Ellis et al., 1976; Rijkers, 1982). Measurement of phagocytosis was greatly facilitated when Allen et al. (1972) demonstrated that cells phagocytizing bacteria exhibit chemiluminescence (CL) in a dose-dependent fashion. The CL assay has since been applied to studies on phagocytic activity of fish cells (Scott and Klesius 1981, Stave et al. 1983, 1984). Although exposure to heavy metals, particularly copper, has been shown to predispose fish to bacterial (Knittel, 1981; Baker et al., 1983), viral (Hetrick et al., 1979), and protozoal (Ewing et al., 1982) infections, the mechanism involved remains unclear. This study was initiated to determine if the phagocytic system might be a point vulnerable to the action of metals. Specifically, we examined the effect of copper (Cu),cadmium (Cd) and aluminum (Al) on the activity of rainbow trout phagocytes *in vitro* as measured by the CL assay.

MATERIALS AND METHODS

Preparation of phagocytes

Adult (1-2 years) rainbow trout (*Salmo gairdneri*) were obtained from the National Fish Health Research Laboratory, Kearneysville, West Virginia. The trout were maintained in a 450 l flow-through tank of carbon-dechlorinated tap water at a temperature of 11-15° C. The trout were fed once daily with Purina trout chow.

The isolation of phagocytes from the pronephros was a modification of the method used by Stave et al. (1983). Briefly, the pronephros was removed from each of 2-3 trout, ground between frosted glass slides in 10 ml of cold oxalate anticoagulant and filtered through glass wool to remove large tissue fragments. The cells were centrifuged at 200x g for 15 min, washed twice in phosphate buffered saline (PBS, pH 7.5) and resuspended in 5 ml of Hanks' balanced salt solution (HBSS) containing 25 mM HEPES buffer, pH 7.5. The phagocytes were counted in a hemacytometer with trypan blue and adjusted to a final concentration of 600,000 cells/ml with HBSS-HEPES. Cells were held at 15° C until used.

Bacteria Employed

Staphylococcus aureus, *Aerococcus viridans*, and *Vibrio anguillarum* strain 43F (Toranzo et al., 1983) were obtained from the departmental culture collection. *Aeromonas hydrophila* and *Yersinia ruckeri* strain 11.47 were kindly supplied by G. L. Bullock, National Fish Health Laboratory, Leetown, West Virginia. The *S. aureus*, *A. hydrophila*, *Y. ruckeri*, and *A. viridans* were grown in Trypticase Soy Broth (TSB, BBL, Cockeysville, Maryland), at 37° C except *A. viridans* which was grown at 23° C. *Vibrio anguillarum* was grown in TSB with 1.5% NaCl at 23° C. Cultures were harvested and washed once with PBS prior to use in the assay. Standard curves relating optical density to colony forming units per ml were used to determine the bacterial concentration in each assay. Washed bacteria were maintained at room temperature and used within 3 hours.

Metals

Stock solutions of $CuCl_2$, $AlCl_3$, and $CdCl_2$ (Sigma) were made in sterile distilled H_2O at metal concentrations of 10 mg/ml. For testing their effects on CL, metals were diluted in PBS to 0.1 the lowest concentration that showed toxicity for a cultured indicator cell line. These levels were 10 ug/ml for Cu and Al, and 1 ug/ml for Cd.

Chemiluminescence Assay

The CL assay used was that described by Stave et al. (1983). Briefly the assay was performed in glass scintillation vials in duplicate and measured using a Beckman LS-3155T scintillation counter in the out-of-coincidence mode. Each vial received 0.5 ml of phagocyte suspension, 0.5 ml of luminol (1.4 ug/ml in PBS, Sigma), and 0.5 ml stimulus or PBS. The stimuli employed were either bacterial suspensions or phorbol myristate acetate (PMA, Sigma) in PBS. The baseline response was defined as the intensity of CL obtained in the absence of any stimulus. The assay was performed at 25° C. Data were stored and analyzed on a IBM 4341 computer and significance determined by the Waller-Duncan K-Ratio T test (Sokol and Rohlf, 1973). Results were considered to be significant at P 0.01.

RESULTS

CL Response To PMA

The CL responses of rainbow trout phagocytes to 3 concentrations of PMA are shown in Fig. 1. The response was dose-related with the highest CL values being obtained with 40 ng/ml, a lesser but significant response to 20 ng/ ml, whereas 10 ng/ml PMA failed to elicit a response above PBS control levels.

CL Response To Bacteria

The ability of 5 species of bacteria to elicit a significant CL response from trout phagocytes was examined (data not shown). Significant responses were obtained only with *S. aureus* and *A. hydrophila*, the responses being essentially equal. *Yersinia ruckeri* produced a marked increase in CL activity but it was of short duration lasting only 20 min. The responses to *A. viridans* and *V. anguillarum* were not significantly different from the baseline responses obtained with cells in the absence of any CL stimulus. *S. aureus* was chosen as the test stimulus organism for the remainder of the study because of the intensity, duration and reproducibility of the CL response that it evoked.

Effects Of Metals On the CL Response

The effect of adding metal ions to the phagocytic cells immediately prior to the assay is shown in Fig. 2. Upon addition of bacteria, Cd-treated cells gave a significantly greater CL response than the positive control (*S. aureus* alone), whereas Al and Cu significantly decreased CL activity. Cu was the more active of the two metals, depressing the CL response to levels of the

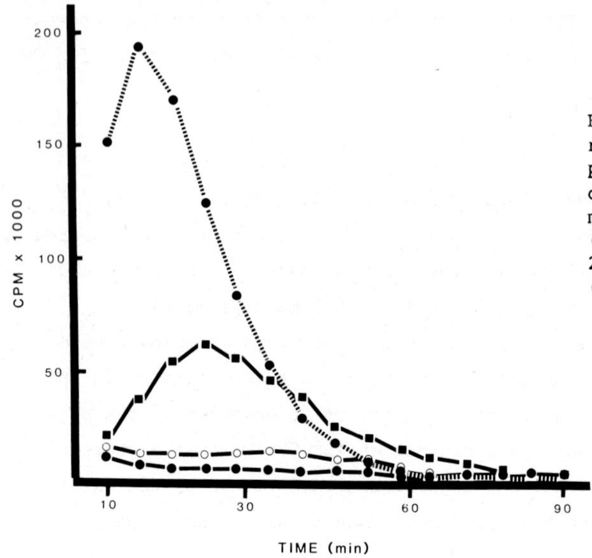

Fig. 1. chemiluminescent response of rainbow trout phagocytes to different concentrations of phorbol myristate acetate (PMA): (●), 40 ng/ml; (■), 20 ng/ml; (○), 10 ng/ml; (●), PBS

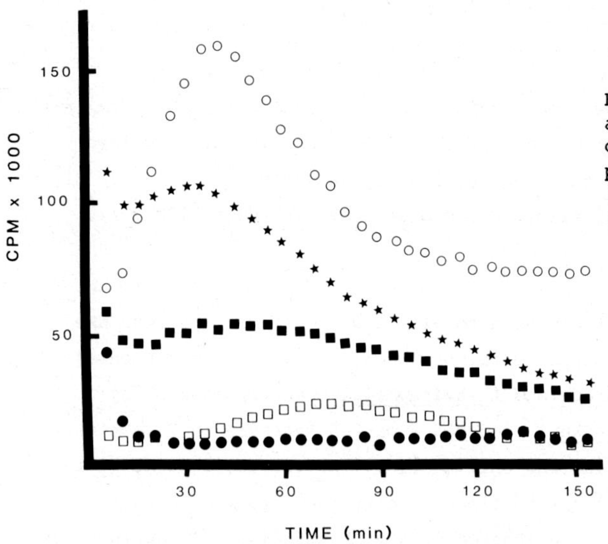

Fig. 2. Effect of Cd, Al, and Cu on the chemiluminescent response of trout phagocytes to S. aureus, (○), Cd; (■), Al; (□), Cu; (★), S. aureus; (●), PBS.

negative controls. Aluminum at the same concentration as Cu gave significant but incomplete suppression of response. Incubation of phagocytic cells with metal ions for one hour prior to the assay gave very similar CL response patterns (Fig. 3). While viability still seemed not to be affected, incubation of the cells with metals for 24 hours prior to the assay gave similar results with Al and Cu, both giving suppressive effects on the CL response, with Cu again being the more effective ion (Fig.4). However, the results with Cd were different from that obtained with the shorter exposure times. Instead of

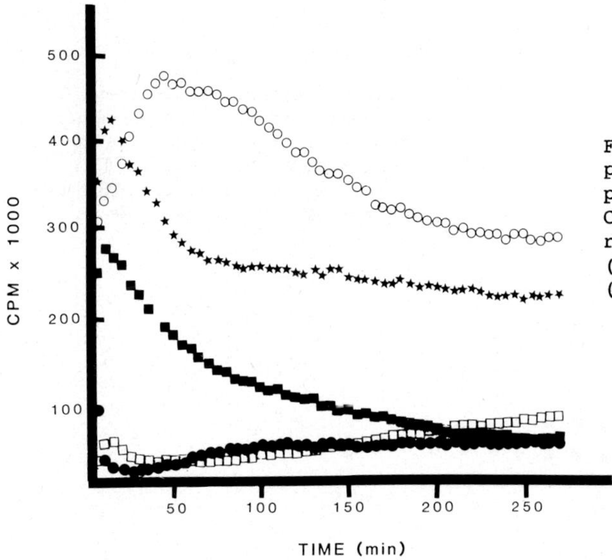

Fig. 3. Effect of 1 hr pretreatment of trout phagocytes with Cd, Al, and Cu on the chemiluminescent response to S. aureus. (○), Cd; (■), Al; (□), Cu; (★), S. aureus; (●), PBS.

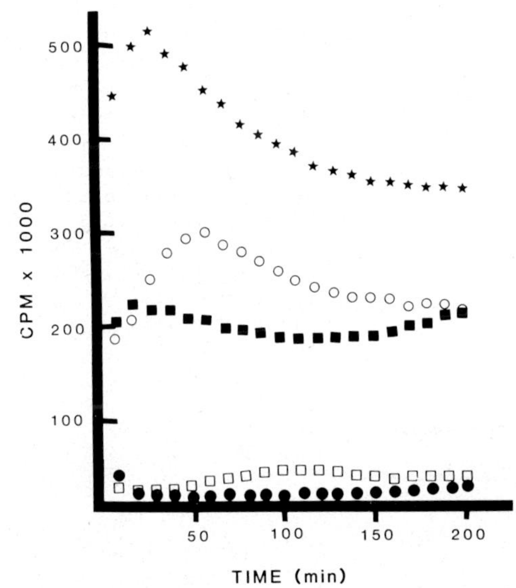

Fig. 4. Effect of a 24 hour pretreatment of trout phagocytes with Cd, Al, and Cu on the chemiluminescent response to S. aureus. (○), Cd; (■), Al; (□), Cu; (★), S. aureus; (●), PBS.

being stimulatory, this exposure suppressed the CL response to levels that were not significantly different from that seen with Al.

Because Cu was the most effective metal in depressing the CL response, its effect was further tested by incubating the cells with different Cu concentrations for one hour prior to the assay (Fig. 5). Clearly, the responses noted were dose-related. Concentrations of 10 and 1 ug/ml depressed the Cl response to that of the negative controls. A concentration of 0.1 ug/ml caused a reduction in response when compared to the S. aureus control, but the response to 0.01 ug/ml was not different from the control. In another experiment, phagocytes were allowed to initiate a response to S. aureus before Cd or Cu was added (Fig. 6). The addition of Cu caused an

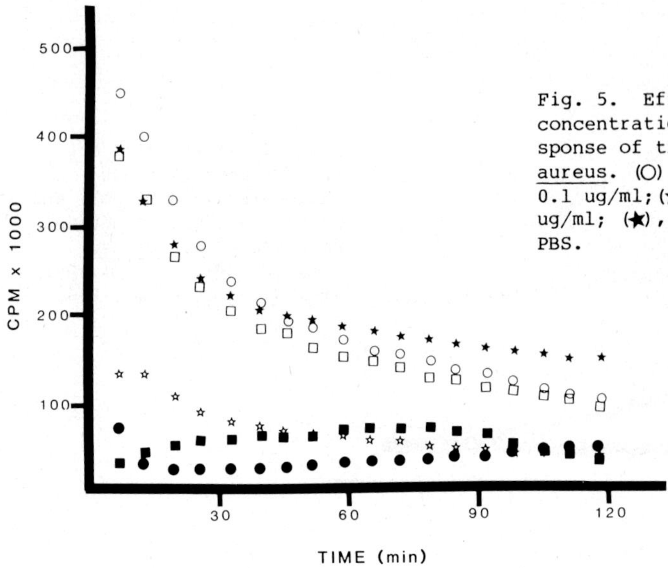

Fig. 5. Effect of different Cu concentrations on the CL response of trout phagocytes to *S. aureus*. (○), 0.01 ug/ml; (□), 0.1 ug/ml; (☆), 1 ug/ml; (■), 10 ug/ml; (★), *S. aureus*; (●), PBS.

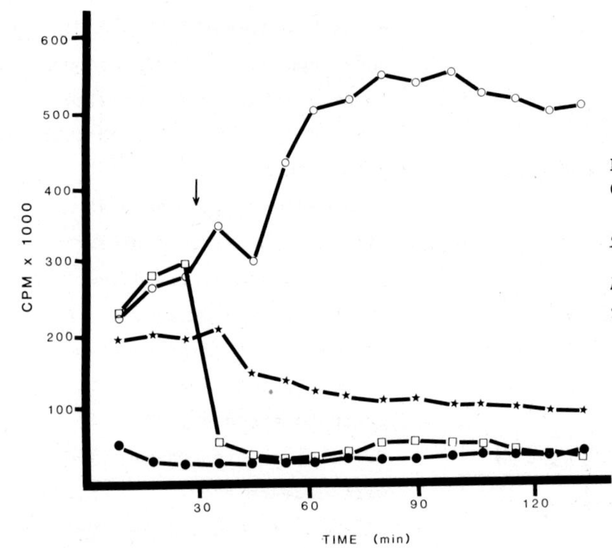

Fig. 6. Effect of adding Cu and Cd to cells eliciting a Cl response to *S. aureus*; (○), Cd; (□), Cu; (★), *S. aureus*; (●), PBS. Arrow denotes time of addition of metal.

immediate decrease in CL to that seen with the negative controls, whereas the addition of Cd again appeared stimulatory as the intensity of CL gradually increased over a 60 min period.

DISCUSSION

The CL response of rainbow trout phagocytes to PMA and bacterial stimuli was found in this study to be comparable to that exhibited by striped bass

(Stave et al., 1983), and is most clearly shown by the dose dependent response to PMA. From our past results, the varied response of phagocytic cells to different bacterial genera was not unexpected. No special significance can be drawn from these results, however, as only a limited range of bacterial concentrations were used for each trial. The strong and reproducible response to *S. aureus* makes a suspension of this organism a good alternative to PMA as a standard stimulus.

Copper exposure has been found to predispose fish to infection upon challenge with viral (Hetrick et al., 1979) or bacterial pathogens (Knittel, 1981). The suppression of CL, which we found associated with Cu exposure, could result in a loss in the ability of phagocytic cells to clear pathogens and may account for this increased susceptibility. Although the effects of Cu have been shown to be complex (Roales and Pearlmutter, 1977; Olson and Christensen, 1980) the reduced phagocytic ability appears to be an important summary effect. Schreck and Lorz (1978) showed that Cu exposure of coho salmon juveniles markedly increases their serum cortisol levels. We have found that administration of hydrocortisol by injection to striped bass similarly suppresses CL responses (Stave and Roberson, 1985). Taken together, it appears that the action of copper is similar to that of other "model" stressants (Wedemeyer, 1974). Fish may adapt to low levels of Cu (Hetrick, 1979; Knittel, 1981) suggesting that the effects are influenced by endocrine fluctuation, acute phase inflammatory substances, or other regulatory substances. Such an interpretation may be incomplete, however, in that Cu also seems to exert a direct suppressive effect on phagocytic cells, suggested by the cessation of CL upon addition of Cu to the stimulated cells.

The contrasting CL responses accompanying exposure to Cd and Cu gives us an opportunity to test the validity of the CL model for predicting increased susceptibility to infection after an *in vivo* exposure or challenge. If Cu increases susceptibility to infection, then Cd for the ranges of doses and exposure and times in which CL is actually increased above the control response, could decrease susceptibility to infection. For longer exposure times to Cd for which CL is suppressed, susceptibility would increase if there is correlation between the CL response and infection of fish ambiently exposed to the metal.

Acknowledgment--This work was supported by EPA Grant No. R811278-01-0.

REFERENCES

Allen, R. C., Sternholm, R. L., and Steele, R. H., 1972. Evidence for generation of an electronic excitation state(s) in human polymorphonuclear leukocytes and its participation in bactericidal activity. Biochem. Biophys. Res. Comm., 47: 679-684.

Baker, R. J., Knittel, M. D., and Fryer, J. L., 1983. Susceptibility of chinook salmon and rainbow trout to infection with *Vibrio anguillarum* following sublethal copper exposure. J. Fish Dis., 6: 267-275.

Ellis, A. E., Munro, A. L. S., and Roberts, R. J., 1976. Defense mechanisms in fish. I. A study of the phagocytic system and the fate of intraperi toneally injected particulate material in the plaice (*Pleuronectes platessa* L.). J. Fish Biol., 8: 67-78.

Ewing, M. S., Ewing, S. A., and Zimmer, M. A., 1982. Sublethal copper stress and susceptibility of Channel catfish to experimental infections with *Icthyophthirius multifiliis.* Bull. Environ. Contam. Toxicol., 28: 674-681.

Finn, J. P., and Nielson, N. O., 1971. The inflammatory response of rainbow trout. J. Fish Biol., 3: 463-478.

Hetrick, F. M., Knittel, M. D., and Fryer, J. L., 1979. Increased suscepti bility of rainbow trout to infectious hematopoietic necrosis virus after exposure to copper. Appl. Environ. Microbiol., 37: 198-201.

Knittel, M. D., 1981. Susceptibility of steelhead trout *Salmo gairdneri* Richardson to redmouth infection *Yersinia ruckeri* following exposure to copper. J. Fish Dis., 4: 33-40.

Olson, D. L., and Christensen, G. M., 1980. Effects of water pollutants and other chemicals on fish acetylcholinesterase (*in vitro*). Environ. Res., 21: 327-335.

Rijkers, G. T., 1982. Non-lymphoid defense mechanisms in fish. Dev. Comp. Immunol., 6: 1-13.

Roales, R. R., and Perlmutter, A., 1977. The effects of sublethal doses of methylmercury and copper, applied singly and jointly, on the immune response of the blue gourami to viral and bacterial antigens. Arch. Environ. Contam. Toxicol., 5: 325-331.

Schreck, C. B., and Lorz, H. W., 1978. Stress response of coho salmon (*Oncorhynchus kisutch*) elicited by cadmium and copper and potential use of cortisol as an indicator of stress. J. Fish Res. Bd. Can., 35: 1124-1129.

Scott, A. L., and Klesius, P. H., 1981. Chemiluminescence: A novel analysis of phagocytosis in fish. Develop. Biol.Stand., 49: 243-256.

Sokol, R. R., and Rohlf, F. J., 1973. *Introduction to Biostatistics*. W. H. Freeman and Co., San Francisco.

Stave, J. W., Roberson, B. S., and Hetrick, F. M., 1983. Chemiluminescence of phagocytic cells isolated from the pronephros of striped bass. Dev. Comp. Immunol., 7: 269-276.

Stave, J. W., Roberson, B. S., and Hetrick, F. M., 1984. Factors affecting the chemiluminescent response of fish phagocytes. J. Fish Biol., 25: 197-206.

Stave, J. W., and Roberson, B. S., 1985. Hydrocortisone suppresses the chemiluminescent response of striped bass phagocytes. Dev. Comp. Immunol., 9: 77-84.

Toranzo, A. E., Barja, J. L., Potter, S. A., Colwell, R. R., Hetrick, F. M., and Crosa, J. H., 1983. Molecular factors associated with the virulence of marine vibrios isolated from striped bass in the Chesapeake Bay. Infect. Immun., 39: 1220-1227.

Wedemeyer, G. A., and Wood, J. W., 1974. Stress as a predisposing factor in fish diseases. U. S. Dept. of Interior Publ., FDL-38, USFWS.

Veterinary Immunology and Immunopathology, 12 (1986) 251–262
Elsevier Science Publishers B.V., Amsterdam — Printed in The Netherlands

PARADOXICAL EFFECTS OF CADMIUM EXPOSURE ON ANTIBACTERIAL ANTIBODY RESPONSES IN TWO FISH SPECIES: INHIBITION IN CUNNERS (*TAUTOGOLABRUS ADSPERSUS*) AND ENHANCEMENT IN STRIPED BASS (*MORONE SAXATILIS*)

RICHARD A. ROBOHM

Experimental Biology Branch, Northeast Fisheries Center, NMFS, NOAA, Milford, CT, 06460, USA

ABSTRACT

Robohm, R.A., 1986. Paradoxical effects of cadmium exposure on antibacterial antibody responses in two fish species: inhibition in cunners (*Tautogolabrus adspersus*) and enhancement in striped bass (*Morone saxatilis*). Vet. Immunol. Immunopathol., 12: 251-262.

Previous work in a marine fish, the cunner (*Tautogolabrus adspersus*), showed that endocytosis of bacteria by cells in the liver and spleen was affected by 96-h exposure of the fish to cadmium at a concentration of 12 μg/mℓ; however, antibody response to sheep erythrocytes was not affected. Since the latter finding was questionable because of short immunization times, and data from more than a single fish species were desirable, both the cunner and an anadromous fish, the striped bass (*Morone saxatilis*), were examined for antibody responses against the bacterium *Bacillus cereus* in Freund's complete adjuvant during a 6- to 8-wk time period. Exposure to 12 μg/mℓ cadmium caused significant inhibition of serum antibody titers ($P<0.007$) in cunners. Paradoxically, antibody response in striped bass exposed to 10 μg/ mℓ cadmium was enhanced sixfold. This enhancement was weaker but still evident when the antigen was injected 48 d after cadmium exposure. Peritoneal exudate cells from cadmium-exposed striped bass also showed more active migration through microporous filters than cells from non-exposed fish. Since the 96-h cadmium LC_{50} was 26 μg/mℓ for cunners and 20 μg/mℓ for striped bass, the differences in antibody response could not be explained on the basis of differences in cadmium toxicity. Although geometric mean liver cadmium levels after exposure at 15°C were higher in cunners (163.8 ± 1.2 μg/gm) than in striped bass (64.4 ± 1.2 μg/g), cunners exposed to cadmium at 2°C had lower cadmium levels (46.4 ± 1.2 μg/g) which were still effective in inhibiting antibody production at 8°C. On the other hand, striped bass not exposed to cadmium showed a strong, exponential rise in serum antibody when the temperature at immunization, 14°C, was reduced to 9°C; whereas cunners held in the same tanks exhibited a weaker, biphasic serum antibody response. Regardless of the cause (innate differences in cellular response, or better stress adaptability in an anadromous fish), the data show that chemical-stress effects on the immune system of one fish species cannot be extrapolated to another species.

0165-2427/86/$03.50 © 1986 Elsevier Science Publishers B.V.

INTRODUCTION

In recent years the effects of the heavy metal cadmium (Cd^{2+}) on physiological processes in mammals have become the subject of numerous studies. Cd^{2+} is known to (1) either activate or inhibit a large number of enzyme systems, (2) bind to both human and bovine albumin and mercaptalbumin where it competes with zinc for the same sulfhydryl or imidazole groups, (3) inhibit mitochondrial respiration in pulmonary alveolar macrophages, and (4) markedly affect the conformation of polyriboadenylic acid and the physical properties of DNA (reviewed by Vallee and Ulmer, 1972). Cd^{2+} also stimulates or inhibits enzyme systems in killifish (Jackim *et al.*, 1970), cunners (MacInnes *et al.*, 1977), striped bass (Dawson *et al.*, 1977), and winter flounder (Gould, 1977). Because of these multiple physiological effects it was suspected that Cd^{2+} would interfere with immune responses in fish. Robohm and Nitkowski (1974) examined two elements of the immune system of a marine fish, the cunner (*Tautogolabrus adspersus*), after 96-h exposure to 12 μg Cd^{2+}/mℓ. Processing of intracardially injected bacteria was significantly affected by pre-exposure to Cd^{2+}; bacteria were sequestered more rapidly but killed more slowly within the liver and spleen. On the other hand, antibody production against intraperitoneally-injected sheep erythrocytes appeared to be unaffected. Since the latter finding was questionable because of short immunization times and data from more than a single fish species were desirable, both the cunner and an anadromous fish, the striped bass (*Morone saxatilis*), were examined for antibody responses against the bacterium *Bacillus cereus* during a 6- to 8-wk time period.

This report will show that pre-exposure to Cd^{2+} inhibits serum antibody in cunners, but enhances antibody production in striped bass.

METHODS

Collection and maintenance of fish

Striped bass were received from the Edenton National Fish Hatchery, U.S. Department of the Interior, Fish and Wildlife Service, Edenton, NC, at 8 months of age, maintained in aerated flowing seawater (24 ± 2°/oo salinity), and used in this study at 1-2 years of age (18-75 g). They were fed daily (three times weekly at temperatures below 10°C) with a varied diet (depending upon availability) of chopped clams, grass-shrimp, or gelatin cubes containing freeze-dried zooplankton and minced, pasteurized fish. This was supplemented with Purina trout chow.

Cunners captured in baited traps in a local marine estuary were maintained in flowing seawater for 4 months and fed on a regimen like that of the striped bass. Fish of 12-18 cm length (29-134 g), 2-3 years of age based on length criteria (Chao, 1973), were used in this study.

Cadmium exposure

The seawater temperature in a 500 ℓ fiberglass tank containing striped bass or cunners was raised from 5°C to 14°C during a 3-d period by passing seawater through a series of glass condensers warmed with well-water at a constant 15°C temperature. Fish were held at 14°C for 60 d prior to cadmium exposure. Glass tanks were filled with 60 ℓ of seawater which had been passed through a nylon filter of 10 µ pore size and aerated for 24 h while the temperature equilibrated with ambient at 16-17°C. $CdCl_2 \cdot 2^1/_2H_2O$ (ACS grade analytical reagent) was dissolved in filtered seawater and added to half the tanks for a final Cd^{2+} concentration of 12 µg/mℓ for cunners and 10 µg/mℓ for striped bass. All fish survived this exposure level. Four cunners or six to eight striped bass in each static, aerated tank were exposed either to no Cd^{2+} or the stated cadmium concentration for 96 h with half the tank water replaced midway (48 h) through the exposure period. Fish were returned to the 14°C seawater tank for 1 d prior to antigen injection.

For a portion of the cunner study, filtered, aerated seawater was added to 60 ℓ glass aquaria in a walk-in refrigerator and allowed to equilibrate at 2°C. Cd^{2+} at 12 µg/mℓ final concentration was introduced into half the tanks and fish exposed for 96 h as before. These fish were returned to 5°C seawater for 1 d prior to immunization.

Fish immunization and antibody assay

Bacillus cereus was grown for 18-22 h at 26°C in trypticase soy broth, (TSB) treated with 0.3% (final concentration) formalin for 24 h, washed 2X in 0.85% NaCl, and re-suspended to 0.5 to 1.0 x 10^9 cells/mℓ. The cell suspension was emulsified in an equal portion of Freund's complete adjuvant, and 0.1 mℓ injected i.p. into each fish. Striped bass received about 0.5 x 10^8 cells and cunners about 1.0 x 10^8 cells one day after termination of Cd^{2+} exposure. However, half the striped bass were not immunized until 43 d after termination of Cd^{2+} exposure. Blood was drawn into a Pasteur pipette after severing the spinal column and dorsal aorta behind the gills. Antibody levels were determined by bacterial agglutination assays in microtiter plates containing serial twofold dilutions of fish serum in buffered saline, pH 7.3 (Robohm *et al.*, 1979).

Migration of striped bass peritoneal exudate cells (PEC)

The ability of PEC to migrate through microporous filters toward a chemotactic or chemokinetic stimulus was assayed in blind-well chambers. The culture medium used in the chambers consisted of the following in distilled-deionized water: 9.0% Gibco 10X basal medium Eagle (with Earl's base, with L-glutamine, and without sodium carbonate), 8.6 mM additional NaCl, 7.3 mM $NaHCO_3$, 10% heat-inactivated fetal calf serum, 20 units/mℓ heparin, and buffered at pH 7.35 with 11.1 mM tris-(hydroxymethyl)-aminomethane, hydrochloride. This medium (final osmolality 306) will be referred to, for convenience, as BMEF (basal medium Eagle with fetal calf serum).

Prior to sacrifice each fish was injected i.p. with 0.5 mℓ of BMEF. After 60-70 min, blood was taken and the peritoneal cavity opened by incision. The peritoneum was rinsed with 0.5 mℓ BMEF and the fluid placed in a 1.5 mℓ polyethylene centrifuge tube. PEC were centrifuged at 300 X G for 5 min, washed once with BMEF, reconstituted to volume in BMEF, counted in a hemocytometer, and diluted to 1 x 10^6 PEC/mℓ in BMEF (6 wk after Cd^{2+} exposure fewer PEC were present and it was necessary to use cell suspensions at 1 x 10^5/mℓ). A migration stimulus consisting of *B. cereus*, which had been grown in TSB 24 h at 26°C, refrigerated for 1 to 10 d, and washed 2X in Hanks balanced salt solution was resuspended in BMEF at 2.7 x 10^8/mℓ. Blind-well chambers were assembled according to an established procedure (Altman *et al.*, 1975) with 0.2 mℓ of *B. cereus* suspension (5 x 10^7 bacteria) in the lower chamber and 0.1 mℓ of PEC (1 x 10^5 or later 1 x 10^4 cells) in the upper chamber. The chambers were separated by a 10 mm d polycarbonate filter with 5.0 μ pores. Two chambers with migration stimulus and one without (random migration control) were used for each fish. The top of each chamber was covered with tape perforated with 4 holes from a 25-gauge needle. Chambers were incubated for 90 min at 22°C in a humid atmosphere and filters removed, dried and stained according to an established procedure (Altman *et al.*, 1975).

The migrated cells on the bottom side of each filter were counted by oil immersion microscopy. All the cells within a row of microscopic fields across each membrane were counted and multiplied by a factor to give the total number of migrated cells. Percent cell migration for each group of 3 fish (2 replicates each) was calculated as geometric mean no. migrated cells/total cells in upper chamber x 100.

RESULTS

Effects of cadmium on antibody response

When cunners were acclimated and exposed to 12 µg/mℓ Cd^{2+} at two temperatures, then immunized with *B. cereus*, the resulting serum antibody responses were depressed at both high and low holding temperatures (Fig. 1). The temperatures in Figure 1 are the result of a 3°C rise in temperature of the incoming water (from 5°C to 8°C). This also caused the condenser-heated water to rise from 14°C to 15°C. At 15°C the inhibition by Cd^{2+} was evident both 4 wk and 6 wk after immunization. At 8°C titers were not only reduced because of the reduced temperature, but there was also an inhibition seen in the Cd^{2+}-treated fish at the 4-wk time period. Variation among fish did not allow a reliable statistical evaluation of this experiment; therefore, additional fish were exposed to Cd^{2+}, injected with antigen, held at 16°C, and analyzed for serum antibody at 5 wk post-immunization. Figure 2 shows that antibody response in cunners was significantly inhibited by Cd^{2+} exposure ($P<0.007$, two-tailed Student's t distribution).

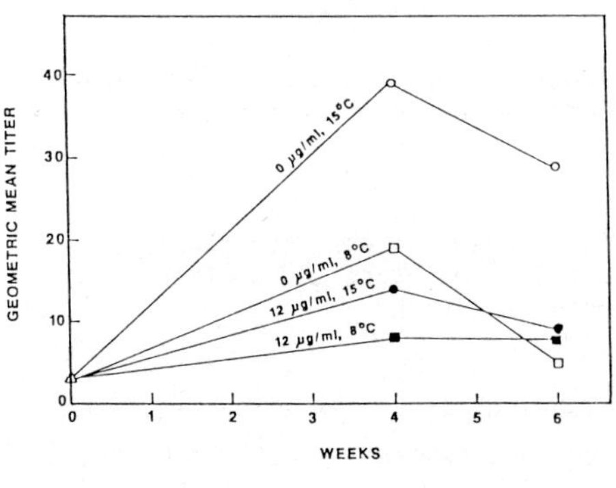

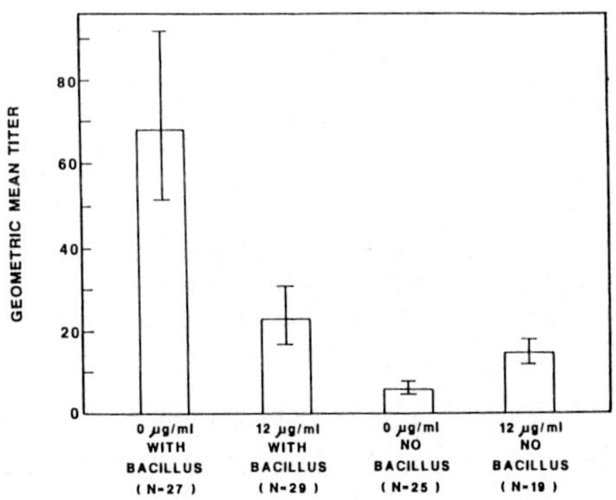

Fig 1. Interactive effects of temperature and 96-h Cd^{2+} exposure on inhibition of antibody to *B. cereus* in cunners. 0 point represents 10 fish; other points, 5 or 6 fish.

Fig. 2. Corroboration of of antibody inhibition caused by 96-h exposure of cunners to 12 µg/mℓ Cd^{2+}. Histogram shows agglutinin titers after 5 wk in flowing seawater at 16°C. Brackets show 95% confidence intervals.

Striped bass were exposed to 10 μg/mℓ Cd^{2+} and split into two groups. The first group was injected with B. cereus 5 d after starting Cd^{2+} exposure (1 d after Cd^{2+} termination) and serum antibody response followed for 56 d while the holding temperature increased from 14°C to 16.5°C (Fig. 3). The second group was injected with antigen 48 d after starting Cd^{2+} exposure (43 d after Cd^{2+} termination) and followed for an additional 56 d while water temperature increased from 16.5°C to 24°C (Fig. 4). Figure 3 shows a sixfold enhancement of antibody response by day 56 in Cd^{2+}-exposed fish. This enhancement was weaker, but still evident when the bacterial antigen was injected 43 d after termination of Cd^{2+} exposure (Fig. 4).

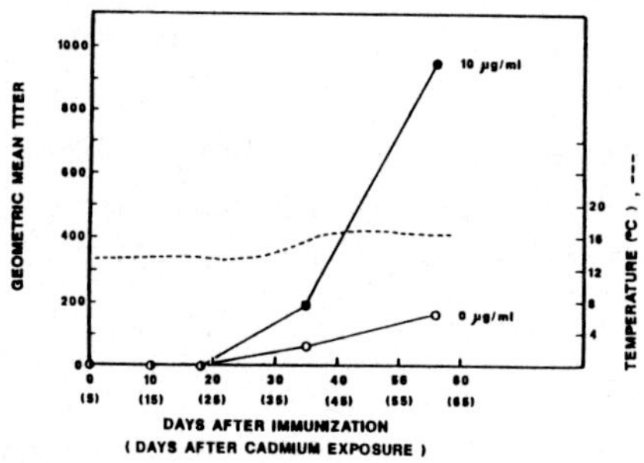

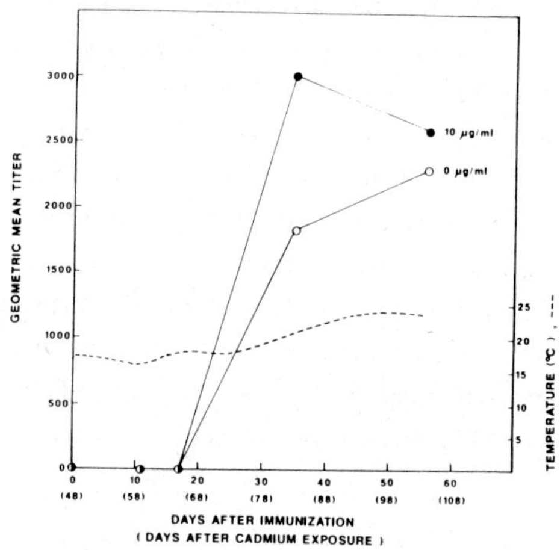

Fig. 3. Enhancement of serum antibody response when striped bass were immunized with B. cereus five d after start of Cd^{2+} exposure (one d after termination of exposure). Each point represents 3 fish.

Fig. 4. Minimal enhancement of serum antibody response when striped bass were immunized with B. cereus 48 d after start of Cd^{2+} exposure (43 d after termination of exposure). Each point represents 3 fish.

Figure 5 is a comparison of the two fish species at the same time intervals, 28 d and 42 d, post immunization. When not exposed to Cd^{2+} both striped bass and cunners had about the same serum antibody levels at the 28 d point (reciprocal geometric mean titers of 40 and 39, respectively). On the other hand, after Cd^{2+} exposure the antibody level was markedly enhanced in striped bass (titer of 120) and depressed in cunners (titer of 14). By 42 d these differences were even more dramatic; however, antibody response in the non-exposed striped bass was also stronger and still in the process of rising while that in the cunners was beginning to fall. It is apparent striped bass were better responders than cunners to this antigen.

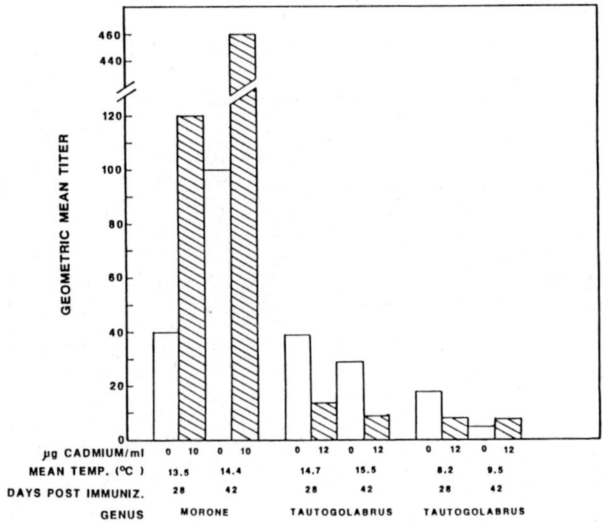

Fig. 5. Comparison of the effects of Cd^{2+} on antibody responses in cunners and striped bass. Serum antibody levels examined at comparable time periods.

Effect of cadmium exposure on migration of PEC

An analysis of the migration of striped bass PEC through polycarbonate filters is given in Figure 6. These PEC were obtained from the same fish that were immunized with B. cereus. Figure 6 shows that PEC from Cd^{2+}-exposed fish in Group 1 had a strong increase in migration beginning at 40 d after exposure (35 d after immunization). PEC activity was nearly as strong in Group 2 at 70 d after exposure (17 d after immunization). Fish with no Cd^{2+} exposure had only a weak response by 56 d in Group 1, while those in Group 2 started with a weak response at 70 d which then rapidly peaked a 83 d (35 d after immunization) and declined to background level at 104 d. The most logical interpretation of Figure 6 is that striped bass PEC were primed for increased activity toward a chemotactic stimulus by pre-exposure to Cd^{2+}. A bacterial infection, which killed a number of striped bass in a neighboring tank and one fish in the experimental tank, prompted treatment of water in the experimental tank with 50 µg/gal of oxytetracycline during 5 d of the experimental period (bracketed lines in Fig. 6). While the infection eventually stimulated a strong increase in migrating PEC in the control fish, the response was late and short-lived. On the other hand, the response in Cd^{2+}-treated fish occurred sooner and was more prolonged. The response appeared to be unconnected with immunization by B. cereus because it began in the Cd^{2+}-exposed fish of Group 1 at day 35 after antigenic stimulation, but was already high in Group 2 at day 17 after antigenic stimulation.

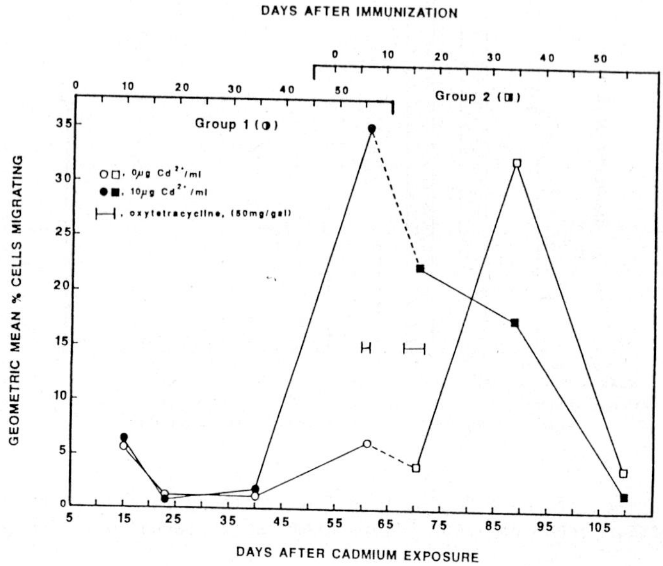

Fig. 6. Increased migration of striped bass PEC after 96-h Cd^{2+} exposure. Each point represents duplicate migration assays from 2 or 3 fish.

Other comparisons

Additional evidence along two lines was sought to explain the apparent differences in antibody response caused by Cd^{2+} exposure in the two fish species: (1) possible species differences in the concentration point at which Cd^{2+} becomes a physiological toxicant (and the related body burden in each species), and (2) possible species differences in cellular interactions which could influence antibody synthesis. The 96-h Cd^{2+} concentration at which 50% of the fish were killed (LC_{50}) was compared for the two species using the Reed-Muench (1938) method for calculating endpoints. Serial twofold reductions in Cd^{2+} concentration were tested for each fish species - 19 fish per concentration for cunner endpoints and 8 fish per concentration for striped bass endpoints. The LC_{50} values for cunners and striped bass were 25.9 µg/mℓ and 19.9 µg/mℓ, respectively. Since each species was exposed to Cd^{2+} at about one-half its LC_{50} value (12 µg/mℓ for cunners and 10 µg/mℓ for striped bass), the differences in antibody response after Cd^{2+} exposure cannot be due to relative sensitivity to metabolic poisoning by Cd^{2+}.

TABLE 1

Liver cadmium levels in striped bass and cunners after 96-h cadmium exposure.

Conditions during exposure		Geometric mean liver cadmium levels ($\mu g/g \pm$ S.E.M.) calculated on a wet (W) or dry (D) basis		
		Cunners		Striped bass
$\mu g\ Cd^{2+}/m\ell$	°C	W	D	D
10	16	-[a]	-	64.4 ± 1.2 (2)[b]
12	16	47.7 ± 1.5 (5)	163.8 ± 1.4 (5)	-
12	2	14.0 ± 1.2 (5)	46.4 ± 1.2 (5)	-
0	16	< 1.3 ± 1.3 (9)	< 4.0 ± 1.3 (9)	< 0.2 ± 0.0 (3)
0	2	< 1.7 ± 1.4 (5)	< 5.4 ± 1.3 (5)	-

[a] -, not done
[b] (n), number of livers analyzed

Table 1 shows that Cd^{2+} levels in the liver of cunners exposed at 16°C were higher (geometric mean of 163.8 µg/g dry wt) than those of striped bass (geometric mean of 64.4 µg/g dry wt). However, the table also shows that the uptake in cunners exposed to Cd^{2+} at 2°C was lower (geometric mean of 46.4 µg/g dry wt) than that observed in striped bass. Since cunners with these lower levels exhibited inhibition of serum antibody production at 8°C like cunners at 15°C (see Fig. 1), Cd^{2+} body burden could not be the cause for the observed differences in antibody response between cunners and striped bass.

Evidence along the second line consists of a single experiment in which cunners and striped bass were held in the same tank at 14°C for 30 d then injected i.p. with bacteria in Freund's complete adjuvant and observed for antibody responses for an additional 60 d during which the ambient water temperature declined to 9°C. Figure 7 shows that striped bass injected with *Aeromonas salmonicida* had a steady, nearly exponential increase in serum antibody levels which peaked at 40 d. The bar shows the antibody level achieved at 30 d in a separate study when fish were injected with *A. salmonicida* and held at 9°C ± 1°C. The response pattern in cunners injected with *B. cereus* was quite different; figure 8 shows that it was biphasic. After an initial increase at the warmest temperature, it peaked at 20 d and began to decline roughly in parallel with the declining temperature. After the temperature reached 9°C, the antibody level increased again with a second peak at 40 d. The experiment showed that a cell (or cells) involved in antibody production responds differently to temperature perturbation in the two species.

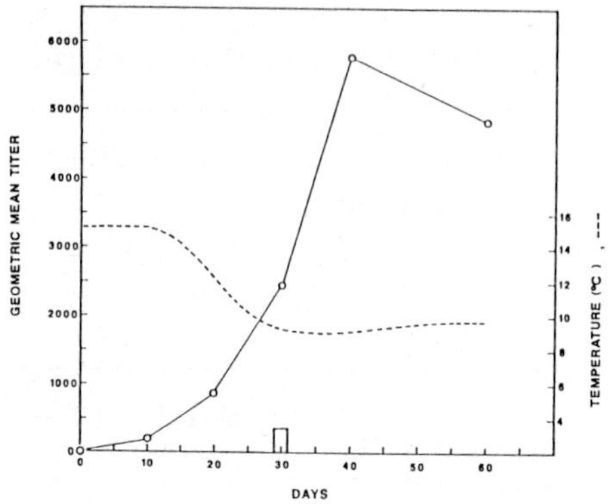

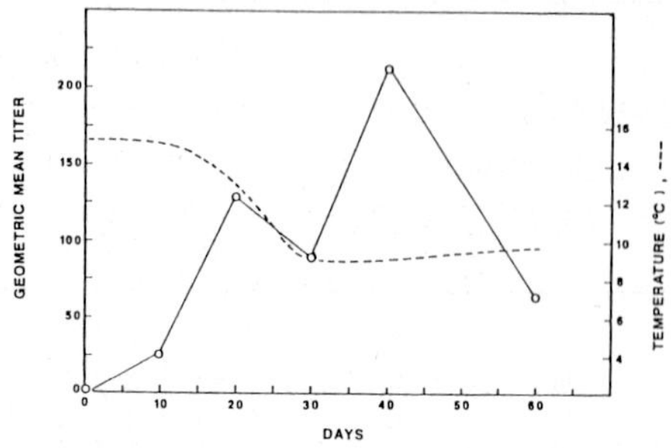

Fig. 7. Increase in serum antibody response in striped bass when the temperature declined from 14° to 9°C. Fish were immunized with *A. salmonicida* in Freund's complete adjuvant. Each point represents 4 fish. Bar represents values from a separate experiment (N=19) in which temperature remained at 9 ± 1°C throughout.

Fig. 8. Biphasic serum antibody response in cunners when the temperature declined from 14°C to 9°C. Fish were immunized with *B. cereus* in Freund's complete adjuvant. Each point represents 4 fish.

DISCUSSION

The reduced antibody response in Cd^{2+}-exposed cunners was consistent with studies showing that this heavy metal interferes with multiple biochemical reactions in living organisms. Therefore, it was surprising that similar Cd^{2+} exposure enhanced the antibody response in striped bass. This difference could not be explained as a difference in susceptibility to Cd^{2+} toxicity since each species was exposed to about half its LC_{50} dose, nor to relative Cd^{2+} retention since cunners at 2°C retained less Cd^{2+} than striped bass but still had reduced antibody levels. However, antibody production in striped bass appeared to be less affected by temperature reduction (Fig. 7) than that in cunners (Fig. 8). Cuchens and Clem (1977) and Avtalion (1981) have shown that T-helper cell function in fish is temperature-dependent. While the evidence in the current study is by no means definitive (particularly since different bacterial antigens were used in the two species), it suggests that T-helper cells in striped bass may be less affected by temperature perturbation than T-helper cells in cunners. If the same holds true for the effects of Cd^{2+}, it could explain why antibody production in striped bass is not inhibited. Certainly there is additional support for the idea that Cd^{2+} exposure affects T-helper cells. Koller *et al*. (1975) found T-helper cell involvement in mice exposed to Cd^{2+} in drinking water. Nevertheless, this explanation still fails to account for the marked antibody enchancement seen in striped bass.

This enhancement could be associated with the activation found in one group of immune response system cells, the PEC, of striped bass (Fig. 6). It would have been difficult to obtain similar PEC migration data in cunners without a better understanding of the required physiological conditions. The results in striped bass were apparently achieved because of a serendipitous co-stimulation by a bacterial infection in the fish population.

Antibody enhancement in striped bass could also be associated with innate physiological responses of anadromous fish. After examination of a number of physiological studies in fish, Calabrese *et al*. (1982) concluded that anadromous species, like striped bass and coho salmon, adapt more readily to trace-metal exposure than strictly marine fish, such as cunners and winter flounder. The idea of adaptability may be connected to a more specific control mechanism described by Stebbing (1981a) in his studies of growth in the colonial hydroid, *Campanularia flexuosa*. When the organism is exposed to various inhibitory substances, including heavy metals, the control mechanism initially overcompensates before settling in at approximately the rate of non-exposed organisms. However, when the inhibitor is removed, there is a transient stimulation having an intensity related to the counter-response which the control mechanism has been exerting to achieve equilibrium. Stebbing (1981b) cites evidence from the literature for this phenomenon in a wide variety of organisms. Although the current experiments were not designed to test for the presence of a similar control mechanism in striped bass, there is suggestive evidence in the fact that antibody enhancement is not as great when antigen is administered 43 d after Cd^{2+} exposure (Fig. 4).

The mechanisms which would explain why striped bass respond immunologically to Cd^{2+} stress in a different way than cunners, require additional study. The most salient conclusion which can be drawn from this work is that chemical-stress effects on the immune system of a single fish species cannot be extrapolated to another species.

ACKNOWLEDGEMENTS

I thank W. Rose, V. Blazer and P. Valente for their excellent technical assistance, R. Greig and G. Sennefelder for Cd^{2+} analysis, V. Van Etten for typing, and R. Riccio for editorial assistance.

REFERENCES

Altman, L.C., Boetcher, D.A., and Goodwing, R.H. Jr. 1975. The use of chemotactic chambers and Nuclepore polycarbonate filters in the study of leukocyte chemotaxis. In: Leukocyte Chemotaxis. Nuclepore Corporation, Pleasanton, CA, pp. 5-9.

Avtalion, R.R. 1981. Environmental control of the immune response in fish. In: C.P. Straub (Editor), CRC Critical Reviews in Environmental Control. CRC Press, Inc., Boca Raton, FL, pp. 163-188.

Calabrese, A., Gould, E., and Thurberg, F.P. 1982. Effects of toxic metals in marine animals of the New York Bight: some laboratory observations. In: G.F. Mayer (Editor), Ecological Stress and the New York Bight: Science and Management. Estuarine Federation, Columbia, S.C., pp. 281-297.

Chao, L.N. 1973. Digestive system and feeding habits of the cunner, *Tautogolabrus adspersus*, a stomachless fish. Fishery Bull. 71: 565-586.

Cuchens, M. and Clem, L.W. 1977. Phylogeny of lymphocyte heterogeneity. II. Differential effects of temperature on fish T-like and B-like cells. Cellular Immunol. 34: 219-230.

Dawson, M.A., Gould, E., Thurberg, F.P., and Calabrese, A. 1977. Physiological response of juvenile striped bass, *Morone saxatilis*, to low levels of cadmium and mercury. Chesapeake Sci. 18: 353-359.

Gould, E. 1977. Alteration of enzymes in winter flounder, *Pseudopleuronectes americanus*, exposed to sublethal amounts of cadmium chloride. In: F.J. Vernberg, A. Calabrese, F.P. Thurberg, and W.B. Vernberg (Editors), Physiological Responses of Marine Biota to Pollutants. Academic Press, New York, pp. 209-223.

Jackim, E., Hamlin, J.M., and Sonis, S. 1970. Effects of metal poisoning on five liver enzymes in the killifish (*Fundulus heteroclitus*). J. Fish. Res. Board Can. 27: 383-390.

Koller, L.D., Exon, J.H., and Roan, J.G. 1975. Antibody suppression by cadmium. Arch. Environ. Health. 30: 598-601.

MacInnes, J.R., Thurberg, F.P., Greig, R.A., and Gould, E. 1977. Long-term cadmium stress in the cunner, *Tautogolabrus adspersus*. Fishery Bull. 75: 199-203.

Reed, L.J. and Muench, H. 1938. A simple method of estimating fifty percent endpoints. Am. J. Hyg. 27: 493-499.

Robohm, R.A. and Nitkowski, M.F. 1974. Physiological response of the cunner, *Tautogolabrus adspersus* to cadmium. IV. Effects on the immune system. NOAA Tech. Rep. NMFS SSRF-681: 15-20.

Robohm, R.A., Brown, C., and Murchelano, R.A. 1979. Comparison of antibodies in marine fish from clean and polluted waters of the New York Bight: Relative levels against 36 bacteria. Appl. Environ. Microbiol. 38: 248-257.

Stebbing, A.R.D. 1981a. The kinetics of growth control in a colonial hydroid. J. Mar. Biol. Assoc. U.K. 61: 35-63.

Stebbing, A.R.D. 1981b. Hormesis--stimulation of colony growth in *Campanularia flexuosa* (Hydrozoa) by copper, cadmium and other toxicants. Aquatic Toxicol. 1: 227-238.

Vallee, B.L. and Ulmer, D.D. 1972. Biochemical effects of mercury, cadmium, and lead. Annu. Rev. Biochem. 41: 91-128.

Veterinary Immunology and Immunopathology, 12 (1986) 263—280
Elsevier Science Publishers B.V., Amsterdam — Printed in The Netherlands

INTERACTIONS OF 2,3,7,8-TETRACHLORODIBENZO-P-DIOXIN (TCDD) WITH IMMUNE RESPONSES OF RAINBOW TROUT

J.M. SPITSBERGEN[1], K.A. SCHAT[2*], J.M. KLEEMAN[3] and R.E. PETERSON[3,4]

[1]DEPARTMENTS OF VETERINARY PATHOLOGY AND

[2]AVIAN AND AQUATIC ANIMAL MEDICINE, CORNELL UNIVERSITY, ITHACA, NEW YORK 14853, USA

[4]SCHOOL OF PHARMACY AND [3]ENVIRONMENTAL TOXICOLOGY CENTER, UNIVERSITY OF WISCONSIN, MADISON, WISCONSIN 53706, USA

ABSTRACT

J.M. Spitsbergen, K.A. Schat, J.M. Kleeman and R.E. Peterson, 1986. Interactions of 2,3,7,8-Tetrachlorodibenzo-p-dioxin (TCDD) with immune responses of rainbow trout. Vet. Immunol. Immunopathol., 12: 263-280.

Chlorinated dioxins, as typified by the most potent isomer, TCDD, are immunosuppressive in mammalian species and can enhance the susceptibility to a number of diseases. In recent years chlorinated dioxins have been detected in fish in many freshwater and marine habitats. Thus far, the effects of these chemicals on the immune responses of fish have not been examined. We studied the influence of TCDD on the defense mechanisms of rainbow trout. Yearling trout were injected intraperitoneally with the vehicle, 0.1, 1.0 or 10 µg/kg of TCDD. Interactions with the humoral immune response to sheep red blood cells (SRBC) were assessed by the Jerne plaque assay using head kidney and spleen leukocytes. Serum antibody was measured by complement-mediated lysis of SRBC in a chromium release assay. Effects of TCDD on the cellular immune responses were evaluated by the response of thymic and splenic lymphocytes to Con A and PWM. In addition, the phagocytic activity of peritoneal macrophages was examined _in vitro_.

Trout which received 0.1 or 1.0 µg/kg TCDD remained clinically normal, and defense mechanisms were unaltered in these fish. Trout which received 10 µg/kg of TCDD became hypophagic and exhibited fin necrosis, ascites and suppression of hematopoiesis. In this treatment group, Con A-induced blastogenesis of thymic and splenic lymphocytes was not significantly changed, however, suppression of the

*To whom correspondence should be addressed.

0165-2427/86/$03.50 © 1986 Elsevier Science Publishers B.V.

PWM-induced response of splenic lymphocytes occurred. No statistically significant alterations occurred in humoral immune responses, and phagocytic activity of peritoneal macrophages was not decreased.

The dose-response curve for various biologic effects of TCDD in the rainbow trout appears different from that in sensitive mouse strains. The 30-day, single-dose, parenteral LD_{50} for TCDD in the C57BL mouse is 100 μg/kg, and TCDD suppresses both cell-mediated and humoral immune responses at 1-2 μg/kg in this mouse strain. In the rainbow trout, however, immunosuppression was evident only at doses of TCDD approaching the 80-day, single-dose, parenteral LD_{50} of 20 μg/kg.

INTRODUCTION

Chlorinated dioxins and structurally related compounds such as chlorinated dibenzofurans, polychlorinated biphenyls and polybrominated biphenyls are immunosuppressive in mammals and can enhance the susceptibility to a number of diseases (Kerkvliet, 1984; Vos, 1977). The integrity of disease resistance and immune responses is frequently the most sensitive parameter altered by toxicant exposure in mammals (Dean et al., 1982). In the mouse, TCDD, the most potent chlorinated dioxin, has markedly altered cell-mediated immune (CMI) responses at doses substantially below those causing clinical disease, histopathologic lesions, or even liver microsomal enzyme induction (Clark et al., 1983; Clark et al., 1981). Because TCDD is the most biologically active chemical in the family of isosteric halogenated aromatic hydrocarbons, it has served as a prototype, and its effects on disease resistance and immunocompetence have been studied extensively in a variety of mammalian species.

A single intraperitoneal dose of 1 and 1.2 ug/kg of TCDD decreased the humoral immune response to sheep red blood cells in adult B6C3F1 and C57BL/6 mice, respectively (Vecci et al., 1983; Dean and Lauer, 1984). With regard to CMI responses, a single intraperitoneal dose of 1 ug/kg of TCDD suppressed the proliferative responses of B6C3F1 lymphocytes to T-cell and B-cell mitogens, as well as to allogeneic leukocytes (Dean and Lauer, 1984). An intraperitoneal dose of TCDD of 4 ng/kg decreased the cytotoxic T cell activity in adult C57BL/6 mice (Clark et al., 1983). Chronic dietary exposure to TCDD at levels below those causing clinical illness decreased delayed-type hypersensitivity to dinitrofluorobenzene and suppressed the primary and secondary humoral immune responses to tetanus toxoid and sheep red blood cells (Hinsdill et al., 1980). Four weekly oral doses of 1 ug/kg of TCDD increased the mortality of C57BL/6 mice following challenge with Salmonella (Thigpen et al., 1975). An intraperitoneal dose of TCDD as low as 0.4 ug/kg augmented the mortality of adult C57Bl/6 mice following challenge with Herpes simplex II virus (Clark et al., 1983). Chronic exposure of adult Swiss mice to dietary TCDD at levels causing no overt toxicity (10 ppb) increased mortality following challenge with Salmonella or Listeria (Hinsdill et al., 1980). Perinatal exposure of B6C3F1 mice to relatively low levels of TCDD increased the susceptibility to challenge with Listeria or syngeneic tumor cells (Luster et al., 1980). Although various aspects of cellular and humoral immune responses appear to be quite sensitive to perturbation by TCDD, a number of parameters of macrophage function appear to be quite resistant to impairment following animal exposure to dioxin (Mantovani et al., 1980; Vos et al., 1978).

In recent years chlorinated dioxins have been detected in fish in many freshwater and marine habitats (Stalling et al., 1983; Ryan et al., 1983). As in all mammalian species studied (McConnell, 1980), in fish species which have been investigated, TCDD causes thymic involution (Spitsbergen et al., 1984). But thus far, the effects of chlorinated dioxins on the immune responses of fish have not been evaluated.

We studied the influence of TCDD on a panel of defense mechanisms of rainbow trout. Although rainbow trout are among the most sensitive species to lethal effects of TCDD and to pathologic effects of TCDD on epidermal tissues (Spitsbergen et al., 1984), we have found that rainbow trout are relatively resistant to immunosuppressive effects of TCDD.

MATERIALS AND METHODS

Fish Maintenance

Yearling 100-250 g Shasta strain rainbow trout, *Salmo gairdneri*, were maintained in a flow through system of 100 l stainless steel tanks. Through each tank, a flow rate of at least one liter per kg fish weight of 17 ± 1°C dechlorinated tap water was maintained. Fish tanks were housed in stainless steel cabinets lighted from 0600 to 2200 hr by two five watt incandescent bulbs. Fish were fed Silver Cup pelleted feed at a rate of 2% of their body weight per day. Fish were acclimated to the laboratory conditions for 3 weeks before initiation of experiments.

TCDD Administration

Fish were anesthetized in benzocaine solubilized in ethanol, then were weighed and administered either a sham injection or 0, 0.1, 1.0 or 10 ug/kg of TCDD (> 99% purity, Dow Chemical Co., Midland, MI) in acetone/corn oil (5/95, v/v). An intraperitoneal injection of 0.1 ml of vehicle per 100 g of fish weight was used.

Immunization

Two weeks after TCDD treatment, fish were anesthetized in benzocaine and a 1 ml preimmunization serum sample was drawn by cardiac puncture. Sheep red blood cells (SRBC) were stored in Alsever's solution at 4 C for up to 4 wk. Erythrocytes were washed 4 times in sterile phophate buffered saline (PBS), then resuspended in PBS. Fish were administered 0.2 ml of washed 10% SRBC intramuscularly (i.m.) anterior to the dorsal fin. To study the secondary responses to SRBC, certain fish received a second i.m. injection of 0.2 ml of 10% SRBC 2 wk following the first injection.

Serum Collection

At selected time points, fish from each treatment group were anesthetized and blood was collected by cardiac puncture or from the caudal vein. Blood was allowed to clot in glass tubes at 20°C for approximately 30 min. followed by 30-60 min. on ice. The blood was centrifuged for 5 min. at 700 g and serum was withdrawn. The serum was heat-inactivated for 30 min. at 45°C, and stored at -80°C until assayed.

<u>Preparation of Lymphoid Cell Suspensions</u>

Head kidney, spleen and thymus were placed separately into 10 ml volumes of ice-cold Leibovitz's L-15 medium (Gibco, Chagrin Falls, Ohio) containing 30 mg/l of crude deoxyribonuclease I (DNAse) (Sigma Chemical Co., St. Louis, MO). The presence of DNAse minimized cell clumping (Spitsbergen, unpublished data). To form single cell suspensions, the organs were teased through a 60 um mesh autoclavable screen (Tetko, Inc., Elmsford, N.Y.). Cell suspensions were spun at room temperature for 10 min. at 400 g and washed once in 5 ml Leibovitz's medium containing DNAse. Mononuclear cells in the suspensions were counted using a hemocytometer, and viability of cells was determined using trypan blue.

<u>Jerne Plaque Assay</u>

An adaptation of the slide modification of the Jerne plaque assay previously used with rainbow trout tissues (Anderson et al., 1979) was utilized. One or two fish per treatment group were sacrificed and assayed at selected time points 14-30 days after primary immunization and 6-16 days after secondary immunization.

Lymphoid cells were suspended in 5 ml Leibovitz's medium containing 2% heat-inactivated fetal calf serum (Leibovitz's-2%), and, where appropriate, 1/10 or 1/100 dilutions of the cells were prepared in Leibovitz's-2%. Glass slides were coated with a thin layer of 1% agarose using a cotton-tipped applicator. Ten to 200 ul of lymphocyte suspension and 0.2 ml of 20% washed SRBC in Leibovitz's-2% were added to 0.2 ml of 37°C Leibovitz's-2% containing 1% agarose. This mixture was agitated gently and poured onto an agarose-coated slide. The slides were incubated for 4 hr at 20°C in humid chambers. The slides were then inverted onto shallow plexiglass troughs containing pooled control rainbow trout serum diluted 1/10 in PBS as a source of complement. Plaques were enumerated following a 2 hr incubation of the trough at 20°C. Duplicate or triplicate slides were counted. Appropriate dilutions and aliquots of cell suspensions were used so that, except in the case of low responders, 100-1000 plaques were counted per organ assayed.

Chromium Release Assay

Serum antibody was quantitated by complement-mediated lysis of SRBC in a chromium release assay. The methods utilized were as previously described (Spitsbergen and Schat, in press 1985).

Mitogen Stimulation

Two fish per treatment group per day were sacrificed on days 16-20 after administration of TCDD. Aliquots of splenic and thymic cell suspensions were centrifuged at 400 g x 10 min and resuspended at a concentration of 10^7 cells per ml in Leibovitz's L-15 medium containing 20% heat-inactivated human serum and 4% heat-inactivated (30 min at 45° C) pooled lake trout serum. To each well of a round bottom microtiter plate was added 50 ul of cell suspension (5×10^5 cells) plus 50 ul of serum-free Leibovitz's medium with or without appropriate amounts of concanavalin A (Con A) or pokeweed mitogen (PWM) (Sigma Chemical Co., St. Louis, MO). For each mitogen, a range of mitogen concentrations was used for each organ culture (20,50,100 ug/ml Con A and 25,250,500 ug/ml PWM). Cultures were prepared in triplicate. Plates were sealed in plastic bags and incubated for 3 days at 20^oC. At this time 0.5 uCi of tritiated thymidine (2 Ci/mmol, New England Nuclear, Boston, MA) in 50 ul of Leibovitz's medium was added to each well of the microtiter plate. The plates were again sealed in plastic bags and incubated for 2 days at 20^oC. Cells were washed with physiological saline and collected on glass filter papers with a semiautomatic processor (Otto Hiller Co., Madison, WI). Radioactivity was assayed by liquid scintillation counting, with a 5 min. counting period per sample. Results were expressed as specific cpm calculated by subtraction of cpm in non-mitogen stimulated cultures from the cpm of stimulated cultures.

Phagocytosis

The phagocytic activity of peritoneal macrophages was assessed using a modification of the technique described by

Blazer (1982). Peritoneal macrophages were collected at the time of sacrifice from the fish used for the mitogen stimulation experiment. The peritoneal cavity of each fish was lavaged with 10 ml of ice-cold calcium-magnesium-free Hank's balanced salt solution containing 30 mg/l of DNAse. Cells in the suspension were counted using a hemocytometer. Cells were pelleted by centrifugation at 400 g x 10 min, and were resuspended at a concentration of 10^6/ml in Leibovitz's medium containing 10% heat-inactivated calf serum (Leibovitz's-10%). A sterile round coverslip was added to each well of a 24-well (2 cm^2 area per well) plate (Falcon, Oxnard, CA), and 1 ml of cell suspension (10^6 cells) was seeded per well. The plate was sealed in a plastic bag and incubated at 20°C overnight. The medium on the cells was replaced with Leibovitz's-10% and 20 ul of 5% washed SRBC in Leibovitz's medium was added per well. The plates were agitated to disperse the SRBC, and incubated for 30, 60 or 120 min. at 20°C. Coverlips were rinsed for 10 seconds in hypotonic ammonium chloride buffer, rinsed for 10 seconds in PBS, then fixed and stained using a Diff Quik staining set (American Scientific Products, McGraw Park, Ill.). One hundred macrophages were counted per coverslip, and the number of these cells containing particles as well as the number of particles per phagocyte were recorded.

Statistical Analysis

Data were analyzed using analysis of variance (Sokal and Rolf, 1981). For groups of treatment means having nonhomogenous variances, a $\log_{10}$ transformation or $\log_{10}$ (Y + 1) was used prior to performing the analysis of variance. Treatment means were compared using orthogonal contrasts or the Bonferroni test (Gill, 1978).

Safety Precautions

Safety precautions for handling of and disposal of TCDD were as described elsewhere (Kleeman et al., in press).

RESULTS

Clinical Signs of Toxicity and Gross Pathology

Throughout the experiment fish which received vehicle, 0.1 or 1.0 ug/kg of TCDD remained clinically normal. Within

2 weeks after the injection of 10 ug/kg of TCDD, rainbow trout became hypophagic, the majority exhibited necrosis of the margins of fins, and approximately half had ascites. Fish in the high dose group also exhibited a suppression of hematopoiesis in the head kidney, with consequent peripheral leukopenia and thrombocytopenia (Spitsbergen et al., in preparation).

Cellularity of Lymphoid Organs

The cellularity of splenic and head kidney cell suspensions was evaluated using tissues obtained from Shasta strain fish from 2 different hatcheries, designated hatchery A and Hatchery B (Table I). Following fish exposure to 10 ug/kg of TCDD, numbers of splenic lymphoid leukocytes were significantly decreased in fish from hatchery A. At this dose of TCDD, splenic lymphoid cells were decreased, but not significantly, in tissues of fish from hatchery B. In head kidney of fish from both hatcheries and in thymus, numbers of lymphoid leukocytes were markedly reduced in animals which received 10 ug/kg of TCDD.

Humoral Immune Responses

When compared to sham- and vehicle-treated trout, those which received TCDD lacked statistically significant differences in antibody-forming cells per 10^6 splenic or head kidney lymphoid leukocytes, in the primary response to SRBC (Table II). An upward trend in number of plaque-forming cells per 10^6 splenic or head kidney leukocytes was apparent in the treatment group receiving 10 ug/kg of TCDD. Because of the wide variability between the responses of individual outbred rainbow trout, the means in this treatment group were not statistically different from those of sham or vehicle controls. In the primary response to SRBC, serum antibody titers in treatment groups which received TCDD were not significantly different from those in control groups at the time points examined (Table III), although a downward trend in the serum titer occurred in the group which received 10 ug/kg of TCDD.

In the secondary response to SRBC, significant treatment-related differences in antibody-forming cells per

Table I. Effects of TCDD on cellularity of lymphoid organ suspensions of rainbow trout

Dose TCDD (ug/kg)	No. of lymphoid leukocytes x 10^7				
	Hatchery A[a]		Hatchery B[b]		
	Head kidney	Spleen	Head kidney	Spleen	Thymus
0 (Sham)	13.6±2.7[c]	4.6±1.2	...[d]	6.6±1.3	22.9±6.6
0 (Vehicle)	14.1±2.2	4.9±0.9	15.0±1.7	4.7±1.1	13.5±2.7
0.1	21.1±3.2	6.2±1.3	...	9.4±2.7	14.8±3.3
1.0	12.9±1.9	4.7±1.2	...	4.0±0.5	6.1±2.5**
10	3.4±0.9**	2.3±0.7	3.4±0.7**	1.9±0.6*	4.5±0.8**

[a]1 or 2 fish per treatment group sampled on days 28-42 after injection of TCDD.
[b]2 fish per treatment group sampled on days 16-20 after injection of TCDD.
[c]Means are averages of data from 10 fish. Mean ± SEM.
[d]... = not done.
**Significantly different from vehicle control ($p < 0.001$).
*Significantly different from vehicle control ($p < 0.05$).

Table II. Effects of TCDD on antibody-forming cells per 10^6 lymphoid leukocytes in rainbow trout

Immunization	Organ	Days after 1° immunization	Days after 2° immunization	Dose TCDD (ug/kg) 0 Sham	0 Vehicle	0.1	1.0	10
Primary	Spleen	14-30[a]	...[b]	10±5[c]	6±3	7±4	7±2	39±16
	Kidney	14-30	...	19±5	22±8	27±9	25±8	60±29
Secondary	Spleen	20-30	6-16	190±44	187±79	347±99	516±190	...
	Kidney	20-30	6-16	699±147	622±159	888±275	892±275	...

[a]One or two fish per treatment group assayed per day on selected days. Means are averages over the entire sampling period.
[b]... = not tested.
[c]Ave. ± SEM. Ten fish assayed per treatment group.

Table III. Effect of TCDD on serum antibody titers of rainbow trout to SRBC quantitated by chromium release assay

Immunization	Days after Immunization	No. of fish	Dose TCDD (ug/kg) 0 Sham	0 Vehicle	0.1	1.0	10
Primary	14-30[a]	10	185±98[b]	199±105	223±102	166±62	75±31
	42	9-11	135±92	103±34	59±14	122±35	...[c]
	70	5-6	18±12	38±23	25±12	52±18	...
Secondary	6-16[a]	10	2048±477	1782±468	2106±777	1750±543	...
	28	9-11	1370±392	1897±679	2020±821	3226±1089	...
	72	4-6	352±96	574±280	716±301	683±306	...

[a]One or two fish per treatment group sampled per day on selected days. Means are averages over the entire sampling period.

[b]Serum antibody titers of unimmunized fish were less than or equal to 8. Mean ± SEM.

[c]... = not tested.

10^6 lymphoid leukocytes were not evident, although upward trends in numbers of plaque-forming cells per 10^6 leukocytes were noted for both splenic and head kidney preparations in treatment groups which received 0.1 or 1.0 ug/kg of TCDD. Significant differences between treatment groups were not noted in serum antibody titers in the secondary response to SRBC (Table III).

Lymphocyte Blastogenesis

Statistically significant differences in Con A-induced lymphocyte blastogenesis in thymic or splenic cultures were not noted among treatment groups (Table IV). PWM-induced stimulation of splenic cultures was suppressed in the group which received 10 ug/kg of TCDD. TCDD did not appear to alter the optimal mitogen concentrations for blastogenesis (data not shown).

The interaction of TCDD with Con A-induced lymphocyte blastogenesis was assessed using splenic lymphocytes from yearling Shasta strain rainbow trout obtained from a second hatchery (Hatchery A). Fourteen animals were sampled per treatment group at selected times 4-12 weeks after receiving TCDD. Triplicate mean specific cpm $\pm$ SEM for vehicle and 1 ug/kg treatment groups were 2663 $\pm$ 326 and 1479 $\pm$ 302, respectively. These means were significantly different ($p < .025$).

Phagocytosis

Neither the percentage of glass-adherent mononuclear cells which took up SRBC, nor the numbers of SRBC within 100 mononuclear cells were significantly altered by exposure of fish to TCDD (Table V).

DISCUSSION

Unlike the situation in the mouse system where the humoral immune response peaks sharply on a given day and falls off precipitously (Mitchell, 1974), the humoral immune response of the rainbow trout to sheep erythrocytes is characterized by a broad peak which extends over a period of a few weeks (Anderson et al., 1984; Blazer, 1982; Spitsbergen and Schat, 1985). This characteristic of the rainbow trout allowed us to sample a small number of fish

Table IV. Effects of TCDD on lymphocyte blastogenesis in rainbow trout[a]

Mitogen	Organ	Dose TCDD (ug/kg)				
		0		0.1	1.0	10
		(Sham)	(Vehicle)			
Con A	spleen[b]	1834±437[c]	1303±343	2366±766	1467±358	643±207
	thymus	1467±447	1248±417	757±218	980±326	1454±321
PWM	spleen	1209±269	955±242	1200±253	1039±277	366±89*

[a]Ten fish sampled per treatment group, 2 each day on days 16-20 after receiving TCDD.

[b]Mean CPM ± SEM for unstimulated splenic and thymic lymphocyte cultures were 247±25 and 212±12, respectively. No statistically significant differences were evident between treatment groups in mean CPM of unstimulated splenic or thymic cultures.

[c]Triplicate mean specific CPM±SEM. Data reflect the response of individual fish lymphocyte cultures at the optimal concentration of mitogen (50 or 100 ug/ml for Con A and 25 or 250 ug/ml for PWM).

*Significantly different from vehicle control ($p < 0.05$).

Table V. Effects of TCDD on phagocytic activity of peritoneal macrophages of rainbow trout[a]

Dose TCDD (ug/kg)	% Phagocytes[b]	Particles per 100 macrophages
0[c]	61 ± 8[d]	281 ± 64
1.0	57 ± 6	253 ± 53
10.0	66 ± 8	369 ± 92

[a]One hour assay.

[b]Percent of glass-adherent mononuclear cells containing particles.

[c]Vehicle control.

[d]Mean ± SEM. Ten individuals per treatment group assayed.

from each treatment group on selected days over a period up to 2 weeks for assessment of the humoral response to SRBC using the Jerne plaque assay. The variation in response between individuals in a given treatment group assayed on a particular day was generally as great as the differences between individuals in a given treatment group which were assayed on different days. Therefore, we were able to combine the data regarding individuals from a particular treatment group, although the data were generated over several days. These combined data were used in comparing treatment groups with one another.

As reported previously (Anderson et al, 1983), the primary immune response of the rainbow trout to SRBC as measured by the Jerne plaque assay was dramatically lower than that of the mouse (Dean and Lauer, 1984).

With an 80-day, single-dose, parenteral LD_{50} of approximately 20 ug/kg, the rainbow trout is among the more sensitive of species with regard to lethal effects of TCDD. And, as in certain mammalian species, sublethal exposure of rainbow trout to TCDD results in characteristic lesions in epithelial tissues (Spitsbergen et al., in preparation). However, unlike sensitive mouse strains, rainbow trout are relatively resistant to immunosuppressive effects of TCDD. Humoral immune responses of the rainbow trout were not significantly impaired even at TCDD doses approaching the LD_{50}. Con A-induced thymocyte blastogenesis was unaffected even at 10 ug/kg, and PWM-induced splenic lymphocyte blastogenesis was suppressed only at 10 ug/kg. Although statistically significant differences were not evident in numbers of antibody-forming cells per 10^6 lymphoid leukocytes when comparing control to dioxin-treated fish, upward trends were evident in the numbers of plaque-forming cells per 10^6 leukocytes in both kidney and spleen in the 10 ug/kg treatment group in the primary response to SRBC. Upward trends were also apparent in numbers of antibody-forming cells per 10^6 leukocytes in both kidney and spleen at 0.1 and 1.0 ug/kg in the secondary response to SRBC.

Such effects may reflect an inhibition of suppressor cell activity such as that seen in mammalian species administered relatively low doses of various immunosuppressive agents (Turk and Parker, 1982; Turk and Parker, 1984). An alternate explanation for the data at 10 ug/kg is that rainbow trout antibody-forming cells are selectively spared in the TCDD-induced reduction of cellularity in the head kidney. Larger treatment groups would probably be necessary to detect subtle or moderate treatment effects using outbred rainbow trout which exhibit such high individual variability.

The data regarding TCDD effects on mitogen stimulation in the rainbow trout further reflects the variability among outbred hatchery strains of rainbow trout. The Con A-induced splenic lymphocyte blastogenesis of one hatchery strain of Shasta rainbow trout was not suppressed by TCDD at a dose of 1 ug/kg, whereas that dose of TCDD suppressed the splenic lymphocyte blastogenesis in Shasta trout from another hatchery. Since Con A-induced lymphocyte blastogenesis in mammalian species often reflects stimulation of T suppressor cells, the suppresion of Con A-induced lymhocyte blastogenesis may further support the suggestion of inhibited suppressor cell activity indicated in our humoral immune response studies in the rainbow trout (Dwyer and Johnson, 1981).

The general failure of TCDD to suppress immune responses of rainbow trout at doses below those causing clinical toxicity parallels the findings regarding effects of a number of other pharmacologic immunomodulators in the rainbow trout. Cyclophosphamide suppresses humoral immune responses of rainbow trout only at doses approaching those causing lethality (Anderson, 1982; Maisse and Dorson, 1976; Sakai, 1982). A dosage regimen of azathioprine (Imuran^{R}) which totally eliminates the primary humoral immune response to SRBC in mice (100 mg/kg) only augments the primary humoral response as measured by the Jerne plaque assay in the rainbow trout (Spitsbergen, unpublished data). Among immunosuppressive drugs, only corticosteroids (Kenalog 40^{R})

have been reported to suppress humoral immune responses of rainbow trout at doses below those causing clinical toxicity (Anderson et al, 1982). And such doses of corticosteroids have failed to suppress humoral immune responses in other studies (Chen et al., 1983). Even *in vitro*, rainbow trout lymphocytes seem to be relatively more resistant to certain immunosuppressive agents than are lymphocytes of mammals. Concentrations of cyclosporin A which eliminate Con A-induced lymphocyte blastogenesis in murine thymocytes and splenocytes only moderately suppress mitogenesis of rainbow trout lymphocytes (Spitsbergen, unpublished data). Although the defense mechanisms against disease in rainbow trout are fundamentally similar to those of mammals (Corbel, 1975; Ingram, 1980), the processes involved in immunoregulation seem to be somewhat different from those occurring in mammals, at least with regard to modulating effects of exogenous agents on the complex interactions of the cells regulating and effecting immune responses. Much additional work remains to clarify these immunoregulatory and effector processes in fish and to elucidate the ways in which exogenous chemicals interact with these mechanisms.

ACKNOWLEDGEMENTS

This work was sponsored in part by the New York and Wisconsin Sea Grant Institutes under grants from the Office of Sea Grant, National Oceanic and Atmospheric Administration (NOAA), United States Department of Commerce. Support was also received from the National Institute of Environmental Health Sciences, National Research Service Award #42 USC 2891-1 42 CFR 66 from the Department of Pathology, New York State College of Veterinary Medicine, Cornell University, grant #5T32 ES07105. Additional support was contributed by Return a Gift to Wildlife funded by voluntary donations by New York taxpayers with their annual state income tax returns. We also acknowledge the excellent technical assistance of Tim Miller, Curtis Helm and Jean Johnson.

REFERENCES

Anderson, D.P., Roberson, B.S. and Dixon, O.W., 1979. Cellular immune response in rainbow trout *Salmo gairdneri* Richardson to *Yersinia ruckeri* O-antigen monitored by the passive haemolytic plaque assay test. J. Fish Dis. 2:169-178.

Anderson, D.P., Roberson, B.S. and Dixon, O.W., 1982. Immunosuppression induced by a corticosteroid or an alkylating agent in rainbow trout (*Salmo gairdneri*) administered a *Yersinia ruckeri* bacterin. Dev. Comp. Immunol. Suppl. 2:197-284.

Anderson, D.P., Merchant, B., Dixon, O.W., Schott, C.F. and Lizzio, E.F., 1983. Flush exposure and injection immunization of rainbow trout to selected DNP conjugates. Dev. Comp. Immunol. 7:261-268.

Anderson, D.P., van Muiswinkel, W.B., Roberson, B.S., 1984. Effects of chemically induced immune modulation on infectious diseases of fish. In: Kende, M., Gainer, J. and Chirigos, M. (Editors), Chemical Regulation of Immunity in Veterinary Medicine. Alan R. Liss, Inc., N.Y., N.Y., pp. 187-211.

Blazer, V.S., 1982. The effects of marginal deficiencies of ascorbic acid and alpha-tocopherol on the natural resistance and immune response of rainbow trout (*Salmo gairdneri*). Ph.D. Thesis. University of Rhode Island. Kingston, R.I.

Chen, M.F., Rohovec, J.S. and Fryer, J.L., 1983. Effect of methotrexate, Kenalog, and cyclophosphamide on the antibody response of steelheads to *Aeromonas salmonicida*. Trans. Amer. Fish. Soc. 112:561-564.

Clark, D.A., Gauldie, J., Szewczuk, M.R. and Sweeney, G., 1981. Enhanced suppressor cell activity as a mechanism of immunosuppresion by 2,3,7,8-tetrachlorodibenzo-p-dioxin. Proc. Soc. Exp. Biol. Med. 168:290-299.

Clark, D.A., Sweeney, G., Safe, S., Hancock, E., Kilburn, D.G. and Gauldie, J., 1983. Cellular and genetic basis for suppression of cytotoxic T cell generation by haloaromatic hydrocarbons. Immunopharmacology 6:143-153.

Corbel, M.J., 1975. The immune response in fish: a review. J. Fish Biol. 7:539-563.

Dean, J.H., Luster, M.I. and Boorman, G.A., 1982. Methods and approaches for assessing immunotoxicity: an overview. Environ. Health Perspect. 43:27-29.

Dean, J.H. and Lauer, L.D., 1984. Immunological effects following exposure to 2,3,7,8-tetrachlorodibenzo-p-dioxin: a review. In: Lowrance, W.W. (Editor), Public Health Risks of the Dioxins. William Kaufman, Los Altos, California. p. 275-294.

Dwyer, J.M. and Johnson, C., 1981. The use of concanavalin A to study the immunoregulation of human T cells. Clin. Exp. Immunol. 46:237-249.

Gill, J.L., 1978. Design and analysis of experiments in the animal and medical sciences. Vol. I. Iowa State University Press, Ames, IA. p. 159-185.

Hinsdill, R.D., Couch, D.L. and Speirs, R.S., 1980. Immunosuppression in mice induced by dioxin (TCDD) in feed. J. Environ. Pathol. Toxicol. 4:401-425.

Ingram, G.A., 1980. Substances involved in the natural resistance of fish to infection--a review. J. Fish Biol. 16:23-60.

Kerkvliet, N.I., 1984. Halogenated aromatic hydrocarbons (HAH) as immunotoxicants. In: Kende, M., Gainer, J. and Chirigos, M. (Editors), Chemical Regulation of Immunity of Veterinary Medicine. Alan R. Liss, Inc. N.Y., N.Y. p. 369-387.

Kleeman, J.M., Olson, J.R., Chen, S.M. and Peterson, R.E. In press. Metabolism and disposition of 2,3,7,8-tetrachlorodibenzo-p-dioxin (TCDD). Toxicol. Appl. Pharmacol.

Luster, M.I., Boorman, G.A., Dean, J.H., Harris, M.W., Luebke, R.W., Padarathsingh, M.L. and Moore, J.A., 1980. Examination of bone marrow, immunologic parameters and host susceptibility following pre- and postnatal exposure to 2,3,7,8-tetrachlorodibenzo-p-dioxin (TCDD). Int. J. Immunopharmacology 2:301-310.

Maisse, G. and Dorson, M., 1976. The agglutinin response of rainbow trout to Aeromonas salmonicida. Effect of temperature, adjuvant and an immunosuppressive agent. Ann. Rech. Veter. 7:307-313.

Mantovanai, A., Vecci, A., Luini, W., Sironi, M., Candiani, G.P., Spreafico, F., and Garattini, S., 1980. Effect of 2,3,7,8-tetrachlorodibenzo-p-dioxin on macrophage and natural killer cell-mediated cytotoxicity in mice. Biomedicine 32:200-204.

McConnell, E.E., 1980. Acute and chronic toxicity, carcinogenesis, reproduction, teratogenesis and mutagenesis in animals. In: Kimbrough, R.D., (Editor), Halogenated Biphenyls, Terphenyls, Naphthalenes, Dibenzodioxins and Related Products. Elsevier/North-Holland Biomedical Press. New York. p. 109-150.

Mitchell, M.S., 1974. Evaluation of immunosuppressive agents. In: Sartorelli, A.C. and Johns, D.G. (Editors), Antineoplastic and Immunosuppressive Agents. Part I. Spring-Verlag. New York. p. 555-571.

Ryan, J.J., Lau, P.Y., Pilon, J.C. and Lewis, D., 1983. 2,3,7,8-tetrachlorodibenzo-p-dioxin and 2,3,7,8-tetrachlorodibenzofuran residues in Great Lakes commercial and sport fish. In: Choudhary, G., Keith, L.H. and Rappe, C., (Editors), Chlorinated Dioxins and Dibenzofurans in the Total Environment. Butterworth Publishers. Boston. p. 87-97.

Sakai, D.K., 1982. Immunological roles of sensitive lymphocytes and resistant lymphocytes against cyclophosphamide in rainbow trout immune system reorganized by adoptive transfer. Bull. Japan. Soc. Sci. Fish. 48:1059-1064.

Sartorelli, A.C. and Johns, D.G., 1974. Antineoplastic and Immunosuppressive Agents. Springer-Verlag. New York.

Sokol,R.R. and Rohlf, F.J. Biometry. W.H. Freeman and Company. San Francisco. 859 p.

Spitsbergen, J.M., Kleeman, J.M. and Peterson, R.E., 1984. Toxicity of 2,3,7,8-tetrachlorodibenzo-p-dioxin (TCDD) in freshwater fish. Toxicologist 4:190.

Spitsbergen, J.M. and Schat, K.A., in press, A chromium release assay for the assessment of spontaneous and immune hemolysis of heterologous erythrocytes by sera of rainbow trout. Dev. Comp. Immunol.

Stalling, D.L., Smith, L.M., Petty, J.D., Hogan, J.W., Johnson, J.L. Rappe, C. and Buser, H.R., 1983. Residues ofchlorinated dibenzo-p-dioxins and dibenzofurans in Laurentian Great Lakes fish. In: Tucker, R.E., Young, A.L. and Gray, A.P., (Editors), Human and Environmental Risks of Chlorinated Dioxins and Related Compounds. Plenum Publishing Corporation. p. 221-240.

Thigpen, J.E., Faith, R.E., McConnell, E.E., and Moore, J.A., 1975. Increased susceptibility to bacterial infection as a sequela of exposure to 2,3,7,8-tetrachlorodibenzo-p-dioxin. Infect. Immun. 12:1319-1324.

Turk, J.L. and Parker, D., 1982. Effect of cyclophosphamide on immunological control mechanisms. Immunological Rev. 65:99-113.

Turk, J.L. and Parker, D., 1984. Drugs that increase delayed hypersensitivity reactions. Trends in Pharmacological Sciences 5:472-474.

Vecci, A., Sironi, M., Canegrati, M.A., Recchia, M. and Garattini, S., 1983. Immunosuppressive effects of 2,3,7,9-tetrachlorodibenzo-p-dioxin in strains of mice with different susceptibility to induction of aryl hydrocarbon hydroxylase. Toxicol. Appl. Pharmacol. 68:434-441.

Vos, J.G., 1977. Immune suppression as related to toxicology. CRC Crit. Rev. Toxicol. 5:67-101.

Vos, J.G., Kreeftenberg,, J.G., Engel, H.W., Minderhoud, A. and van Noorlejansen, L.M., 1978. Studies on 2,3,7,8-tetrachlorodibenzo-p-dioxin-induced immune suppression and decreased resistance to infection: endotoxin hypersensitivity, serum zinc concentrations and effect of thymosin treatment. Toxicology 9:75-86.

Veterinary Immunology and Immunopathology, 12 (1986) 281—286
Elsevier Science Publishers B.V., Amsterdam — Printed in The Netherlands

FISH AND ANTIBIOTICS: PHARMACOKINETICS OF SULPHADIMIDINE IN CARP (CYPRINUS CARPIO)

J.L. GRONDEL[1], J.F.M. NOUWS[2] and O.L.M. HAENEN[1]

1 Department of Experimental Animal Morphology and Cell Biology, Agricultural University, P.O. Box 338, 6700 AH Wageningen, The Netherlands

2 R.V.V.-District 6, P.O. Box 40010, 6504 AA Nijmegen, The Netherlands

ABSTRACT

Grondel, J.L., Nouws, J.F.M. and Haenen, O.L.M., 1986. Fish and Antibiotics: Pharmacokinetics of sulphadimidine in carp (*Cyprinus carpio*). Vet. Immunol. Immunopathol., 12: 281-286.

Pharmacokinetics, metabolism and clearance of sulphadimidine (SDM) were studied after a single intraperitoneal injection of SDM in carp at 20^oC. SDM was acetylated and hydroxylated to a small extent. The main metabolite was N_4-acetyl derivative amounting only 2% of the total drug dose excreted; hydroxylation was less important (0.41% of the dose). The elimination half-life for SDM in carp was 17.5h. The clearance values for SDM and its metabolites were equivalent. The importance of pharmacokinetic studies in different fish species is discussed.

INTRODUCTION

In large-scale fish culture, disease outbreaks can cause a substantial loss of animals. Antimicrobial drugs, often used as food additives, are employed for prophylactic and therapeutic purposes. In practice the dosage employed is often extrapolated from mammals. This may result in unwanted side effects. As reported in previously presented papers (Anderson *et al*., 1984, Grondel and Boesten, 1982, Grondel *et al*., 1985a, Grondel and Muiswinkel van, 1985b, Muiswinkel van *et al*., 1984, Rijkers *et al*., 1981) antibiotics may interfere with the immune system. Furthermore, the induction of bacterial resistance and the occurrence of drug residues in edible tissues can be a serious problem. A rational and optimal plan for antimicrobial therapy for fish is needed.

0165-2427/86/$03.50 © 1986 Elsevier Science Publishers B.V.

Sulphadimidine (SDM) is the most widely used sulphonamide for prophylactic and therapeutic purposes administered to a wide range of species. SDM can be metabolized by hydroxylation and by the

acetylation-deacetylation pathway (Vree _et al_., 1983, Vree _et al_., 1984, Vree and Hekster, 1985). The hydroxy metabolites are microbiologically active and they may be potentiated by trimethoprim (Nouws _et al_., 1984). In this paper we will present pharmacokinetics and metabolism of SDM in carp (_Cyprinus carpio_) following intraperitoneal administration.

MATERIALS AND METHODS

Drugs

Sodium sulphadimidine^R (33.3%) was obtained from A.U.V. (Cuyk, The Netherlands). N_4-acetylsulphadimidine (N_4-SDM), 6-hydroxymethyl-sulphadimidine (SCH_2OH) and 5-hydroxysulphadimidine (SOH) were synthesized and isolated according to Vree _et al_.(1984) and Vree and Hekster (1985).

Experimental set up

Carps, 6-8 months of age, were bred in our laboratory and kept in aquaria with aerated running tapwater at a temperature of 20°C. Animals were fed daily with pelleted dry food (K30, Trouw & Co., Putten, The Netherlands) by means of a "Scharflinger" automatic feeder. For the experiment animals, weighing 179 ± 12 gram, were kept individually in tanks with stagnant aerated tapwater (20°C). Water samples were taken at 4 and 12 h intervals followed by replacement of tapwater (20°C).

Sodium sulphadimidine (SDM) in solution was administered intraperitoneally to five carp (100mg/fish). Heparinized blood samples (0.2 ml) were taken from the caudal vein at regular time intervals, centrifuged and frozen (-20°C) pending HPLC analysis.

HPLC analysis

Deglucuronidation, protein binding determination, sample preparation and HPLC analysis were performed as described by Nouws _et al_. (1986a,b). SDM, its N_4-SDM metabolite, and the two hydroxymetabolites were determined simultaneously in the samples. Pharmacokinetic analysis was performed by standard procedures (Baggot,1977).

RESULTS

Figure 1 shows the plasma disposition of SDM for one carp. Two hours after a single SDM injection (75 mg/kg) a maximum plasma concentration (C_{max}) was observed (124 ug/ml). In carp SDM was hydroxylated and acetylated to a small extent. The metabolite concentrations in plasma slowly increased and reached their maximum concentrations between 10 and 20h post SDM injection. Beyond 20h p.i. the plasma concentrations of SDM and its metabolites were essentially parallel. The plasma elimination half-life for SDM was 17.5 ± 5.8 hours (n=5) measured over a period of 48 hours after SDM injection. The total drug recovery in the water within 48h was 64.4% of the dose applied. The main metabolite was N_4-SDM

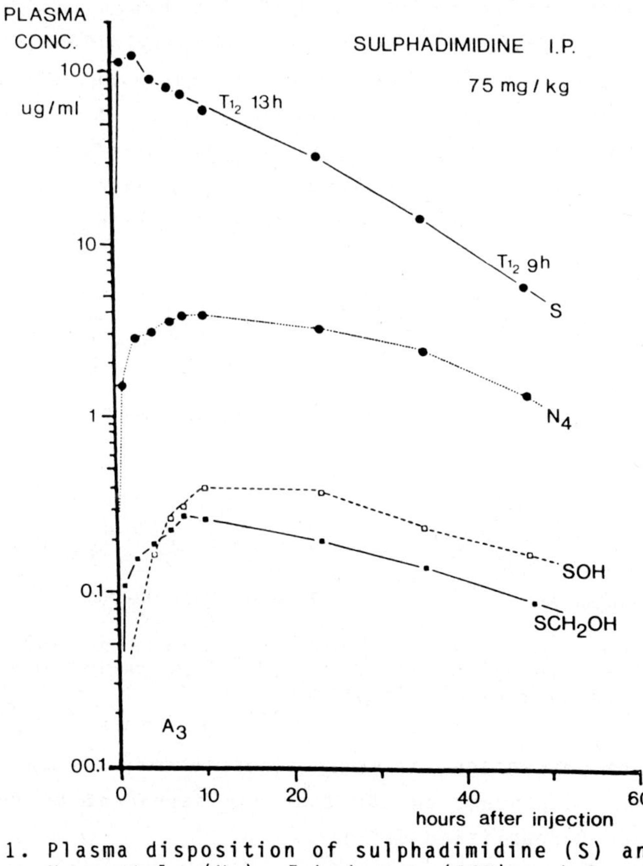

Fig. 1. Plasma disposition of sulphadimidine (S) and its metabolites N_4-acetyl- (N_4), 5-hydroxy- (SOH) and 6-methylhydroxy-sulphadimidine (SCH_2OH) in plasma of a carp following intraperitoneal administration of SDM (75 mg/kg).

and composed only 2% of the total drug dose excreted. Hydroxylation was less important; 0.18% was excreted within 48h as SOH and 0.23% as SCH_2OH. The clearance values of SDM, N_4-SDM and the hydroxymetabolite SCH_2OH were equivalent: 0.29, 0.39 and 0.22 ml/kg/min (n=5) respectively. Plasma protein binding data were obtained from carp kept in tanks with stagnant water and in tanks continuously refreshed with running tapwater (20°C). The percentages plasma protein binding of SDM, N_4-SDM and SCH_2OH were 41.2 (n=6), 14.7 (n=2) and 33.8 (n=5), respectively.

DISCUSSION

After i.p. injection SDM was absorbed quickly. The plasma elimination half-life is approximately 17.5 hours. SDM can be metabolized by hydroxylation as well as by acetylation (Fig. 2). Both the 5-hydroxysulphadimidine and the 6-hydroxymethylsulphadimidine metabolites were detected. However, in carp SDM was mainly converted into N_4-SDM, which is in contrast to the observations in mammals. In cows and calves SDM is extensively hydroxylated into hydroxy derivatives and to a lesser extent acetylated into N_4-SDM (Nouws *et al*., 1986a).

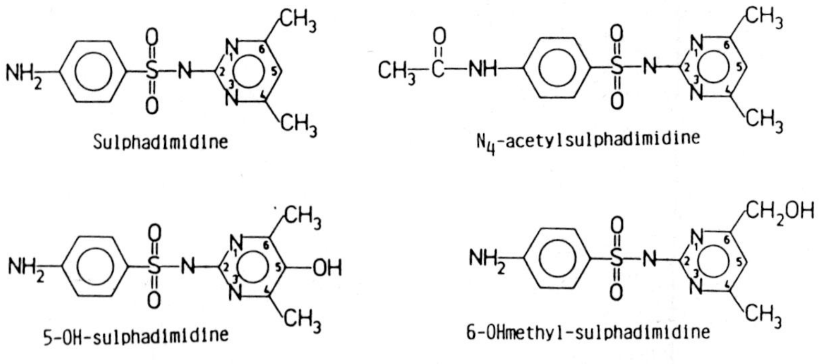

Fig. 2. Molecular structures of sulphadimidine and of its 5-hydroxy-4,6-dimethyl-pyrimidine, 6-hydroxymethyl-4-methyl-pyrimidine and N_4-acetyl metabolite.

Furthermore, the percentages of metabolites in carp plasma appeared to be neither dependant on the dose nor dependant on replacement of tapwater (unpublished data).

The N_4-SDM and hydroxymetabolites showed concentration-time curves running parallel to SDM beyond 20h p.i.. The clearance values were equivalent and the elimination was predominantly by a passive diffusion process. It was also observed that an acetylation-deacetylation equilibrium exists (results not shown).

The pharmacokinetic data were obtained from fish kept under optimal laboratory circumstances: healthy fish, all of a certain weight, constant water temperature and one species (*Cyprinus carpio*). However, differences in the pharmacokinetic behaviour can be expected for SDM with respect to age, temperature, species and disease status. Recently, obvious differences in half-life times for oxytetracycline were observed between rainbow trout (kept at 12°C) and carp (kept at 20°C) (unpublished data). However, for chloramphenicol the elimination half-life values for both rainbow trout and carp were equal (unpublished data).

For some species pharmacokinetic data are scarce or even absent. It is well-known that between mammalian species the kinetic data on tissue distribution, plasma dispositon and drug persistence in the body can differ markedly. Similarly, extreme differences between fish species may be expected with respect to the pharmacokinetic behaviour of drugs.

It has to be emphasized that a multidisciplinary approach is needed to optimize large-scale fish culture. Immunological, pharmacological, environmental and microbiological research has to be extended over a wide range of species to support the effective management of fish culture.

REFERENCES

Anderson, D.P., Muiswinkel van, W.B. and Roberson, B.S., 1984. Effects of chemically induced immune modulation on infectious diseases of fish. In: M. Kende, J. Gainer and M. Chirigos (eds.), Chemical regulation of immunity in Veterinary Medicine. A.R. Lisse Inc., New York, pp. 187-211.

Baggot, J.D., 1977. Principles of drug disposition in domestic animals. W.B. Saunders Co, Philadelphia/Toronto, London.

Grondel, J.L. and Boesten, H.J.A.M., 1982. The influence of antibiotics on the immune system. I. Inhibition of the mitogenic leukocyte response *in vitro* by oxytetracycline. Dev.Comp.Immunol., Suppl. 2, pp. 211-216.

Grondel, J.L., Gloudemans, A.G.M. and Muiswinkel van, W.B., 1985a. The influence of antibiotics on the immune system. II. Modulation of fish leukocyte responses in culture. Vet. Immunol. Immunopathol., 9: 251-260.

Grondel, J.L. and Muiswinkel van, W.B., 1985b. Immunological defence mechanisms as a target for antibiotics. In "Comparative Veterinary Pharmacology, Toxicology and Therapy, 3rd EAVPT congress, Ghent", Abstracts, p. 145.

Muiswinkel van, W.B., Anderson, D.P., Lamers, C.H.J., Egberts, E., Loon van, J.J.A. and IJssel, J.P., 1984. Fish immunology and fish health. Fish Immunology, M.J. Manning & M.F. Tatner, eds., Proceedings of the Plymouth Meeting 1983, Academic Press, London.

Nouws, J.F.M., Vree, T.B. and Hekster, Y.A., 1984. In vitro antimicrobial activity of hydroxy and N_4-acetyl-sulfonamide metabolites. The Veterinary Quarterly, 7: 70-72.

Nouws, J.F.M., Vree, T.B., Baakman, M., Driessens, F., H.J. Breukink and Mevius, D., 1986a. Age and dosage dependency in the plasma disposition and renal clearance of sulphamethazine and its N_4-acetyl and hydroxy metabolites in calves and cows. Am. J. Vet. Res., in press.

Nouws, J.F.M., Vree, T.B., Baakman, M., Driessens, F., Vellenga, L. and Mevius, D., 1986b. Pharmacokinetics, renal clearance, tissue distribution and residue aspects of sulphadimidine and its N_4-acetyl metabolite in pigs. The Veterinary Quarterly, 7, in press.

Rijkers, G.T., Oosterom van, R. and Muiswinkel van, W.B., 1981. The immune system of cyprinid fish. Oxytetracycline and the regulation of humoral immunity in carp. Vet. Immunol. Immunopathol., 2: 281-290.

Vree, T.B., Tijhuis, M., Baakman, M. and Hekster, Y.A., 1983. Analysis of N_4-trideuteroacetylsylphamerazine and its metabolites sulphamerazine and N_4-acetylsulphamerazine in man by means of high-performance liquid chromatography and mass spectrometry. Biomed. Mass. Spectrom., 10: 114-119.

Vree, T.B., Tijhuis, M., Nouws, J.F.M. and Hekster, Y.A., 1984. Identification, isolation, chromatography, and preliminary pharmacokinetics of 4-hydroxysulfamerazine in dogs. Pharmac. Weekbl., Sci. Ed., 6: 80-87.

Vree, T.B. and Hekster, Y.A., 1985. Pharmacokinetics of sulfonamides revisited. Antibiotics and Chemotherapy, 34: 1-208.

Veterinary Immunology and Immunopathology, 12 (1986) 287–296
Elsevier Science Publishers B.V., Amsterdam — Printed in The Netherlands

EFFECT OF AN IMMUNOPOTENTIATOR ON *AEROMONAS SALMONICIDA* INFECTION IN RAINBOW TROUT (*SALMO GAIRDNERI*)

T. KITAO AND Y. YOSHIDA

Dept. of Fisheries, Faculty of Agriculture, Miyazaki Univ., 7710 Kumano, Mayazaki 889 - 21, Japan

ABSTRACT

Kitao, T., Yoshida, T., 1986. Effect of an Immunopotentiator on *Aeromonas salmonicida* Infection in Rainbow Trout (*Salmo gairdneri*). Vet. Immunol. Immunopathol., 12: 287-296.

The immunoactive peptide FK-565 (heptanoyl-y-D-glutamyl-(L)-meso-diaminopimelyl-(D)-alanine) was found to induce protection against intraperitoneal *Aeromonas salmonicida* infection in rainbow trout (*Salmo gairdneri* Richardson). The survival rate was as high as 60% when FK-565 was given intraperitoneally as a single dose (lmg/kg) one day before bacterial challenge. A non-specific stimulation of phagocytic cells by FK-565 at an early stage of the bacterial infection may contribute to the resistance observed. The phagocytic activity of peritoneal phagocytic cells as well as phagocytic cells of the pronephros were stimulated by FK-565 *in vivo* and *in vitro*, respectively, as compared to untreated control fish. Furthermore, decreased activity of phagocytic cells previously immunosuppressed with cyclophosphamide was rapidly restored by application of FK-565.

INTRODUCTION

Chemotherapy as well as specific immunotherapy have both contributed to the control of many infectious diseases in man and animals. It is well known that phagocytes play an important role in the host defense mechanisms and it has been reported that immunostimulants, various microbial products such as Bacille Calmette-Guerin (BCG; Sher et al., 1975), *Corynebacterium parvum* (Sher et al., 1975; Berd, 1978), endotoxin (Dubos and Schaedler, 1956), glucan (Reynolds et al., 1980), krestin (Mayer and Drews, 1980), phospholipids (Fanve and Hevin, 1979), *Nocardia rubra* cell wall skeleton (Masuno et al., 1979), and the synthetic compounds, azimexon (Bicker et al., 1979), muramyl dipeptide and its analogs (Parant et al., 1980; Fraser-Smith et al., 1983; Saiki et al., 1983) and levamisole (Fisher et al., 1974) activate phagocytic functions.

Recently, in the course of extensive screening for immunostimulants, a lactoyl tetrapeptide (FK-156) was isolated from cultures of *Streptomyces olivaceogriseus* sp. nov. (Hemmi et al., 1981; Gotoh et al., 1982a; Gotoh et

0165-2427/86/$03.50 © 1986 Elsevier Science Publishers B.V.

al., 1982b; Hemmi et al.,m 1982; Kawai et al., 1982) at Fujisawa Pharmaceutical Co., Ltd. (Osaka, Japan) and a related peptide, FK-565, was synthesized and shown to be active against microbial infection in mice (Hemmi et al., 1982; Mine et al., 1983a; Mine et al., 1983b; Yokota et al., 1983). The present investigation was initiated to study the effects of FK-565 on phagocytic cells in normal and experimentally immunosuppressed rainbow trout.

MATERIALS AND METHODS

Fish

One year old rainbow trout (80-120g) were obtained from a local commercial farmer. The fish were kept in flow-through tanks holding 200 liters of dechlorinated tap water at 18-20°C. Five fish were used for each experimental and control group.

Bacterium employed

Aeromonas salmonicida strain MZ8501, isolated recently from rainbow trout suffering from furunculosis, was used throughout the experiments. The organism was grown in Mueller- Hinton broth (Difco) at 20°C. Log phase cultures were harvested by centrifugation for 10 min. at 3,000 x g, washed twice with phosphate buffered saline (PBS), and suspended in Eagle's minimum essential medium (MEM; Nissui Seiyaku Co., Tokyo) at a concentration giving an optical density of 0.4 at 620 nm, which represented approximately 10^8 cells per ml.

Immunosuppressants and preparation of immunosuppressed fish

Cyclophosphamide (Endoxan, Shionogi & Co., Ltd.) and hydrocortisone (Wako Chemical Ltd.) were used as immunosuppressants. Fish were given three injections of cyclophosphamide intraperitoneally at a dose of 100 mg/kg 5 days, 4 days and 3 days before the experiment. Hydrocortisone was given at 40 mg/kg following the same procedure.

Effect of FK-565 on A. salmonicida infection

A single dose of FK-565 (1 mg/kg) was given intraperitoneally to groups of rainbow trout at 7, 5, 3 or 1 day(s) before challenge with 10^4 cells of *A. salmonicida*. The effect of FK-565 on the bacterial infection was estimated by the survival rate of fish 6 days after injection.

Phagocytosis assay of peritoneal cells

Fish treated one day previously with FK-565, as well as untreated controls, were injected intraperitoneally with 10^8 cells of formalin killed *A. salmoni-*

cida. After 2 hr., fish were bled from the caudal vein and sacrificed. Four ml of cold MEM containing 5% fetal calf serum (Difco) and 10 units of heparin per ml were injected into the peritoneal cavity. Peritoneal fluid was harvested after slight massaging of the abdomen and filtered through glass wool. The filtrate was centrifuged for 10 min. at 800 x g. Packed cells were suspended in one ml of Eagle's MEM. The cell suspension was smeared on a glass slide, fixed with absolute methyl alcohol, and stained with Giemsa solution. The number of phagocytized cells per 1,000 peritoneal cells was counted microscopically (Sakai, 1984).

Phagocytosis assay of pronephros cells

Fish treated for 24 hr. with FK-565 and untreated control fish were exsanguinated by bleeding from the caudal peduncle. The procedure used for isolating phagocytic cells from the pronephros of rainbow trout was that described by Stave et al. (1983). Viable phagocytic cells, including neutrophils and macrophages, were adjusted to a concentration of 10^7 cells per ml in MEM. One ml of the pronephros phagocytic cells and 1 ml containing about 10^8 cells of formalin killed *A. salmonicida* were mixed in a siliconized plastic tube, sealed with a rubber stopper, and incubated in 5% CO_2 for 2 hr. at 20°C. Following the incubation, cells phagocytized by the pronephros phagocytic cells were enumerated by the method described above.

Effect of FK-565 on intracellular killing by phagocytic cells collected from the peritoneal cavity and pronephros

FK-565 was given intraperitoneally to rainbow trout at 1 mg/kg one day before the experiment. Two hr. prior to sacrificing, 0.5ml of 0.5% glycogen was inoculated into the peritoneal cavity. Phagocytic cells were collected from the peritoneal cavity and pronephros, and viable cells were suspended in Eagle's MEM at a concentration of 10^6 cells per ml. One ml of cell suspension and 1 ml containing 10^8 virulent *A. salmonicida* were placed in a siliconized plastic tube and closed with a rubber stopper. The mixture was incubated for 2 hr. at 20°C, after which the phagocytic cells were disrupted by the addition of 1% sodium dodecyl sulfate solution to a final concentration of 0.1%. The lysis was performed at 4°C. Intracellular killing of *A. salmonicida* by phagocytic cells was measured by viable cell count method described by Van Furth et al. (1978).

Restorative effect of FK-565 on phagocytic cells and number of peripheral leukocytes in immunosuppressed rainbow trout

Two intraperitoneal injections of FK-565 (1 mg/kg) were given to previously immunosuppressed rainbow trout, 3 days and 1 day before the experiment. The phagocytic activity of the peritoneal and pronephros cells was determined as described above. In addition, a comparison was made of the number of peripheral leukocytes in the caudal vein blood of FK-565 treated and untreated fish.

Statistics

Statistical analyses were performed by the Student's *t* test.

RESULTS

Experiments with normal fish

The results of treating rainbow trout with FK-565 prior to infection with *A. salmonicida* are shown in Table 1 and Fig. 1. All groups of fish treated with FK-565 had significantly greater survival rates than the untreated controls. When FK-565 was given 7, 5, or 3 days before challenge, 40% of the fish survived, compared to no survivors in the control group. The optimal protection (60% survival) was seen in the group receiving FK-565 one day before challenge, indicating that the protection is conferred fairly rapidly. The phagocytic activities of both peritoneal and pronephros cells from fish pretreated with FK-565 were also significantly enhanced compared to similar cells from untreated fish (Tables 2 and 3).

TABLE 1.
Time-dependence of the protective effect of FK-565 on *Aeromonas salmonicida* infection of rainbow trout

Treatment (Day)	Survival (%)
-7	40
-5	40
-3	40
-1	60
Control	0

Fish were given 1 mg/kg of FK-565, intraperitoneally, 7, 5, 3, or 1 day(s) prior to injection of 1 X 10^4 *A. salmonicida* cells

Comparative results on killing activity of the peritoneal and pronephros phagocytic cells from fish pretreated with FK-565 and untreated control fish are shown in Table 4. After incubation, the number of living bacteria inside peritoneal phagocytic cells from fish pretreated with FK-565 was 1.8 x 10^6 compared to 4.5 x 10^6 in the untreated controls. Similarly, the number of living bacteria in pronephros phagocytic cells from treated fish was 8 x 10^6,

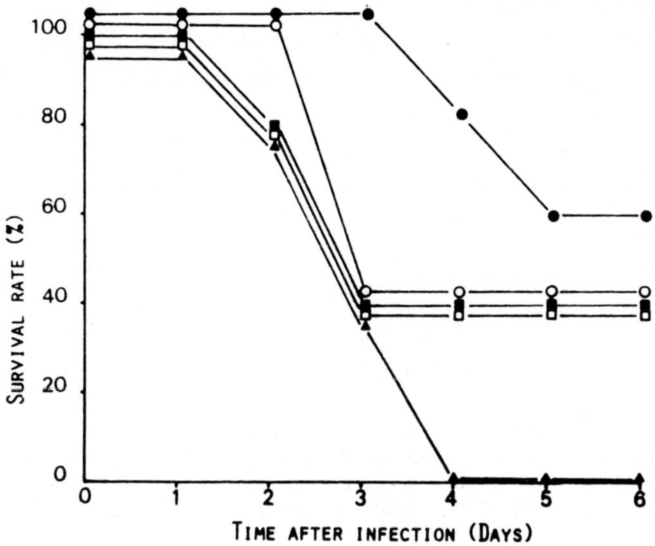

Fig. 1. Time-dependence of the protective effect of FK-565 on Aeromonas salmonicida infection in rainbow trout. Fish were given intraperitoneally 1 mg/kg of FK-565 on 7 days (□–□), 5 days (■–■), 3 days (○–○), and 1 day (●–●) before an infection. Untreated control; (▲–▲).

TABLE 2.

Phagocytic activity of peritoneal phagocytic cells from rainbow trout treated with FK-565

Treatment	Phagocytic activity[a]
FK-565	141.3[b] ± 14.5
Control	84.0 ± 9.2

Peritoneal phagocytic cells were obtained from rainbow trout 1 day after intraperitoneal injection of 1 mg/kg of FK-565.
[a] Number of phagocytized bacteria/1,000 peritoneal phagocytic cells.
[b] Significantly different ($p<0.05$) from control group.

compared to 2.2×10^7 in the control group. These data clearly demonstrate the enhancement of the killing activity of peritoneal and pronephros phagocytic cells from rainbow trout treated with FK-565, as compared to those isolated from untreated animals.

Experiments with immunosuppressed fish

The restorative effect of FK-565 on the number of peripheral leukocytes and the phagocytic activity of peritoneal and pronephros cells from fish

TABLE 3.

Phagocytic activity of pronephros phagocytic cells from rainbow trout treated with FK-565

Treatment	Phagocytic activity[a]
FK-565	153.5[b] ± 8.0
Control	84.7 ± 9.0

Pronephros phagocytic cells were obtained from rainbow trout one day after intraperitoneal injection of 1 mg/kg of FK-565.
[a] Number of phagocytized bacteria/1,000 pronephros phagocytic cells.
[b] Significantly different ($p<0.05$) from control group.

TABLE 4.

Effect of FK-565 on intracellular killing of *Aeromonas salmonicida* by phagocytic cells collected from the peritoneal cavity and pronephros of rainbow trout

Treatment	No. of viable *A. salmonicida* Peritoneal Phagocytes	Pronephros Phagocytes
FK-565	1.8 (± 1.2) x 10^6*	8.0 (± 6) x 10^6*
Control	4.5 (± 1.3) x 10^6	22 (± 10) x 10^6

* Significantly different ($p<0.05$) from control groups.

TABLE 5.

Restorative effect of FK-565 on the number of peritoneal leukocytes in immunosuppressed rainbow trout.

Treatment	No. of peripheral leukocytes/ml
None (Normal)	5.3 (± 0.4) X 10^4
Cyclophosphamide	2.5 (± 0.4) X 10^4*
Cyclophosphamide + FK-565	3.7 (± 0.5) X 10^4**
None (Normal)	5.1 (± 0.2) X 10^4
Hydrocortisone	3.1 (± 0.5) X 10^4*
Hydrocortisone + FK-565	4.0 (± 0.5) X 10^4**

* Significantly different ($p<0.05$) from normal fish.
** Significantly different ($p<0.1$) from normal fish.

immunosuppressed by cyclophosphamide and hydrocortisone are demonstrated in Tables 5 and 6. As shown in Table 5, the number of peripheral leukocytes (2.5×10^4 and 3.1×10^4 per ml) previously reduced by immunosuppressants were partially restored to normal levels (3.7×10^4 and 4.0×10^4 per ml) following application of FK-565. Similarly, the phagocytic activity of immunosuppressed phagocytic cells (49.5, 68.0, 59.5 and 65.0 phagocytized cells per 1,000 phagocytic cells) was also restored to almost the normal level (67.5, 91.5, 92.5 and 87.0 cells per 1,000 phagocytic cells) following FK-565 treatment. (Table 6).

TABLE 6.
Restorative effect of FK-565 on phagocytosis of *Aeromonas salmonicida* by peritoneal and pronephros phagocytic cells from immunosuppressed rainbow trout.

Treatment	Phagocytic activity	
	Peritoneal cells	Pronephros cells
None (Control)	84.0 ± 10.0	105.0 ± 14.8
Cyclophosphamide	49.5* ± 2.1	68.0* ± 6.8
Cyclophosphamide + FK-565	67.5 ± 17.7	91.5 ± 1.0
None (Control)	102.5 ± 17.6	96.0 ± 11.0
Hydrocortisone	59.5* ± 10.6	65.0* ± 7.1
Hydrocortisone + FK-565	92.5 ± 16.4	87.0 ± 7.0

* Significantly different ($p<0.05$) from control fish.

DISCUSSION

It has been reported that the synthetic immunoactive peptide FK-565 protects mice against microbial infection after parenteral or oral application (Mine et al., 1983a). Similarly, we have found that FK-565 induced a strong protective activity against *Aeromonas salmonicida* infection in both normal and immunosuppressed rainbow trout after parenteral application. The protection against *A. salmonicida* infection by FK-565 inoculated intraperitoneally at a single dose of 1 mg/kg only one day before microbial challenge indicates that the host defense mechanisms were enhanced by FK-565 within a short time after its administration.

It is well known that phagocytic cells play an important role in defense against microbial infection of fish (Finn and Nielson, 1971; Avtalion and Shahrabani, 1975; Ellis et al., 1976; Braun-Nesje et al., 1982; Rijkers, 1982; Griffin, 1983). Phagocytosis and killing of *A. salmonicida* by phagocytic cells isolated from the peritoneal cavity and the pronephros of rainbow trout pretreated with FK-565 were investigated by using the assay described by Van Furth et al. (1978) and Griffin (1983). The data obtained shows that phagocytic activity as well as killing rates are significantly different between FK-565 pretreated and untreated control fish.

On the other hand, there are numerous reports on the immunosuppression of fish caused by cyclophosphamide (Chen et al., 1983; Stave et al., 1983), hydrocortisone and its analogs (Bullock and Stuckey, 1975; Knittel, 1981; Anderson et al., 1982; Rickering and Dukston, 1983; Anderson et al., 1984; Stave and Roberson, 1985), and oxytetracycline (Rijkers et al., 1980). Our data obtained in immunosuppressed rainbow trout confirm previous findings that the number of peripheral leukocytes and the phagocytic activity of the peritoneal and pronephros phagocytic cells can be restored to the normal level by FK-565.

A potential application of immunopotentiators such as FK-565 may be to prevent fish diseases caused by microorganisms and to restore the defense mechanisms in immunosuppressed or immunocompromised fish in fish farms (Rijkers et al., 1980; Knittel, 1981; Anderson et al., 1984). Future studies will address the questions as to whether FK-565 exhibits a protective effect when given orally and if it has a stimulatory effect on the humoral antibody response of treated fish.

ACKNOWLEDGEMENTS

The authors would like to thank Professor F. M. Hetrick, Department of Microbiology, University of Maryland, and Dr. D. P. Anderson, National Fish Health Research Laboratory, U.S.A., for their critical review of the manuscript and numerous comments. The authors also are indebted to Fujisawa Pharmaceutical Co., Ltd., Osaka, Japan, for providing the immunoactive peptide, FK-565.

REFERENCES

Anderson, D. P., Roberson, B. S. and Dixon, O. W. 1982. Immunosuppression induced by a corticosteroid or alkylating agent in rainbow trout (*Salmo gairdneri*) administered a *Yersinia ruckeri* bacterin. Dev. Comp. Immunol. Sup., 2: 197-204.

Anderson, D. P., Van Muiswinkel, W. B. and Roberson, B. S. 1984. Effects of chemically induced immune modulation on infectious disease of fish. In: Chemical regulation of immunity in veterinary medicine, M. Keude, J. H. Gainer, and M. Chirigos (Editors). Alan R. Liss, Inc., New York, pp. 187-211.

Avtalion, R. R. and Shahrabani, S. 1975. Studies on phagocytosis in fish. I. *In vitro* uptake and killing of living *Staphylococcus aureus* by peritoneal leucocytes of carp (*Cyprinus carpio*). Immunology, 29: 1181-1187.

Berd, D. 1978. Effects of *Corynebacterium parvum* on immunity. Pharmacol. Ther., A 2: 373-395.

Bicker, V., Ziegler, A. E. and Hebold, G. 1979. Investigation of a new immunostimulant compound. J. Infect. Dis., 139: 389-395.

Braun-Nesje, R., Bertheussen, K., Kaplan, G. and Seljelid, R. 1981. Salmonid macrophages: Separation, in vitro culture and characterization. J. Fish Dis., 4: 141-151.

Braun-Nesje, R., Kaplan, G. and Seljelid, R. 1982. Rainbow trout macropages in vitro: Morphology and phagocytic activity. Dev. Comp. Immunol., 6: 281-291.

Bullock, G. L. and Stuckey, H. M. 1975. Aeromonas salmonicida: detection of asymptomatically infected trout. Prog. Fish Culturist, 37: 237-239.

Chen, M. F., Rohovec, J. S. and Fryer, J. L. 1983. Effect of methotrexate, kenalog, and cyclophosphamide on the antibody response of steelhead to Aeromonas salmonicida. Trans. Am. Fish Soc., 112: 561-564.

Dubos, R. and Schaedler, R. W. 1956. Reversible changes in the susceptibility of mice to bacterial infections. J. Exp. Med., 104: 53-65.

Ellis, A. E., Munroe, A. L. S. and Roberts, R. J. 1976. Defense mechanisms in fish. 1. A study of the phagocytic system and the fate of intraperitoneally injected particulate material in the plaice (Pleuronectes platessa L.). J. Fish Biol., 8: 67-78.

Fanve, R. M. and Hevin, B. 1974. Immunostimulation with bacterial phospholipid extracts. Proc. Nat. Acad. Sci., 71: 573.

Finn, J. P. and Nielson, N. O. 1971. The inflammatory response of rainbow trout. J. Fish Biol., 3: 463-478.

Fisher, G. W., Oi, V. T., Kelley, J. L., Pogore, J. K., Bass, J. W., Wagner, F. S. and Gordon, B. L. 1974. Enhancement of host defense mechanisms against gram-positive pygonic coccal infections with levotetramisole (levamisole) in neonatal rat. Ann. Allergy, 33:193-198.

Fraser-Smith, E. B., Eppstein, D. A., Larsen, M. A. and Matthews, T. R. 1983. Protective effect of muramyl dipeptide analog encapsulated in or mixed with liposomes against Candida albicans infection. Infect. Immun., 39: 172-178.

Gotoh, T., Nakahara, K., Iwai, M., Aoki, M. and Imanaka, H. 1982a. Studies on a new immunoactive peptide, FK-156. I. Taxonomy of the producing strains. J. Antibiotics, 35: 1280-1285.

Gotoh, T., Nakahara, K., Nishimura, T., Hashimoto, M., Kino, T., Kuroda, Y., Okuhara, M., Kohsaka, M., Aoki, M. and Imanaka, H. 1982b. Studies on a new immunoactive peptide, FK-156. II. Fermentation, extraction and chemical and biological characterization. J. Antibiotics, 35: 1286-1292.

Griffin, B. R. 1983. Opsonic effect of rainbow trout (Salmo gairdneri) antibody on phagocytosis of Yersinia ruckeri by trout leukocytes. Dev. Comp. Immunol., 7: 253-259.

Hemmi, K., Takeno, H., Okada, S., Nakaguchi, O., Kitamura, Y. and Hashimoto, H. 1981. Total synthesis of FK-156 isolated from a Streptomyces as immunostimulating peptide: Application of a novel copper chelate amino protein. J. Am. Chem. Soc., 103: 1181-1187.

Hemmi, K., Aratani, M., Takeno, H., Okada, S., Miyazaki, Y., Nakaguchi, O., Kitamura, Y. and Hashimoto, M. 1982. Studies on a new immunoactive peptide, FK-156. IV. Synthesis of FK-156 and its geometric isomer. J. Antibiotics, 35: 1300-1311.

Kawai, Y., Nakahara, K., Gotoh, T., Uchida, I., Tanaka, M. and Imanaka, H. 1982. Studies on a new immunoactive peptide, FK-156. III. Structure elucidation. J. Antibiotics, 35: 1293-1299.

Knittel, M. D. 1981. Susceptibility of steelhead trout Salmo gairdneri Richardson to redmouth infection Yersinia ruckeri following exposure to copper. J. Fish Dis., 4: 33-40.

Mayer, P. and Drews, J. 1980. The effect of a protein-bound polysaccharide from Coriolus versicolor on immunological parameters and experimental infections in mice. Infection, 8: 13-21.

Mine, Y., Yokota, Y., Wakai, Y., Fukada, S., Nishida, M., Goto, S. and Kuwahara, S. 1983a. Immunoactive peptides, FK-156 and FK-565. I. Enhancement of host resistance to microbial infection in mice. J. Antibiotics, 36: 1045-1050.

Mine, Y., Watanabe, Y., Tawara, S., Yokota, Y., Nishida, M., Goto, S. and Kuwahara, S. 1983b. III. Enhancement of host defense mechanisms against infection. J. Antibiotics, 36: 1059-1066.

Msuno, T., Ito, M., Ogura, T., Hirano, F., Yamawaki, M., Azuma, I. and Yamamura, Y. 1979. Activation of peritoneal macrophage by oil-attached cell-wall skeleton of BCG and Nocardia rubra. Gann, 70: 223-227.

Parant, M., Audibert, F., Chedid, L., Level, M., Lefrancier, P., Choay, J. and Lederer, E. 1980. Immunostimulant activities of lipophilic muramyl dipeptide derivatives and of desmuramyl peptidolipid analogs. Infect. Immun., 27: 826-831.

Pickering, A. D. and Duston, J. 1983. Administration of cortisol to brown trout, Salmo trutta L., and its effects on the susceptibility to Saprolegnia infection and furunculosis. J. Fish Biol., 23: 163-175.

Reynolds, J. A., Kastello, M. D., Harrington, D. G., Crabbs, C. L., Peters, C. J., Jemski, J. V., Scott, G. H. and Luzio, R. D. 1980. Glucan-induced enhancement of host resistance to selected infectious diseases. Infect. Immun., 30: 51-57.

Rijkers, G. T., Teunissen, A. G., Van Oosterom, R. and Van Muiswinkel, W. B. 1980. The immune system of cyprinid fish. The immunosuppressive effect of the antibiotic oxytetracycline in carp (Cyprinus carpio). Aquaculture, 19: 177-189.

Rijkers, G. T. 1982. Non-lymphoid defense mechanism in fish. Dev. Comp. Immun., 6: 1-13.

Saiki, I., Tokushima, Y., Nishimura, K., Yamamura, Y. and Azuma, I. 1983. Activation of macrophages by quinonyl-N-acetyl-muramyl dipeptide. Infect. Immun., 40: 622-628.

Sakai, D. K. 1984. Opsonization by fish antibody and complement in immune phagocytosis by peritoneal exudate cells isolated from salmonid fishes. J. Fish Diseases, 7: 29-38.

Sher, N. A., Chaparas, S. D., Greenberg, L. E. and Bernard, S., 1975. Effect of BCG, Corynebacterium parvum, and methanol-extraction residue in the reduction of mortality from Staphylococcus aureus and Candida albicans infection in immunosuppressed mice. Infect. Immun., 12: 1325-1330.

Stave, J. W., Roberson, B. S. and Hetrick, F. M. 1983. Chemiluminescence of phagocytic cells isolated from the pronephros of striped bass. Dev. Comp. Immunol., 7: 269-276.

Stave, J. W., and Roberson, B. S. 1985. Hydrocortisone suppressed the chemiluminescent response of striped bass phagocytes. Dev. Comp. Immunol., 9: 77-84.

Van Furth, R., Van Zwet, T. L. and Leijh, P. C. J. 1978. In vitro determination of phagocytosis and intracellular killing by polymorphonuclear and mononuclear phagocytes. In: D. M. Weir (Editor), Handbook of experimental immunology: Application of immunological methods, Vol. 3. Blackwell Sci. Public. Oxford, pp. 32.1-32.19.

Yokota, Y., Mine, Y., Wakai, Y., Watanabe, Y., Nishida, M., Goto, S. and Kuwahara, S. 1983. Immunoactive peptides, FK-156 and FK-565. II. Restoration of host resistance to microbial infection in immunosuppressed mice. J. Antibiotics, 36: 1051-1058.

Veterinary Immunology and Immunopathology, 12 (1986) 297—304
Elsevier Science Publishers B.V., Amsterdam — Printed in The Netherlands

MODULARY EFFECTS OF TEMPERATURE ON ANTIBODY RESPONSE AND SPECIFIC RESISTANCE TO CHALLENGE OF CHANNEL CATFISH, *Ictalurus punctatus*, IMMUNIZED AGAINST *Edwardsiella ictaluri*

J. A. Plumb, M. L. Wise and W. A. Rogers. Department of Fisheries and Allied Aquacultures, Alabama Agricultural Experiment Station, Auburn University, Alabama 36849 USA

ABSTRACT

Plumb, J. A., Wise, M. L. and Rogers, W. A. 1986 Modulary effects of temperature on antibody response and specific resistance to challenge of channel catfish, *Ictalurus punctatus*, immunized against *Edwardsiella ictaluri*. Vet. Immunol. Immunopathol., 12: 297-304.

The effects of various temperature treatments on the level of the humoral antibody response in channel catfish immunized with formalin killed *Edwardsiella ictaluri* was determined in laboratory controlled experiments. Immunized fish that were held at 25°C for 30 days and 12°C for an additional 30 days had higher antibody titers, and were more protected upon challenge, than immunized fish held at 25°C for 60 days. Also immunized catfish held at 25°C for 5 or 10 days followed by 12°C water had higher antibody titers than immunized fish held at 12°C or 25°C for 60 days.

In a field experiment carried out during winter and spring (February-May) fingerling channel catfish were vaccinated with *E. ictaluri* using intraperitoneal injection or immersion with either sonicated or whole cell preparations. Following challenge, the fish vaccinated by immersion in the sonicated preparation had 11.8% mortality whereas the groups immersed in whole cell bacterin, injected with the whole cell bacterin in adjuvant, or injected with sonicate showed 24.6, 57.9 and 41.7% mortality, respectively. Although the fish vaccinated by immersion with the sonicated bacteria had lower antibody titers than those vaccinated by the other methods the immersion vaccinates were more protected against challenge with the pathogen.

INTRODUCTION

In recent years the study of fish immunology has been intensified due to the interest in developing vaccines for immunization application in fish culture. The high cost of chemical treatments and legislation restricting its use (Horner, 1983; Herman, 1970) makes immunization an attractive approach to disease control. The most significant advances in fish vaccinations have occurred in salmonid culture where vaccines against vibriosis and enteric redmouth disease are routinely used (Fryer et al., 1976, 1977; Busch, 1982, Tebbit and Goodrich, 1982). The use of vaccines in the catfish culture industry is non-existant because economical and effective vaccines against the most common pathogens of this species have not been developed. The bacterial pathogen *Edwardsiella ictaluri* (Hawke et al., 1981), commonly encountered in

0165-2427/86/$03.50 © 1986 Elsevier Science Publishers B.V.

cultured catfish, may prove to be an excellent candidate for vaccine development.

One of the problems confronting vaccine use in fish is the suppressive effect of low temperature on the humoral immune response of fish (Avtalion, 1981). Incidence of many fish pathogens in the southeastern United States, including E. ictaluri, occurs most frequently during the spring and early summer when water temperatures are rapidly rising (Plumb, 1975, Meyer, 1970). Vaccination during the winter, immediately prior to the expected occurance of a disease, may not appear practicable, however, it might be possible to vaccinate fish in the fall while water temperatures are still warm and induce protective immunity which would last until the following spring. More thorough understanding of the effect of temperature on the immune response of channel catfish would be of great value in implementing such a managment plan.

These experiments were initiated to investigate the effect of temperature modulation which occur during winter, and under controlled laboratory conditions, on the longevity and protectiveness of humoral immunity in channel catfish immunized against E. ictaluri.

MATERIALS AND METHODS

Edwardsiella ictaluri (ATCC# 33202) (Hawke, 1979; Hawke et al., 1981) was grown in 1 L of brain heart infusion (BHI) broth overnight at 25 C with constant shaking. Cells were harvested by centrifugation, resuspended in sterile 0.85% NaCl, and killed with 1% formalin. The bacteria were washed in saline and resuspended to a volume of 6 ml, tested for sterility and 0.1% formalin added for preservation before lyophilization. The lyophilized bacterin was resuspended in a sterile 0.85% NaCl solution so that each 0.1 ml of solution contained 20 mg (dry weight) of bacteria. A 0.5 L BHI broth culture of E. ictaluri was concentrated into 15 ml of saline and sonicated at 8 kilocycles for 1 minute. A 1 L undiluted culture was similarly sonicated. A whole cell vaccine was prepared by the above culture methods, however the cells were killed with 1% formalin.

Channel catfish (Ictalurus punctatus), ranging from 70 to 120 g, each were acclimated to laboratory conditions before experimentation. For the temperature modulation studies each fish was injected intraperitoneally (IP) at a rate of 2.0 mg per kilogram. Non-vaccinated fish were injected IP with sterile 0.85% NaCl. In the winter vaccination study fish were vaccinated by IP injection of a concentrated vaccine of either whole or sonicated cells, or immersed for 5 minutes in a whole or sonicated cell solution.

Blood samples were obtained by venipuncture of the caudal vessels and the sera were stored at 4°C until tested using the microagglutination technique

(Conrath 1972). Sera were heated at 45°C for 30 minutes and then double serially diluted with 0.85% NaCl in microtiter plates. A 0.05 ml of antigen was added to each well to test for agglutination. Plates were covered and read at 24 hr.

Antibody titers were compared using the non-parametric Mann-Whitney test (Zar, 1974). Results from the challenge experiments were analyzed by the Fisher exact test of 2x2 contingency tables when the total sample size was less than 30. All data were analyzed at the 95% confidence level unless otherwise noted.

RESULTS

Results of immunizing channel catfish in January and analysis of their immune response in May are summarized in Tables 1 and 2. These fish were immunized on January 28, 1985 by immersion or IP injection using either a formalin killed whole cell or sonicated *E. ictaluri* preparation, and held at 25°C for 4 days prior to stocking in an earthen pond. The pond temperature ranged from 7°C to 28°C (average 17.3°C). Fish that were vaccinated by immersion had the lowest mortality; 27% for those immersed in the sonicated vaccine and 29% in the whole cell immersed fish (Table 1). Sonicate, whole cell and non-immunized (saline) injected fish had 63%, 68% and 42% mortality respectively, while in the pond. On May 29, 1985, all fish were harvested and sera collected from 20 fish in each group and the remaining survivors challenged with virulent *E. ictaluri* by immersion in a solution containing 3.9 x 10^6 cells per ml for 1 hr. Following challenge of the immunized fish, the sonicate immersed fish had 11.8% mortality (Table 2). The whole cell immersed, sonicate injected, whole cell injected and non-immunized groups had 24.6%, 41.7%, 57.9% and 46% mortality, respectively.

Table 1. Natural mortality occurring during winter time in channel catfish fingerlings, nonvaccinated or vaccinated with sonicated or formalin killed vaccine either by immersion or by intraperitoneal injection.

	Sonicated Vaccine		Whole cell Vaccine		Control
	Immersed	Injected	Immersed	Injected	
Number stocked	120	120	120	120	120
Number harvested	88	44	85	39	70
Percent mortality	27	63	29	68	42

When the immunized fish were removed from the pond their antibody titers were low (Table 2). The sonicated and whole cell immersed fish had titers of 1:2 compared to 1:14, 1:16 and 0, respectively, for the sonicate injected, whole cell injected and non-immunzed groups. Twenty three days after challenge, titers of all groups, including non-immunized fish, increased (Table 2).

Table 2. Results of channel catfish vaccinated on January 28, 1985, and challenged on May 29 by bathing the fish in a solution containing 3.9 x 10^6 E. ictaluri cells per ml for 0.1 hr.

	Sonicated Vaccine		Whole cell Vaccine		
	Immersed	Injected	Immersed	Injected	Non-immunize
Mortality/Total	8/22	10/22	16/65	11/9	23/50
Percent mortality	11.8	41.7	24.6	57.9	46
Mean Antibody Titers (Log_2)					
Pre-challenge[a]	2	4.0	2	5	0
Post-challenge[b]	6.4	7	6.5	6	5.1

[a]Serum collected 4 months after vaccination

[b]Serum collected 23 days after challenge

Figures 1-3 illustrate the immune response of catfish immunized by injection of formalin killed E. ictaluri and then held at 12°C or 25°C for various lengths of time. Channel catfish were injected with E. ictaluri and held at 25°C for 60 days while a second immunized group were held at 25°C for 30 days and then at 12°C for an additional 30 days. During the study period humoral antibody levels were measured and at termination of the experiment the fish were challenged (injection) with two concentrations of virulent E. ictaluri. Upon challenge, fish on which temperature was reduced to 12°C were protected against 0.6 mg and 0.3 mg of virulent bacteria, but the non-immunized fish were not protected (Fig. 1). Fish that were immunized and held at 25°C for 60 days were not resistant to the 0.6 mg challenge. Antibody levels of immunized fish held at the two temperature regimes expressed similar antibody responses through the first 30 days. However, antibody titers of fish maintained at 25°C for 60 days dropped below the titers of fish reduced to 12°C at day 30 (Fig. 2).

To determine the time required at 25°C after vaccination for a humoral response to E. ictaluri, groups of 12 catfish were immunized by injection as previously described. These immunized fish were held for 5 days (Group A), 10 days (Group B) or 0 days (Group C) at 25°C and then temperature reduced to 12°C. Group D was injected with saline and treated as group A to serve as non-immunized control; group E was immunized and held at 25°C for 60 days. Sera were taken from a random sample of 10 fish prior to immunization and at days 30 and 60 post immunization. Fish that were held at 25°C for 5 and 10 days prior

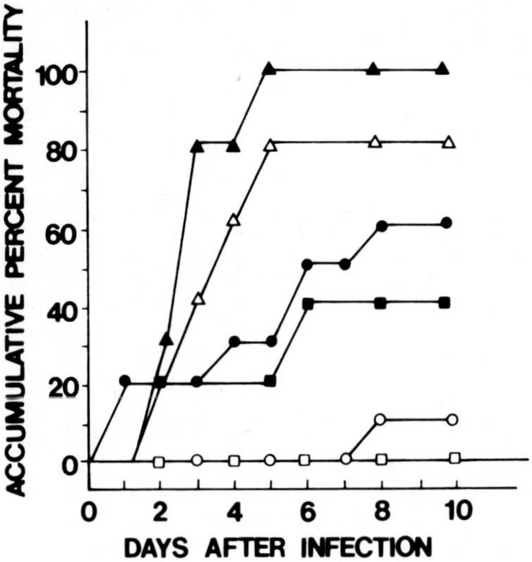

Fig. 1. Accumulative percentage of mortality of vaccinated (open symbols) and nonvaccinated (solid symbols) channel catfish challenged with E. ictaluri. Fish were held at 25°C for 30 days and an additional 30 days at 12°C then challenged with 0.6 mg of bacteria (●,○) or 0.3 mg of bacteria (■,□) or at 25°C for 60 days and challenged with 0.6 mg of bacteria (▲,△).

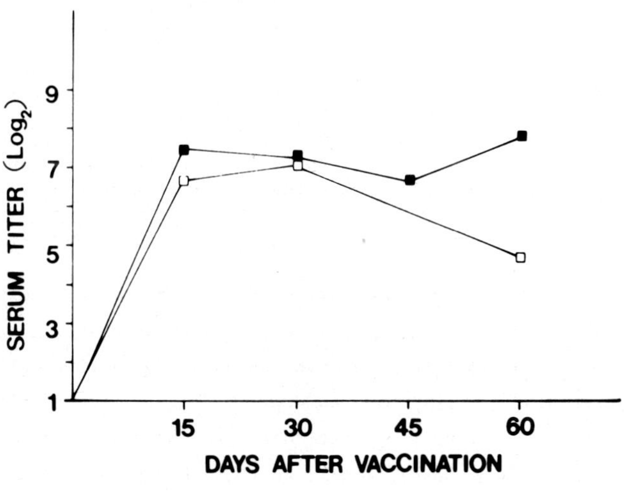

Fig. 2. Antibody titers of channel catfish vaccinated with E. ictaluri and held at 25°C for 30 days and then at 12°C for 30 additional days (■) or held at 25°C for 60 days (□).

to reducing the temperature to 12°C produced significantly higher antibody titers ($P<0.05$) than the other immunized groups (Fig. 3). Antibody titers of fish immunized and held at 12°C for 60 days produced antibody very slowly.

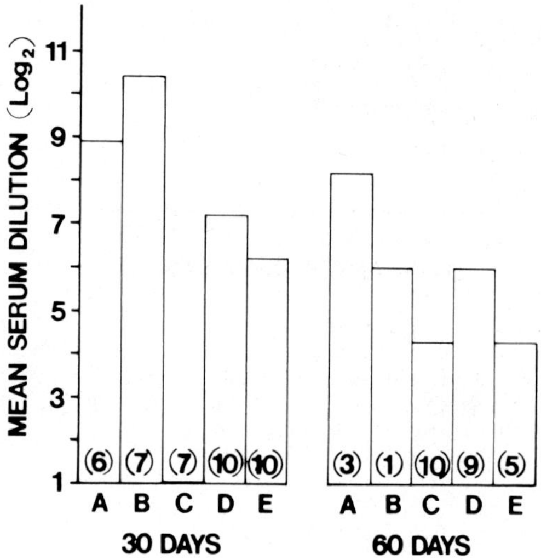

Fig. 3. Temperature effect on antibody titers of channel catfish vaccinated with *E. ictaluri* and bled at 30 and 60 days post vaccinated. A, Vaccinated and held at 25°C for 5 days then at 12°C. B, Vaccinated and held at 25°C for 10 days and then 12°C. C, Vaccinated and held at 12°C for 60 days. D, Saline injected controls with temperature treatment as "B". E, Vaccinated and held at 25°C for 60 days. Number inside of bars is the number of samples.

DISCUSSION

These studies indicate that channel catfish can be immunized by either injection or immersion during cold temperatures, as long as the fish are held in warm water for 4 to 5 days prior to cold water exposure. The fish will develop humoral antibodies and will have some protection against challenge 2 to 4 months later. Data even strongly suggest that a cool temperature is more desirable for maximum antibody level, longer antibody duration, and better protection than continuous exposure to warm temperatures.

Some data collected in these studies concur with previous results, but there are also some contradictions. Saeed (1983) demonstrated that vaccination with lipopolysaccharide and adjuvant was necessary to elicite a protective humoral antibody response. The winter immunization data showed that immunization by injection with adjuvant was not protective but immunization by immersion was protective even though the injection produced higher antibody titers.

In the experiment to demonstrate protective immunity against an injected challenge (Fig. 1) some groups did not show strong protection, however mortality in the vaccinated fish was delayed. These data indicated that immunity was partially protective and the challenge inoculum probably overwhelmed immunity. In the winter vaccination study, the immersion challenge with *E. ictaluri* appeared to serve as a booster vaccination (Table 2). This is demonstrated by the higher antibody titers of immunized fish, which ranged from 1:32 to 1:64, compared to the titers of the control fish which averaged 1:18 (1:8 to 1:32) following challenge. This should be further evaluated using a killed vaccine as a booster.

ACKNOWLEDGEMENTS

This research was supported by USDA/SEA Grant No. 59-2011-1-2-073-0, Southeastern Cooperative Fish Disease Project, and Aquatic Animal Regional Cooperative Research S-168.

REFERENCES

Avtalion, R. R. 1981. Environmental control of the immune response in fish. CRC Critical Rev. Environ. Contr. 11, 163.

Busch, R. A. 1982. Enteric redmouth disease. In: D. P. Anderson, M. Dorson, Ph. Dubouget (Editors). Antigens of Fish Pathogens. Foundation Merieux. Lyons, France, pp. 201-222.

Conrath, T. B. 1972. Handbook of Microtiter Procedures. Dynatech Corporation. Cambridge, Massachusettes.

Fryer, J. L., Rohvec, J. S., Tebbet, G. L., McMicheal, J. S., and Pilcher, K. S. 1976. Vaccination for control of infectious diseases in Pacific salmon. Fish Path. 10:155-164.

Fryer, J. L., Amend, D. F., Harrell, W. L., Novotny, A. J., Plumb, J. A., Rohvec, J. S., Tebbet, G. L. 1977. Development of bacterins and vaccines for control of infectious diseases in fish. Oregon State University Sea Grant Program, Publication Number ORESU-T-77-012. 10 pp.

Hawke, J. P. 1979. A bacterium associated with disease of cultured channel catfish (*Ictaluris punctatus*). J. Fish. Res. Board Can. 36:1508-1512.

Hawke, J. P., McWhorter, A. C., Steigerwalt, A. G. and Brenner, D. J. 1981. *Edwardsiella ictaluri* sp. nov. the causitive agent of enteric septicemia of catfish. Internat. J. Syst. Bacteriol. 31:396-400.

Herman, R. L. 1970. Prevention and control of fish diseases in hatcheries. In: S. F. Snieszko (Editor). A Symposium on Diseases of Fishes and Shellfishes. Special Publication Number 5. American Fisheries Society. Washington, D.C. pp. 3-16.

Horner, R. W. 1983. Chemotherapy. In: F. P. Meyer, J. W. Warren, T. G. Carey (Editors). A guide to Integrated Fish Health Management in the Great Lakes Basin. Special Publication Number 83-2. Great Lakes Fishery Commission. Ann Arbor, Michigan pp. 99-111.

Meyer, F. P. 1970. Seasonal fluctuations in the incidence of disease on fish farms. In: S. F. Snieszko (Editor). A Symposium on Diseases of Fishes and Shellfishes. Special Publication Number 5. American Fisheries Society. Washington D.C. pp. 21-29.

Plumb, J. A. 1975. An 11 year summary of fish disease cases at the Southeastern Fish Disease Laboratory. Proc. Ann. Conf. Southeast. Assoc. Game and Fish Comm. 29:254-266.

Saeed, M. O. 1983. Chemical characterization of the lipopolysaccharide of Edwardsiella ictaluri and the immune response of channel catfish to this fraction and to whole cell antigen with histopathologic comparisons. Doctoral dissertation, Auburn University, Auburn, Alabama. 80 pages.

Tebbit, G. L. and Goodrich, T. D. 1982. Vibriosis and the development of effective vaccines. In: D. P. Anderson, M. Dorsn, Ph. Dubourget (Editors). Antigens of Fish Pathogens. Foundation Merieux. Lyons, France, pp. 225-250.

Zar, J. H. 1974. Biostatistical Analysis. Prentiss Hall, Inc., Englewood Cliffs, New Jersey. 420 pages.

Veterinary Immunology and Immunopathology, 12 (1986) 305—311
Elsevier Science Publishers B.V., Amsterdam — Printed in The Netherlands

EFFECT OF EXOGENOUS CORTICOSTEROIDS ON CIRCULATING VIRUS AND NEUTRALIZING ANTIBODIES IN STRIPED BASS (Morone saxatilis) INFECTED WITH INFECTIOUS PANCREATIC NECROSIS VIRUS.

S.J. WECHSLER[1], P.E. McALLISTER[2], F.M. HETRICK[3] and D.P. ANDERSON[2]

[1]Cooperative Fish and Wildlife Research Unit, 117 Newins-Ziegler, University of Florida, Gainesville, Fl 32611, USA

[2]U.S. Fish and Wildlife Service, National Fish Health Research Center, Box 700, Kearneysville, WV 25430, USA

[3]Department of Microbiology, University of Maryland, College Park, MD 20742, USA

ABSTRACT

Wechsler, S.J., McAllister, P.E., Hetrick, F.M. and Anderson, D.P., 1986. Effect of exogenous corticosteroids on circulating virus and neutralizing antibodies in striped bass (Morone saxatilis) infected with infectious pancreatic necrosis virus. Vet. Immunol. Immunopathol., 12: 305-311.

Corticosteroids have been reported to induce immunosuppression in fish exposed to many types of bacterial antigens. We document a similar phenomenon in fish exposed to infectious pancreatic necrosis virus (IPNV). Fingerling striped bass that were injected with the steroid triamcinolone acetonide (100 mg/kg body weight) 24 hours before receiving intraperitoneal inoculation with IPNV became viremic 3 days post inoculation (dpi) and virus was still detected in the buffy coat cells 14 dpi. In contrast, viremia could not be detected after 7 dpi in fish that received virus but not steroids.

Circulating virus neutralizing antibodies were first detected in steroid treated fish at 10 dpi compared to 7 dpi for the virus injected fish and titers were consistently lower in the steroid group. Steroid treatment of chronic IPNV-carriers did not induce detectable viremia nor alter circulating antibody levels in chronic IPNV-carriers. None of the striped bass demonstrated clinical signs of viral disease.

INTRODUCTION

Corticosteroids have been reported to induce immunosupression in fish exposed to many different types of bacterial antigens; however, few data are available on their effects on the immune response to viral infection of fish.

The goal of the present study was to investigate the effects of corticosteroids on viremia and circulating virus - neutralizing antibodies in striped bass (Morone saxatilis) that were experimentally infected with infectious pancreatic necrosis virus (IPNV).

0165-2427/86/$03.50 © 1986 Elsevier Science Publishers B.V.

We clearly demonstrated that corticosteroids given striped bass before virus inoculation extended the duration of viremia and reduced development of circulating neutralizing antibodies. Steroid administration to long-term virus carriers caused neither viremia nor a change in neutralizing antibodies.

MATERIALS AND METHODS

Cell culture and virus

Chinook salmon embryo (CHSE-214) cells were grown at 18°C in Eagle's minimal essential medium (MEM, Flow Laboratories, McLean, VA) containing 10% fetal bovine serum (Rehatuin, Armour Pharmaceuticals, Tarrytown, NY), 200 IU/mL penicillin and 200 ug/mL streptomycin (P/S, both from Sigma, St. Louis, MO). We used IPNV originally isolated from moribund striped bass (Schutz et al., 1984). It was passaged twice in CHSE-214, aliquots were frozen at -70°C, then thawed and diluted in phosphate buffered saline (PBS, pH 7.2).

Drugs

Fish were anesthetized with tricaine methanesulfonate (MS-222, Crescent Research Chemicals, Paradise Valley, AZ) for all injection and sampling procedures. Triamcinolone acetonide (KENALOG-40; E.R. Squibb and Sons, Inc., Princeton, NJ) was injected i.p. at a dose of 100 mg/kg body weight).

Fish

Striped bass fingerlings obtained from Harrison Lake (VA) National Fish Hatchery were held at 21°C and fed commercial pelleted trout food daily.

Virus plaque assay

Following the procedure of Wolf and Quimby (1973), each sample dilution was inoculated in duplicate wells of 8-well tissue culture plates containing drained CHSE monolayers, incubated for 1 hour at 19°C to allow adsorption of the virus to cells, after which they were overlayed with MEM with and without 1% agarose (SeaKem, FMC Corp., Rockland, ME), 2% newborn calf serum (Flow Laboratories) and 0.16 M Tris buffer. After 48 hours incubation at 18°C, cell sheets were fixed, stained and plaques counted. Virus titers were calculated as plaque forming units (PFU) per mL.

Virus assay of fish tissues

Anterior and posterior kidneys, spleen, and liver were removed, weighed individually, ground to a paste 90 mesh Norton alundum RR (Fisher Sci. Co.). The paste was suspended 1:10 (w/v) dilution in PBS and centrifuged (30 min, 4°C, 1500 G) to sediment debris. The supernatant liquid was diluted in PBS and assayed for virus as described above.

Experimental protocol

Chronic IPNV-carriers were inoculated with 10^5 PFU of virus 7 and 11 months before the onset of this investigation. Two weeks before steroid injection, selected fish were sacrificed and their organs were assayed to confirm 100% incidence of carriers. Groups of unexposed fish were divided into four groups: (1) normal control - injected with PBS, (2) steroid control - injected with steroid followed 24 hours later with PBS, (3) virus control (V)- injected with 10^7 PFU of IPNV and (4) steroid + virus (SV)- injected with steroid 24 hours before inoculation with IPNV. Initially all fish were anesthetized, weighed and a blood sample was taken using a 20 gauge needle to tap the caudal vein. A heparinized microhematocrit capillary tube (American Scientific Products, McGraw Park, IL) was filled. Half of the fish in each group were bled at 3 days post inoculation (dpi) and the other half were bled at 7 dpi. Each fish was bled weekly thereafter. Within 2 hours after the blood samples were collected, they were centrifuged (International Micro-capillary centrifuge, International Equipment Co., Boston, MA) (5 min, 25°C) and processed immediately as described below.

Preparation of blood samples for virus assay

The buffy coat (about 1 uL) was cut from the microhematocrit tube at the interface of cells and plasma, put into 0.5 mL sterile distilled water with P/S, and incubated at 19°C for 1 hour to lyse cells and release virus. Plasma and lysed blood cells were diluted in PBS and immediately assayed for virus.

Neutralization Antibody Assay

Ten microliters of plasma were added to 1.0 mL PBS, heated to inactivate complement, and stored at 4°C. Plasma samples were further diluted 1:500, 1:1000, and 1:5000 in PBS. Equal volumes of diluted virus and sample were mixed, incubated at 19°C for 1 hour and assayed by virus plaque assay. Titers of plasma were recorded as the reciprocal of the dilution that neutralized 50% of virus plaques (Reed and Muench, 1938).

Statistical analysis

A Hewlett-Packard (Ft. Collins, CO) Series 9800 Desk Top computer was used to perform paired T-tests.

RESULTS

Virus recovery from blood samples is documented in Table 1. Virus titers of fish in both virus only (V) and steroid plus virus (SV) groups were of the same magnitude (10^4-10^5 PFU/mL). No fish demonstrated any clinical signs of viral disease.

TABLE 1

Virus recovery from blood samples of fingerlings inoculated with infectious pancreatic necrosis virus following administration of steroids.

Treat-ment	Sample	Days post injection					
		3	7	10	14	17	21
		Percent recovery of virus					
Steroid + IPNV[a]	buffy coat	100	100	0	33	0	0
	plasma	33	0	0	0	0	0
IPNV[b]	buffy coat	33	100	0	0	0	0
	plasma	0	0	0	0	0	0
Controls[c]	buffy coat	0	0	0	0	0	0
	plasma	0	0	0	0	0	0

[a]Fingerlings received Kenalog-40 (100 mg/kg) 24 hours before intraperitoneal inoculation with IPNV.
[b]Fingerlings received phosphate buffered saline (PBS) 24 hours before inoculation with IPNV.
[c]Fingerlings that were not injected or that received injections of PBS.

Levels of circulating virus-neutralizing antibodies were first detected in V fish at 7 dpi (Fig. 1A), concurrent with viremia. At 10 dpi all fish had neutralizing antibodies (Fig. 1B) although titers in V fish were much higher than those in SV fish. There was a noticeable, but not significant, difference in antibody titers in V fish bled at 3 dpi compared with values from fish sampled at 7 dpi.

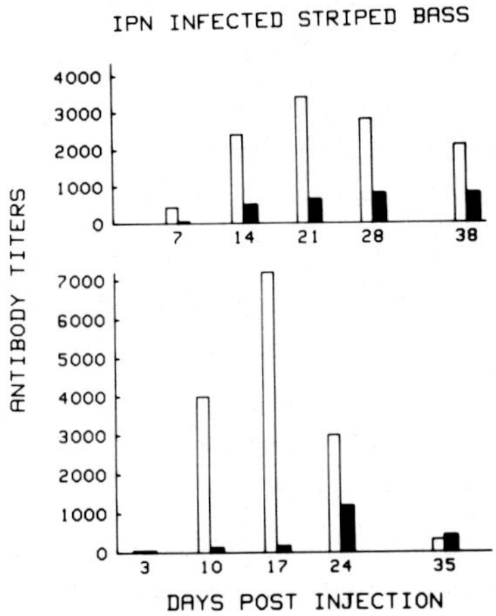

Fig. 1. Comparison of circulating neutralizing antibodies in striped bass injected with IPNV. (□) Fish that received only virus. (■) Fish that received exogenous steroid (100 mg/kg body weight) before inoculation with IPNV. Bar graphs indicate the mean (n = 3) 50% neutralizing antibody titers.

There was 30% mortality in chronic carrier fish inoculated with steroid within the first 2 weeks. Although virus was consistently isolated from the anterior kidneys of fish that died, the titers were low (10^2-10^3 PFU/mL) and of a magnitude similar those obtained from fish assayed prior to steroid injection. No virus was isolated from the blood of carrier fish nor were antibody titers affected (data not shown).

DISCUSSION

Viremia was more persistent in striped bass that received steroids (SV) before inoculation with IPNV than in those (V) which received virus but not steroids. The V group had no detectable virus in the blood after 7 dpi. Brown trout (Salmo trutta) and carp (Cyprinus carpio) have been reported to clear the bacteriophage MS2 in a similar time period (O'Neill, 1980). In contrast, virus was present 14 dpi in SV fish. The semisynthetic corticosteroid Kenalog affects mammalian adrenal function for a least 30 days, although clinical response to the drug usually abates within 2 weeks. The time required for the steroid to be cleared in striped bass has not been determined: however, the SV fish cleared virus from their blood after 15 days following steroid treatment suggesting that the effect of the drug on the humoral response system was diminished by this time.

The lack of virus in the plasma of most samples agrees with the findings of Swanson and Gillespie (1982). Our results from pilot studies also confirm their report that virus is isolated most consistently if the samples are assayed immediately. Unlike the previous authors who purified blood cells over Ficoll, we used a simple separation procedure that permitted virus assay of smaller blood volumes. Detection of virus at concentrations lower than those detected in this study is possible if white blood cells are co-cultured with virus susceptible cells (Yu et al, 1982).

We demonstrated that striped bass infected with IPNV are stimulated to produce circulating neutralizing antibodies, the levels of which can be depressed by exogenous corticosteroids. In V fish circulating neutralizing antibodies were first detected 7 dpi. Antibody levels reached their peak values between 14 and 21 days, thus following the same temporal pattern reported for response of fish exposed to other viruses and bacteriophage (Sigel and Clem, 1965; O'Neill, 1979; O'Neill, 1980). In SV fish, the appearance of antibodies followed a delayed pattern. Antibodies first appeared at 10 dpi, peaked between 21 and 28 days and were significantly reduced in magnitude. A similar corticosteroid induced depression of antibody production has been reported in trout that were exposed to bacterial antigens (Anderson et al., 1982).

Neutralizing antibody titers in striped bass inoculated with IPNV were similar in magnitude to titers reported in IPNV infected trout (Wolf and Quimby, 1969; Yamamoto, 1975). Our long-term (7 to 11 month) IPNV-carriers had no detectable antibodies and adminstration of steroids did not result in changes in circulating virus or antibody levels. When assayed 2 to 3 months after original virus inoculation, fish from this group did have antibodies. Levels of antibodies decreased with time, even though the fish maintained a chronic, low level infection of IPNV that could be isolated from the major immune tissues: anterior kidney, spleen, and leukocytes (unpublished data; Wolf and Quimby, 1969; Yamamoto, 1975b). An unenveloped, RNA virus, IPNV matures intracellularly and is released by lysis of the cell (Hill, 1982). Presumably the virus is not exposed to antibodies until the cytolytic event, thus it can successfully survive within the host cells.

Clearly, exogenous corticosteroids depress the humoral immune response of striped bass but this immunosuppression was not sufficient to cause clinical disease due to infections pancreatic necrosis virus.

REFERENCES

Anderson, D.P, Roberson, B.S. and Dixon, O.W., 1982. Immunosuppression induced by a corticosteroid or an alkylating agent in rainbow trout (Salmo gairdneri) administered a Yersinia ruckeri bacterin. Dev. Comp. Immunol., Supplement 2: 197-204.

Hill, B.J., 1982. Infectious pancreatic necrosis virus and its virulence. In: R.J. Roberts (Editor) Microbial Diseases of Fish, Academic Press, N.Y., pp. 91-114.

O'Neill, J.G., 1979. The immune response of the brown trout, Salmo trutta, to MS2 bacteriophage: immunogen concentration and adjuvants. J. Fish Biol., 15: 237-248.

O'Neill, J.G., 1980. Temperature and the primary and secondary immune responses of three teleosts, Salmo trutta, Cyprinus carpio and Notothenia rossii, to MS2 bacteriophage. Dev. Immunol., 10: 123-130.

Schutz, M., May, E.B., Kraeuter, J.N. and Hetrick, F.M., 1984. Isolation of infectious pancreatic necrosis virus from an epizootic in cultured striped bass Morone saxatilis. J. Fish Dis., 7: 505-507.

Reed, L.J. and Muench, H., 1938. A simple method of estimating fifty per cent endpoints. Am. J. Hygiene, 27: 493 - 497.

Sigel, M.M. and Clem, L.W., 1965. Antibody response of fish to viral antigens. Ann. NY Acad. Sci., 126: 662-677.

Swanson, R.N. and Gillespie, J.H., 1982. Isolation of infectious pancreatic necrosis virus from the blood and blood components of experimentally infected trout. Can. J. Fish. Aquat. Sci., 39: 225-228.

Wolf, K. and Quimby, M.C., 1969. Infectious pancreatic necrosis: clinical and immune response of adult trouts to inoculation with live virus. J. Fish. Res. Board Can., 26: 2511-2516.

Wolf, K. and Quimby, M.C. 1973. Fish virology: procedures and preparation of materials for plaquing fish viruses in normal atmosphere. U.S. Fish Wildlife Service Fish Disease Leaflet 35: 1-13.

Yamamoto, T., 1975. Infectious pancreatic necrosis (IPN) virus carriers and antibody production in a population of rainbow trout (Salmo gairdneri). Can. J. Microbiol., 21:1343-1347.

Yamamoto, T., 1975b. Frequency of detection and survival of infectious pancreatic necrosis virus in a carrier population of brook trout (Salvelinus fontinalis) in a lake. J. Fish. Res. Board Can., 32: 568-570.

Yu, K. K-Y., MacDonald, R.D. and Moore, A. R., 1982. Replication of infectious pancreatic necrosis virus in trout leucocytes and detection of the carrier state. J. Fish Dis., 5: 401-410.

Veterinary Immunology and Immunopathology, 12 (1986) 313—320
Elsevier Science Publishers B.V., Amsterdam — Printed in The Netherlands

FUNCTIONAL EVALUATION OF MACROPHAGES IN FISH FROM A POLLUTED ESTUARY

B. A. WEEKS and J. E. WARINNER

Virginia Institute of Marine Science, College of William and Mary, Gloucester Point, Virginia 23062, USA

ABSTRACT

Weeks, B. A. and Warinner, J. E., 1986. Functional evaluation of macrophages in fish from a polluted estuary. Vet. Immunol. Immunopathol., 12: 313-320.

The chemotactic and phagocytic efficiencies of macrophages from spot, *Leiostomus xanthurus* and hogchoker, *Trinectes maculatus* are reported here. Fish were captured from the York and Ware Rivers, two relatively nonpolluted rivers, and from a reach of the Elizabeth River, known to be contaminated with high concentrations of polynuclear aromatic hydrocarbons (PAHs). Kidney cell types were separated by density gradient centrifugation and single cell suspensions of macrophages were used for *in vitro* studies. Chemotactic activity was measured in Boyden chambers using *Escherichia coli* as the chemotactic stimulus. The percentage of macrophages migrating was maximal at 90 min but was markedly reduced in Elizabeth River fish (spot, 33%; hogchoker, 56%) as compared to clean water controls (spot, 55%; hogchoker, 85%). Macrophage phagocytosis of bacteria was quantified by the microscopic enumeration of the proportion of phagocytes which contained intracellular bacteria. Phagocytic activity reached maximum values within 120 min and remained relatively constant for the remainder of the experiment. Phagocytic activity was reduced significantly in the fish obtained from the Elizabeth River. Values at 120 min were 74% and 19% for spot from the control and PAH-contaminated sites, respectively. Comparable values for hogchoker were 88% and 32%. The results suggest that defective macrophage function is related to exposure to PAH-contaminated sediments.

INTRODUCTION

Interest in the effect of environmental stresses on health and disease in fish has increased in recent years (Couch, 1975; Haensly et al., 1982; Middaugh et al., 1977, 1980; Overstreet and Howse, 1977; Pierce et al., 1980; Rowe et al., 1983 a,b; Solangi and Overstreet, 1982). Neff and Anderson (1981) considered the responses of marine animals to petroleum and several specific hydrocarbons.

Acutely toxic substances often operate directly on some control mechanism in the affected organism causing death quickly. In contrast, sublethal or low concentrations of these same toxicants may exert a chronically debilitating effect which lowers host resistance to disease. The reticuloendothelial system is an important defense mechanism because of its phagocytic capacity to destroy pathogenic material. Since macrophages are an important part of the

0165-2427/86/$03.50 © 1986 Elsevier Science Publishers B.V.

immune system in fish (Ellis et al., 1976), it is of interest to determine the effect of toxic substances on the normal chemotactic and phagocytic activities of macrophages.

Two species of fish, spot (*Leiostomus xanthurus* Lacépède) and hogchoker (*Trinectes maculatus* Block and Schneider) were selected because they are bottom-feeders in close contact with sediments. Areas chosen for capture of fish were the York and Ware Rivers, two relatively nonpolluted rivers, and the highly polluted Elizabeth River.

The Elizabeth River is recognized as the most heavily contaminated estuary in the lower Chesapeake region. The river is contaminated with aromatic and aliphatic hydrocarbons especially in a reach of the Southern Branch polluted by creosote spills which have been incorporated into the bottom sediments. An analysis of these sediments shows high concentrations of polynuclear aromatic hydrocarbons (PAHs) (Huggett et al., 1985).

Evidence has been obtained to indicate that fish exposed to this environment develop gross abnormalities including fin erosion, skin lesions and cataracts. Spot collected from the most heavily PAH-contaminated location in the Elizabeth River exhibited hyperplasia of gill tissue and necrosis of pancreatic tissues of the liver. Spot exposed to contaminated Elizabeth River sediments and sediment-exposed overflow water in the laboratory developed symptoms which ranged from almost total fin loss, severe skin lesions, cataracts, gill hyperplasia, and liver-pancreatic necrosis, to death (Hargis et al., 1984).

MATERIALS AND METHODS

Fish

The two species of fish, spot (10-100 g) and hogchoker (10-60 g), were captured by trawl net on several occasions from October 1983 through October 1984. Fish to be used in experiments were collected from the Southern Branch of the Elizabeth River where PAH contamination is most pronounced and from the relatively nonpolluted York and Ware Rivers. Fish were held in tanks of running York River water at ambient temperature until use (3-7 days). Fish were fed Zeigler's trout chow (No. 3, starter pellets) daily. Salinities and water temperatures were roughly equivalent in the three river systems ranging from 13-23 ppt and 4-25°C seasonally.

Isolation of Kidney Macrophages

Fish were sacrificed and kidneys were aseptically removed and transferred to 5 ml Minimal Essential Medium (MEM) (GIBCO) supplemented with 0.33% glucose, 500 U/ml penicillin, 0.3 mg/ml streptomycin, 0.1 U/ml heparin and

10% fetal calf serum. The kidney tissue was homogenized and clumps of cells were allowed to settle in a 10 ml plastic test tube (American Scientific Products). Macrophages were separated from the cell suspension using a modification of the technique of Braun-Nesje et al. (1981) (Weeks and Warinner, 1984). Percoll gradients were prepared with densities of 1.040, 1.045, 1.050 and 1.060 g/ml and centrifuged at 400xg for 20 min at 4°C. The macrophage fractions were removed from the gradients with pasteur pipettes and washed in MEM; viability and cell concentration were determined by trypan blue exclusion. Macrophage identity was based on nonspecific esterase stain, morphological characteristics using light microscopy and phagocytosis of *Escherichia coli* as confirmed by electron microscopy (Weeks and Warinner, 1984).

Chemotaxis Assay

Chemotaxis was measured by a modification of the Boyden microscopic filter technique (Boyden, 1962; Weeks and Kavas, 1979) using a double chamber apparatus. The upper chamber contained 1×10^5 macrophages suspended in 0.2 ml supplemented MEM and the lower chamber contained a 0.2 ml formalin killed suspension of *E. coli* (1×10^8 bacteria) in teleost buffered saline with 10% v/v human serum. Chambers were separated by millipore membranes of 5 μm or 8 μm pore size which allowed chemotactically-stimulated macrophages to migrate from the upper to the lower surface of the filter. Chambers were incubated in triplicate at 15°C. Membranes were removed at 30, 60, 90, and 120 minute intervals, fixed with methanol and stained with Wright's stain. Macrophages were differentially counted on the upper and lower surfaces of the filter. Chemotaxis was represented as the ratio of macrophages on the lower surface of the filter to the total number of macrophages counted (at least 100 cells). Results were expressed as the mean of four experiments ± SEM and differences were evaluated by a one-tailed Student's *t* test.

Phagocytosis Assay

Phagocytosis by fish macrophages was evaluated by the method described by Weeks and Kavas (1979). Macrophage suspensions in supplemented MEM (1×10^6 viable cells in 1.0 ml) were placed on coverslips in Leighton tubes, and the cells were allowed to settle for 60 min at 15°C. To this monolayer of cells was added a suspension of formalin-killed bacteria (1×10^8 *E. coli* in 0.5 ml) and the tubes were incubated for 180 min. At 30 min intervals coverslips were removed from Leighton tubes, rinsed with MEM and stained with Wright's stain. Phagocytosis was quantified by determining the proportion of macrophages which contained intracellular bacteria in a random microscopic count of at least 100 macrophages.

RESULTS

Isolation of Kidney Macrophages

Separation of kidney cells by discontinuous Percoll gradient centrifugation gave rise to four different fractions for spot and five different fractions for hogchoker (Figure 1). The banding patterns observed for York and Ware River control fish were the same as those obtained for experimental Elizabeth River fish of the same species. Macrophages from both control and experimental spot were consistently located in two bands, one at the lower boundary of the 1.040 g/ml density layer and the other at the lower boundary of the 1.050 g/ml density layer. Macrophages from control and experimental hogchoker appeared in one band at the lower boundary of the 1.050 g/ml density layer. Greater than 85% of the cells from the bands between 1.050 and 1.060 were macrophages with the remainder consisting of lymphocytes and red blood cells. The lower density from spot contained 25-30% macrophages.

Chemotaxis

Table 1 shows the effects of the Elizabeth River environment on macrophage chemotaxis and phagocytosis in spot and hogchoker. Chemotactic activity increased at each time interval, reaching maximum values within 90 minutes for both control and experimental fish. Chemotactic activity was reduced significantly ($P<0.05$) in both species of fish obtained from the Elizabeth River. The percentage of cells migrating at 90 minutes for spot was 55 ± 5 for control fish and 33 ± 2 for experimental fish, and comparable values for hogchoker were 85 ± 5 and 56 ± 5.

Phagocytosis

Macrophage phagocytosis in fish taken from the control and experimental rivers is also shown in Table 1. Phagocytic activity increased with time, reached maximum values within 120 min for both control and experimental fish, and remained relatively constant for the remainder of the experiment (180 min). Phagocytic activity was reduced significantly ($P<0.05$) in both species of fish obtained from the Elizabeth River. Percent phagocytosis at 120 minutes for spot was 74 ± 5 and 19 ± 3 for control and experimental fish, respectively. Values at 120 min for hogchoker were 88 ± 4 and 32 ± 5 for control and experimental fish.

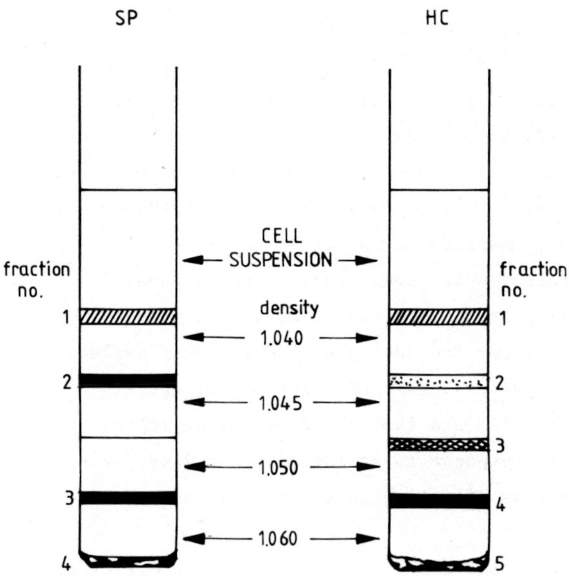

Fig. 1. Schematic representation of Percoll discontinuous density gradients used for cell separation: spot (SP) and hogchoker (HC) obtained from the York River. Solid bands indicate the presence of macrophages. For *in vitro* assays, fraction 3 served as source of spot macrophages; fraction 4 served as source of hogchoker macrophages.

TABLE 1. Effect of environment on macrophage activity

	Control River	Elizabeth River
Chemotaxis % Cells Migrating (at 90 min)		
Spot	55 ± 5	33 ± 2
Hogchoker	85 ± 5	56 ± 5
Phagocytosis % Phagocytosis (at 120 min)		
Spot	74 ± 5	19 ± 3
Hogchoker	88 ± 4	32 ± 5

Each value represents the mean ± SEM of 4 experiments using 6-10 fish per experiment. The Elizabeth River group differed significantly ($P < 0.05$) from the control group.

DISCUSSION

Our results show that two functional aspects of macrophage activity (phagocytosis and chemotaxis) are compromised in fish exposed in the wild to contaminated sediments. Wolke et al. (1985) have reported that the examination of spleens and livers from winter flounder taken from clean and polluted waters showed significant differences in size, number, and pigmentation of macrophage aggregates. Wolke (1984) has also demonstrated that the same response was obtained in the laboratory under conditions of nutritional deficiency and exposure to chemical pesticides. Others have presented evidence that the presence of these pigmented macrophage centers may reflect upsets in homeostasis and early disease processes (Roberts, 1975; Aguis, 1979; Aguis and Roberts, 1981). Wolke's data indicate an increase in the size and number of the aggregates in response to stress, and our data indicate that these macrophages may be less effective in their chemotactic and phagocytic abilities.

There is evidence that macrophages differ in density and size in different teleost species (Braun-Nesje et al., 1981). In our study macrophages from both spot and hogchoker were found in the same density layer, but in spot a second macrophage fraction was found at a lower density. Microscopically these two populations differ in cell size, suggesting that two different populations of macrophages are present in spot. Further work will be required to describe these two cell types.

We have shown that the phagocytic and chemotactic activities of macrophages from fish in the Elizabeth River were markedly reduced as compared to clean water controls. Furthermore, preliminary experiments using control fish exposed to Elizabeth River sediments in the laboratory exhibited the same reduced phagocytic and chemotactic activities. Chemical analyses have shown a gradient of concentrations of PAHs in Elizabeth River sediments, increasing in an upstream direction (Huggett et al., 1985). In a core sample taken in the area of highest contamination, benzo[a]pyrene concentrations in the top 2 cm of sediment approached 100 ug/g while total aromatic hydrocarbon concentrations were about 13,000 ug/g at the 30 cm sediment depth (Lu, 1982). Since sediments from the Elizabeth River site contain high levels of polynuclear aromatic hydrocarbons, it is probable that these toxicants are responsible for the reduced macrophage activities. It remains to be determined if PAH's are indeed the causative agents. Furthermore, the effects of age, nutrition, season, or other factors on macrophage activity need to be ascertained.

ACKNOWLEDGEMENTS

The authors gratefully acknowledge the expert technical assistance of Ms. Maura E. Jansen and Patrice L. Mason. This work is the result of research sponsored in part by NOAA Office of Sea Grant, U. S. Department of Commerce, under Grants No. NA81AA-D-0025 and No. NA85AA-D-SG016 to the Virginia Graduate Marine Science Consortium and Virginia Sea Grant College Program. The U. S. Government is authorized to produce and distribute reprints for governmental purposes notwithstanding any copyright notation that may appear hereon. This article summarizes in part data published in Marine Environmental Research and Journal of Fish Biology. Virginia Institute of Marine Science Contribution No. 1274.

REFERENCES

Aguis, C., 1979. The role of melano-macrophage centres in iron storage in normal and diseased fish. J. Fish Dis., 2:337-343.

Aguis, C. and Roberts, R. J., 1981. Effects of starvation on the melano-macrophage centres of fish. J. Fish Biol., 19:161-169.

Boyden, S. V., 1962. Chemotactic effect of mixtures of antibody and antigen on PMN leukocytes. J. Exp. Med., 115:453-463.

Braun-Nesje, R., Bertheussen, K., Kaplan, G. and Seljelid, R., 1981. Salmonid macrophages: Separation, *in vitro* culture and characterization. J. Fish Dis., 4:141-151.

Couch, J. A., 1975. Histopathological effects of pesticides and related chemicals on the livers of fishes. In: W. E. Ribelin and A. Migaki (Editors), The Pathology of Fishes. University of Wisconsin Press, Madison, pp. 559-584.

Ellis, A. E., Munroe, A. L. S. and Roberts, R. J., 1976. Defense mechanisms in fish. 1. A study of the phagocytic system and the fate of intraperitoneally injected particulate material in the plaice (*Pleuronectes platessa* L.). J. Fish Biol., 8:67-78.

Haensly, W. E., Neff, J. M., Sharp, J. R., Marris, A. C., Bedgood, M. F. and Boem, P. D., 1982. Histopathology of *Pleuronectes platessa* L. from Aber Wrac'h and Aber Benoit, Brittany, France: long-term effects of the *Amoco Cadiz* crude oil spill. J. Fish Dis., 5:365-391.

Hargis, W. J., Jr., Roberts, M. H., Jr., and Zwerner, D. E., 1984. Effects of contaminated sediments and sediment-exposed effluent water on an estuarine fish: Acute toxicity. Mar. Environ. Res., 14:337-354.

Huggett, R. J., Bender, M. E. and Unger, M. A., 1985. Polynuclear aromatic hydrocarbons in the Elizabeth River, Virginia. Environ. Toxicol. Chem. (in press)

Lu, M. Z., 1982. Organic compound levels in a sediment core from the Elizabeth River of Virginia. Master's Thesis, College of William and Mary, School of Marine Science, Gloucester Point, Virginia, 157 pp.

Middaugh, D. P., Crane, A. M. and Couch, J. A., 1977. Toxicity of chlorine to juvenile spot, *Leiostomus xanthurus*. Water Res., 11:1089-1096.

Middaugh, D. P., Burnett, L. E. and Couch, J.A., 1980. Toxicological and physiological responses of the fish, *Leiostomus xanthurus*, exposed to chlorine-produced oxidants. Estuaries, 3:132-141.

Neff, J. M. and Anderson, J. W., 1981. Response of Marine Animals to Petroleum and Specific Petroleum Hydrocarbons. Applied Science Publishers, London. 177 pp.

Overstreet, R. M. and Howse, H. D., 1977. Some parasites and diseases of estuarine fishes in polluted habitats of Mississippi. Ann. NY Acad. Sci., 298:427-462.

Pierce, K. V., McCain, B. B. and Wellings, S. R., 1980. Histopathology of abnormal livers and other organs of starry flounder *Platichthys stellatus* (Pallas) from the estuary of the Duwamish River, Seattle, Washington, USA. J. Fish Dis., 3:81-91.

Roberts, R. J., 1975. Melanin-containing cells of the teleost fishes and their relation to disease. In: W. E. Ribelin and G. Migaki (Editors), The Pathology of Fishes. University of Wisconsin Press, Madison, pp. 399-428.

Rowe, D. W., Sprague, J. B. and Heming, J. A., 1983a. Sublethal effects of treated liquid effluent from a petroleum refinery. I. Chronic toxicity to flat fish. Aquat. Toxicol., 3:149-159.

Rowe, D. W., Sprague, J. B., Heming, T. A. and Brown, I. T., 1983b. Sublethal effects of treated liquid effluent from a petroleum refinery. II. Growth of rainbow trout. Aquat. Toxicol., 3:161-169.

Solangi, M. A. and Overstreet, R. M., 1982. Histopathological changes in two estuarine fishes, *Menidia beryllina* (Cope) and *Trinectes maculatus* (Block and Schneider), exposed to crude oil and its water-soluble fraction. J. Fish Dis., 5:13-35.

Weeks, B. A. and Kavas, A. F., 1979. Macrophage chemotaxis and phagocytosis in guinea pigs: Influence of age and nutrition. J. Reticuloendothel. Soc., 26:502-506.

Weeks, B. A. and Warinner, J. E., 1984. Effects of toxic chemicals on macrophage phagocytosis in two estuarine fishes. Mar. Environ. Res., 14:327-335.

Weeks, B. A., Warinner, J. E., Mason, P. L. and McGinnis, D. S., 1985. Influence of toxic chemicals on the chemotactic response of fish macrophages. J. Fish Biol., (in press).

Wolke, R. E., 1984. Using fish as pollution monitors. University of Rhode Island Marine Resources Information, 136.

Wolke, R. E., Murchelano, R. A., Dickstein, C. D. and George, C. J., 1985. Preliminary evaluation of the use of macrophage aggregates (MA) as fish health monitors. Bull. Environ. Contam. Toxicol., 35:222-227.

Veterinary Immunology and Immunopathology, 12 (1986) 321—330
Elsevier Science Publishers B.V., Amsterdam — Printed in The Netherlands

BLOOD CHANGES IN CARP (*CYPRINUS CARPIO*) INDUCED BY ULCERATIVE *AEROMONAS SALMONICIDA* INFECTIONS

Dolf Evenberg[1], Pieter de Graaff, Willy Fleuren and *Willem B. van Muiswinkel

Institute of Molecular Biology and Dept. of Molecular Cell Biology, University of Utrecht, and* Dept. of Experimental Animal Morphology and Cell Biology, Agricultural University, Wageningen, The Netherlands

ABSTRACT

Evenberg, D., De Graaff, P., Fleuren, W., and Van Muiswinkel, W.B., 1986. Blood changes in carp (*Cyprinus carpio*) induced by ulcerative *Aeromonas salmonicida* infections. Vet. Immunol. Immunopathol., 12: 321-330.

Only recently *Aeromonas salmonicida* has been recognized as a significant bacterial pathogen in ulcerative disease of cyprinid fish. Our attempts to formulate a vaccine based on bacterial surface antigens were unsucessful in conferring reliable protection against lethal challenge. This lead us to study pathological changes in the humoral defense system during ulcerative *A. salmonicida* infection in carp.

High numbers of opportunist pathogens such as *A. hydrophila* and *Pseudomonas sp.* were frequently recovered from the internal organs of moribund fish, in addition to *A. salmonicida*. These findings together with leucopenia in moribund fish suggest that pathogenesis is characterized by a state of immune suppression.

In addition, fish which had sustained a sublethal infection were not protected against a subsequent lethal challenge. However, fish previously injected with a concentrated and inactivated culture supernatant showed protection. Differential blood cell counts did not differ between experimental and control groups during sublethal infection in contrast to serum proteins. Furthermore infected non-immune carp showed a progressive derease of immunoglobulin and total serum protein levels before the day of peak mortality whereas protected carp maintained the immunoglobulin concentration despite a decrease in protein. Our observations suggest the involvement of multiple pathogenic events, affecting different parts of the humoral defense system during ulcerative *A. salmonicida* infection.

The immunosuppressive effects can be minimized by prior vaccination with culture supernatant.

[1] To whom correspondence should be sent at the present address: National Institute of Public Health and Environmental Hygiene, Unit of Immunochemistry, P.O. Box 1, 3720 BA Bilthoven, The Netherlands.

0165-2427/86/$03.50 © 1986 Elsevier Science Publishers B.V.

INTRODUCTION

A. salmonicida is a Gram negative bacterium, which causes a systemic disease known as furunculosis in salmonids (reviews: McCarthy and Roberts, 1980; Paterson, 1983). Only recently *A. salmonicida* has been recognized as a bacterial pathogen in ulcerative disease of cyprinid fish (Bootsma *et al.*, 1978; Shotts *et al.*, 1980). Furthermore, recent evidence indicates that cases of ulcer disease earlier attributed to *Haemophilus piscium* (Snieszko *et al.*, 1950) should now be considered as caused by atypical *A. salmonicida* (Paterson *et al.*, 1980: Trust *et al.*, 1980; Evenberg *et al.*, 1985).

Attempts to immunize carp against experimental infection with atypical *A. salmonicida*, using bacterial surface antigens, were unsuccessful in conferring reliable protection (Evenberg, *et al.*, 1984). Moreover, rainbow trout which did survive an earlier infection were poorly protected against a subsequent challenge (Michel, 1982) suggesting a lack of acquired immunity. Furthermore, contradictory results on vaccination against *A. salmonicida* are reported (reviews: Michel, 1982; Munro, 1984). Clearly, there is a need for a better understanding of the molecular architecture of the pathogen and the interaction with its host, before an improved vaccine can be developed. These considerations led us to study blood changes in carp during an experimental *A. salmonicida* infection.

MATERIAL AND METHODS

Fish

Common scale and mirror carp, *Cyprinus carpio*, 6 to 18 months of age and weighing 50 - 400 g were kept in tanks at an average density of 1 kg fish/200 l.c., at 22 ± 2°C, using continuous flowing tap water (80 l/h). The fish were fed daily with commercial pellets (K_{30}, Trouw). Carp were allowed to acclimatize for several weeks before experimental use.

Bacteria (strains, cultivation and identification)

Virulent, atypical *A. salmonicida* strains V234/81 and 3.111 were respectively isolated from diseased carp and goldfish. The strains were donated by Dr. G. Wiedeman (strain V234/81), Bavarian Animal Health Service, F.R.G. and Dr. R.C. Cipriano (strain 3.111), National Fish Health Research Laboratory, Leetown, U.S.A. Both strains are resistant for ampicillin and polymyxin B. Fresh virulent *A. salmonicida* isolates were obtained after fish passage and preserved without glycerol at -70°C as single colonies punched out of an agar plate. *A. salmonicida* was cultured at 22°C as described by Evenberg *et al.* (1981) using the following peptone-yeast oleate (PYO) medium: Peptone (Difco) 1%; yeast extract, 0.7%; Na Cl, 0.5%; $Na_2HPO_4.2H_2O$, 0.1%; potassium oleate 0.004% and Brij 58 (Serva), 0.04%; pH 7.2. For selective and elective plates 1.2% Difco agar, 0.1 mg/ml Coomassie Brilliant Blue R250 (Bio-Rad), ampicillin (50 ug/ml) and polymyxin B (20 ug/ml) were added, (Evenberg *et al.*, 1985), and used in single step re-isolations of virulent *A. salmonicida*.

To evaluate sepsis, the number of viable bacteria in blood, spleen and kidney was determined by standard drop plate counting on selective plates and blood agar plates. The organs were removed aseptically, weighed, and homogenized at a weight of 10 mg/ml in sterile glycine diluent pH 6.8. The glycine diluent consisted of 240 mM glycine, 30 mM NaCl, 3 mM Na_2HPO_4 and 0.004% potassium oleate and 0.04% Brij 58, to reduce aggregation of autoagglutinating *A. salmonicida*.

Bacteria were identified by their colony morphology, pigmentation, mobility, shape, arrangement, Gram staining, oxidase-catalase reactions and responses to biochemical tests (API 10S, API system S.A., France). Presumptive identification of *A. hydrophila* and *A. salmonicida* was confirmed by comparison with type strains.

Challenge procedure

A logarithmic phase culture was diluted with glycine diluent to appropriate turbidity and 5-10 ul of the bacterial suspension was deposited just under a dorsal scale using a Hamilton microliter syringe. For a sublethal virulent challenge approximately 2×10^4 colony forming units (CFU) per fish were administered and 4×10^5 CFU/fish in a lethal challenge.

Analysis of carp serum

Blood was obtained by caudal vein puncture and allowed to clot at room temperature. Clots were removed by centrifugation and the serum was stored at -20°C. Total serum protein was determined by the biuret method and albumin was quantified by dye binding using bromocresol green. Bovine serum albumin was used as standard. The immunoglobulin (Ig) level was estimated by single radial immunodiffusion (Mancini *et al.*, 1965) using purified carp Ig as standard. To enhance the precipitation 1% poly-ethylene glycol 6000 was added to the agarose (1.5%). The concentration of the rabbit anti-carp Ig serum was 4%. The readings were made after 60 h diffusion at room temperature.

Immunizations

Rabbits were immunized with 100 μg purified carp Ig emulsified in Freund's complete adjuvant, as described before (Overbeeke *et al.*, 1980). The rabbits were bled 8 days after a booster injection. The sera were stored at -20°C prior to use. Carp Ig was kindly donated by Dr. E. Egberts (Agricultural University, Wageningen).

Carp were immunized by an intramusculair (i.m.) injection anterior to the dorsal fin using 0.1 ml of an ultrafiltrated (Millipore, 220 nm), inactivated (0.3% formalin) and 20x concentrated culture supernatant or formalin killed whole cells (10^6/fish).

RESULTS

Infectivity of atypical *Aeromonas salmonicida*

At a challenge dose of approximately 8 x 10^4CFU/fish, strain 3.111 caused no mortality whereas for strain V234/81 this was approximately a 2 x LD_{50} value. However, both strains produced typical carp erythrodermatitis ulcers within 3 days post-infection. Inconsistent and relative low numbers of *A. salmonicida* were re-isolated from the lesion (10^3 - 10^4 bacteria/g muscle tissue). *A.salmonicida* was re-isolated from the organs of only 9 (28%) of 32 diseased fish in contrast to *A.hydrophila* (68%) and *Pseudomonas* sp. (56%). No bacteria were isolated from the organs of control fish. To check the infectivity of *A.hydrophila* and *Pseudomonas* sp. isolated from a diseased fish, carp were challenged similarly, receiving 10^6 CFU/fish. Between day 1-4 post infection the fish showed anorexia and reduced movement. No lesions developed and after a week the fish behaved normal again. These observations indicate that *A.salmonicida* is acting as a primary pathogen but the host is subsequently invaded by secondary pathogens as *A.hydrophila* and *Pseudomonas* species.

Blood changes in carp induced by *A. salmonicida* infection.

The changes in total protein and Ig levels induced by a lethal infection in fish primed with an intramusculair injection with formalin killed cells of *A. salmonicida* strain V234/81, are shown in figures 1A and 1B respectively.

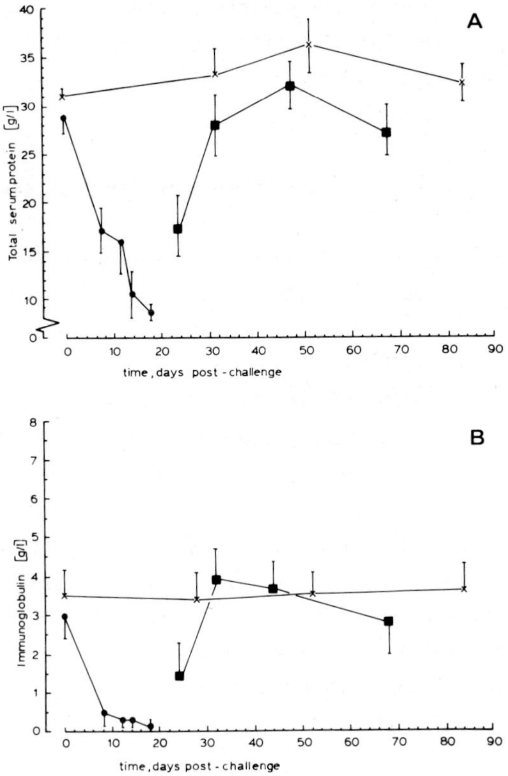

Fig. 1. The changes in total serum protein are depicted in panel A, the changes in immunoglobulin are shown in panel B. All carps received a single i.m.-injection with approx. 10^6 formalin killed A. salmonicida cells (V234/81). A month after the injection, the control group (X) received another injection, and the experimental group was challenged, by inoculating approx. 2×10^5 virulent A. salmonicida (V234/81) under a dorsal scale. (●) moribund fish; (■) surviving fish. Points represent arithmetic mean ± 1 SE (N = 4-6).

It can be seen that within one week a rapid and dramatic fall occurred in protein and particularly in Ig level of moribund fish. In the case of moribund the decrease was 70% in total protein and 90% in Ig at day 12. The surviving carp showed a 40% reduction in protein and 60% reduction in Ig, which gradually became normal from day 28 onwards. The control group showed no significant changes.

In another series of experiments, the serum changes were studied in 5 different groups of carp. Control group 1, received 10 µl glycine diluent under a dorsal scale, while group 2 was challenged sublethally i.e. without any mortalities. The remaining 3 groups were challenged lethally. Group 3 was not immunized, while group 4 was immunized with a single i.m. injection containing inactivated and concentrated culture supernatant. Group 5 was primed by a sublethal infection 6 weeks before the challenge. Table 1 shows the mortality data of the lethal challenge groups. The data on serum protein and Ig are shown in figures 2A and B.

TABLE 1
The survival of carp after a lethal challenge with atypical *Aeromonas salmonicida*.

Groups	Survival/Total[a]	R.P.S.[b]
Control	2/18 (11)	0
Sublethal[c]	3/18 (17) (p ~1)	6
Supernatant[d]	11/18 (61) (p<0.01)	56

Three different groups were lethally challenged by inoculating approximately 4×10^5 CFU of virulent *A. salmonicida* (V234/81)/fish.
[a]Number of surviving animals after 28 days post-infection. Percentage of survival is indicated between parentheses. The level of probability, P, is obtained by standard X^2 (chi-square) calculation (Baily, 1981).
[b]Relative percentage of survival (R.P.S.) is calculated according to Amend (1981).
[c]Fish were infected sublethally with 2×10^4 CFU *A. salmonicida* (V234/81). Six weeks later the fish received a lethal dose at the other side of the body than the healed ulcer.
[d]Fish were i.m. injected with 0,1 ml inactivated and concentrated culture supernatant 1 month before challenge.

Without exception all groups that received a lethal dose again showed a rapid decrease in protein. Interestingly enough, the reduction in the group injected with supernatant occurred approximately 4 days later compared with the unprotected fish. The sublethally infected group showed only a 10% reduction in protein. The observed Ig reduction was the largest (65%) in the non-immunized group, while in the sublethal infected and the protected group the reduction was limited to

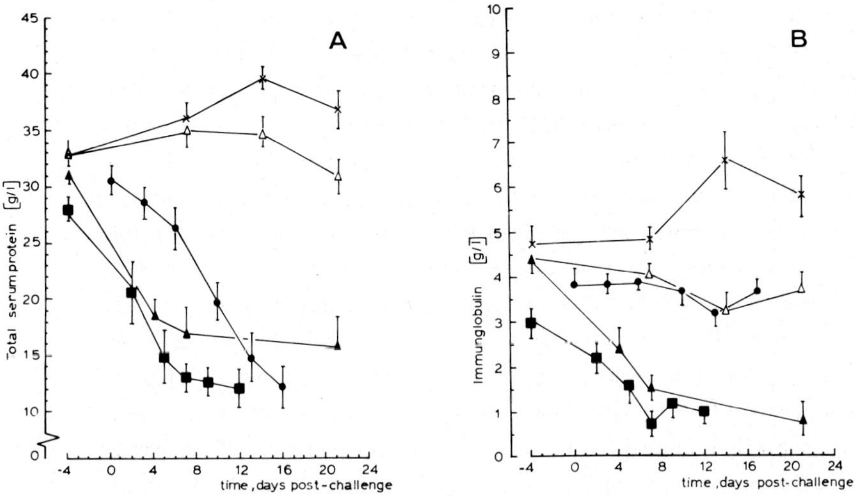

Fig. 2. Total serum protein and immunoglobulin changes induced by virulent, experimental A. salmonicida infection are shown in respectively panel A and panel B. Carp received respectively 10 μl diluent (x); 2 x 10^4 (△) or 4 x 10^5 (●), (■) and (▲) virulent cells of A. salmonicida strain V234/81. Two groups of carp were primed before receiving a lethal challenge, respectively by a sublethal (▲) infection with (2 x 10^4) virulent cells and (●) by i.m. injection with 0.1 ml inactivated and concentrated culture supernatant.

respectively, 26% and 15%. Quantification of the serum albumin level showed that this protein was reduced more slowly than Ig and was maintained at approx. 40% of the total protein. Analysis of carp sera by SDS-polyacrylamide gel electrophoresis confirmed these findings (results not shown). It could be shown in a rechallenge experiment of the survivors of the supernatant group, that protection was solid, 9% (1/11) mortality compared with 100% in the control group (10/10). Furthermore the total protein level showed only a minor decrease of 8% and Ig an increase of 9%. In addition, lesion was less intense and healing more rapid than in controls. This latter observation indicates an enhanced response to the pathogen during rechallenge suggesting the formation of memory. No significant differences in the white blood cell (WBC)/red blood cell (RBC) ratio's of control and sublethal infected group were observed in blood smears. WBC/RBC ratio's were significantly decreased in moribund fish and even in the protected group, i.e. those immunized with bacterial culture supernatant preparation, a gradual decrease in the WBC/ RBC ratio was observed during the course of infection.

DISCUSSION

It is known that isolation of atypical *A. salmonicida* is difficult (Bootsma, 1978; Shotts, 1980). We were able to make an positive identification in approximate 30% of the biopsies. Furthermore, it has been suggested by Chart and Trust (1983) that a restricted ability of atypical *A. salmonicida* strains to sequester iron may contribute to a predominantly non-systemic disease pattern. However, it cannot be excluded that the isolation media we have used may be not optimal. The development of sepsis caused by opportunist pathogens such as *A. hydrophila* suggests that *A. salmonicida* acts as primary pathogen weakening the immune system of the host. In addition, it has been reported that apparent healthy rainbow trout carried a diversity of potential virulent strains of *Aeromonas, Vibrio* and *Pseudomonas* (Nieto *et al.*, 1984). Moreover, sublethal primed carp were not protected against a subsequent lethal challenge, indicating the inability to generate acquired immunity. This also suggests a lack of memory formation. Current studies suggest, that *A. salmonicida* indeed affects the specific immune response of carp (Pourreau *et al.*, in this issue).

The observed clinical disease symptoms, such as scale protrusion, ophtalmia and abominal swelling, are signs of generalized oedema. This is in complete agreement with the observed reduction of serum protein, as a low serum protein level diminishes the osmotic value of the vascular system, which in turn reduces the interstitial fluid resorption (Green, 1978). The mechanism(s) causing the reduction of total serum protein and in particular Ig is (are) not clear, but it is conceivable to be a consequence of the following processes: (i) loss of proteins through vascular leaking caused by increased permeability due to histamine release (Green, 1978; Ellis, 1981a), (ii) impaired synthesis of serum proteins (liver damage) and anorexia in diseased fish, (iii) (non)specific proteolysis of serum proteins (Ellis, 1981b). At the present stage, it is difficult to assess the relative importance of each possibility. However, several lines of evidence do suggest that (un)-specific proteolysis may be a major cause. Recently, Sakai (1985) showed that a protease of *A. salmonicida* was a significant virulence factor. In addition, the bacterium is able to produce a leucocytolysin (Fuller *et al.*, 1977). Furthermore, *in vitro* and *in vivo* experiments with mammals have shown that a sepsis of Gram-negative bacteria can be accompanied by an unspecific degradation of almost all serum proteins (review, Duswald, 1985).

In conclusion, we hypothesize that the protective ability of fish against *A. salmonicida* is highly dependent on maintaining serum proteins and in particular Ig above certain critical levels. Because of the multiple events, the pathogenesis of ulcerative *A. salmonicida* infection is complex and therefore a vaccine should incorporate a diversity of antigens cellular as well as extra-cellular products from *A. salmonicida* and perhaps also some common antigens of *A. hydrophila* and *Pseudomonas*.

ACKNOWLEDGEMENTS

We like to thank all colleagues who provided us with virulent bacterial strains, Dr. E. Egberts for his generous gift of carp Ig, and Dr. R. Bootsma for the experimental fish and permission to use his aquarium facilities. The continuous interest of Dr. B. Lugtenberg is also acknowledged. These investigations were supported (in part) by the Netherlands Technology Foundation (STW).

REFERENCES

Amend, D.F., 1981. Potency testing of fish vaccines. In: International Symposium on Fish Biologics, Serodiagnostics and Vaccines. Developments in Biological standardization 49, 447-454.

Bailey, N.T.J., 1981. Statistical Methods in Biology, 2nd. ed., Hodder and Stoughton, London.

Bootsma, R. and Blommaert, J., 1978. The etiology of *Erythrodermatitis* of carp, *Cyprinus carpia*. In: H.H. Reichenbach-Klinke (Editor). Proceedings of the Munich Fisheries Conference, 26 october-28 october 1976, at Munich, German Fed. Rep., Gustav Fisher Verlag, Stuttgart. Fish and Environment, 5: 20-27.

Chart, H. and Trust, T.J., 1983. Acquisition of iron by *Aeromonas salmonicida*. J. Bacteriol., 156: 758-764.

Chart, H., Shaw, D.H., Ishiguro, E.E. and Trust, T.J., 1984, J. Bacteriol. 158: 16-22. Structural and immunochemical homogeneity of *Aeromonas salmonicida* lipopolysaccharide.

Duswald, K.H., 1985, Zur Pathobiochemie der Leukozyten-Elastase und ausgewählter Plasmaproteine bei Sepsis nach abdominalchriturgische Eingriffen. G-I-T-Verlag Ernst Giebeler, Darmstadt.

Ellis, A.E., Hastings, T.S. and Munro, A.L.S., 1981a. The role of *Aeromonas salmonicida* extracellular products in the pathology of furunculosis. J. Fish Dis. 4: 41-52.

Ellis, A.E., 1981b. In: International Symposium on Fish Biologics: Serodiagnostics and Vaccines, Leetown, W.Va, U.S.A. Develop. Biol. Standard. 49: 337-352. S. Karger, Basel.

Evenberg, D., Van Boxtel, R., Lugtenberg, B., Schurer, F., Blommaert, J., Bootsma, R., 1982. Cell surface of the fish pathogenic bacterium *Aeromonas salmonicida*. I. Relationship between autoagglutination and the presence of a major cell envelope protein. Biochim. Biophys. Acta, 684: 241-248.

Evenberg, D., Bootsma, R. and Lugtenberg, B., 1984. Antigens of the fish pathogens *Aeromonas salmonicida* and their potential as a vaccine candidate. Abstract p. 36-37, 16th Lunteren Lectures on Molecular genetics, "Stragegies in vaccine development", 2-5 October 1984, Lunteren, The Netherlands.

Evenberg, D., Versluis, R. and Lugtenberg, B., 1985. Biochemical and immunological characterization of the cell surface of the fish pathogenic bacterium *Aeromonas salmonicida*. Biochim. Biophys. Acta, 815: 233-244.

Fuller, D.W., Pilcher, K.S. and Fryer, J.L., 1977. A leucocytolytic factor isolated from cultures of *Aeromonas salmonicida*. J. Fish Res. Board Can., 34: 1118-1125.

Green, J.H. 1978. Basic clinical physiology, chap. 7. Tissue Fluid and Lymph, p. 49-52 (3rd ed.). Oxford University Press, U.K.

Hahnel, H.B., Gould, R.W. and Batman, E.S., 1983. Serological comparison of selected isolates of *Aeromonas salmonicida* ssp. *salmonicida*. J. Fish Dis., 6: 1-11.

Mancini, G., Carbonara, A.D. and Heremans, J.F., 1965. Immunochemical quantitation of antigens by single radial immunodiffusion. Immunochem., 2: 235-254.

McCarthy, D.H. and Roberts, R.J., 1980. Furunculosis of fish: the present state of an knowlegde. Adv. in Aquatic Microbiol., 2: 293-341.

Michel, C., 1982. Progress towards furunculosis vaccination. In: R.J. Robberts (Editor), Special publication of the Society for General Microbiology, Academic Press, London. Microbial diseases of fish, 9: 151-171.

Munro, A.L.S., 1984. A furunculosis vaccine, illusion or achievable objective. In: P. De Kinkelin and C. Michel (Editors), From: Symposium on fish vaccination. Office Internat. des Epizooties, p. 97-120, Paris.

Nieto, T.P., Toranza, A.E. and Barja, J.L., 1984. Comparison between the bacterial flora associated with fingerling rainbow trout cultured in two different hatcheries in the North-West of Spain. Aquaculture, 42: 193-254.

Overbeeke, N., Van Scharrenburg, G. and Lugtenberg, B., 1980. Antigenic relationships between pore proteins of *Escherichia coli* K-12. Eur. J. Biochem., 110: 247-254.

Paterson, W.D., Douey, D. and Desautels, D., 1980. Relationship between selected strains of typical and atypical *Aeromonas salmonicida*, *Aeromonas hydrophila* and *Haemophilus piscium*. Can. J. Microbiol., 26: 588-598.

Paterson, W.D., 1983. Furunculosis and other associated diseases caused by *Aeromonas salmonicida*. In: D.P. Anderson, M. Dorson and Ph. Dubourget (Editors), Antigens of Fish Pathogens. Symposium international de Talloires, 10-12 May 1982, Collection Foundation Marcel Merieux, Lyon, France. Development and production for vaccin and serodiagnostics: 119-136.

Sakai, D.K., 1985. Loss of virulence in a protease-deficient mutant of *Aeromonas salmonicida*. Inf. and Imm., 48: 146-152.

Shotts, E.B., Talkington, F.D., Elliot, D.G. and McCarthy, D.H., 1980. Aetiology of an ulcerative disease in goldfish, *Carassius auratus* (L.): characterization of the causative agent. J. Fish Dis., 6: 181-186.

Snieszko, S.F., 1971. Diseases of Fishes, book 2A. In: S.F. Snieszko and H.R. Azelrod (Editors), TFH publication.

Trust, T.J., Ishiguro, E.E. and Atkinson, H.M., 1980. Relationship between *Haemophilus piscium* and *Aeromonas salmonicida* revealed by *Aeromonas hydrophila* bacteriophage. FEMS Microbiol. Lett. 9: 199-201.

Veterinary Immunology and Immunopathology, 12 (1986) 331—338
Elsevier Science Publishers B.V., Amsterdam — Printed in The Netherlands

DOES AEROMONAS SALMONICIDA AFFECT THE IMMUNE SYSTEM OF CARP, CYPRINUS CARPIO L.?

Catherine N. Pourreau, Dolf Evenberg*, Wanda M. de Raadt,
Jan A.N. van Mechelen, and Willem B. van Muiswinkel

Dept. of Exp. Animal Morphology & Cell Biology, Agricultural University,
P.O. Box 338, 6700 AH Wageningen (the Netherlands)
*Dept. of Molecular Cell Biology, University of Utrecht,
P.O.Box 80.056, 3508 TB Utrecht (the Netherlands)

ABSTRACT

Pourreau, C.N., Evenberg, D., De Raadt, W.M., Van Mechelen, J.A.N. and Van Muiswinkel W.B., 1986. Does Aeromonas salmonicida affect the immune system of carp, Cyprinus carpio L.? Vet. Immunol. Immunopathol., 12: 331-338.

Aeromonas salmonicida is a significant bacterial pathogen of cyprinid and salmonid fishes causing the systemic disease furunculosis. Several observations led us to believe that A. salmonicida was able to evade or suppress the immune system of the fish: 1) injection of whole bacteria or surface antigens was unsuccessful at protecting fish against lethal challenges; 2) memory did not develop in survivors of sublethal infections; 3) diseased fish often carried other opportunistic bacterial pathogens in addition to A. salmonicida, and 4) serum protein and particularly immunoglobulin significantly decreased during A. salmonicida infections.
We tested the ability of fish sublethally infected with virulent and avirulent A. salmonicida to mount a humoral immune response to sheep erythrocytes and found fewer plaque forming cells in the pronephros and lower serum anti-SRBC antibodies in infected fish as compared to controls.
We also monitored the cellular immune response of diseased fish by skin allograft rejection and found an enhancement of the response that increased as the disease progressed. However, the extend of inflammation was reduced in infected fish as compared to non-infected animals. At this moment these preliminary observations are difficult to explain. Our future research will focuss more specifically on cell populations that may be affected by A. salmonicida.

INTRODUCTION

Aeromonas salmonicida, the etiologic agent of furunculosis in trout and salmon, carp erythrodermatitis, and ulcerative disease of goldfish, has been a world wide economic threat to intensive culture of these fishes for over fifty years (Herman, 1968, McCarthy and Roberts, 1980, McCraw, 1952). Attempts to protect fish

0165-2427/86/$03.50 © 1986 Elsevier Science Publishers B.V.

against A. salmonicida using oral or immersion vaccines (Paterson and Fryer, 1974, Smith et al., 1980, Udey and Fryer, 1978), injection of surface antigens (Evenberg et al., 1984) or toxoids (Austin and Rogers, 1981, Klontz et al., 1966, Spence et al., 1965) has often been unsuccessful (Paterson, 1981). More specific studies on the interaction between the bacterium and its host have therefore been initiated (i.e. mechanism of bacterial virulence, and defense response of the fish)

We now know that certain strains of A. salmonicida possess an additional cell envelope protein (A-layer), first described by Udey and Fryer (1978), which is important for virulence (Munn et al., 1982, Trust et al., 1980, Udey and Fryer, 1978), autoagglutination (Evenberg et al., 1982), and protection of underlying cell wall components from bactericidal activity of fish serum (Munn et al., 1982, Paterson, 1981). The bacteria produce toxins in vivo which have proteolytic (Mellegaard, 1983, Munro et al., 1980, Shieh and McLean, 1975, Sheeran and Smith, 1981, Tajima et al., 1984), haemolytic (Karlsson, 1962, Munro et al., 1980, Nomura and Saito, 1982, Titball and Munn, 1981), and leucocytolytic activities (Fuller et al., 1977, Munro et al., 1980).

Fish respond immunologically to the bacterium and its extracellular products (ECP) by producing specific antibodies directed against cell surface antigens and extracellular products (Anderson, 1974, Anderson et al., 1979, Cipriano, 1982, Krantz et al., 1963, Michel, 1979, Udey and Fryer, 1978, Weber and Zwicker, 1979). However the presence of agglutinins is not necessarily indicative of protection (Cipriano, 1982, 1983, Michel, 1979). Normal fish serum is also capable of neutralizing the extracellular products (ECP) via activation of complement by extracellular proteases (Sakai, 1984).

Recent observations by Evenberg et al. (in this issue) led us to believe that the bacterium was able to suppress the immune response of the fish: 1) injection of surface antigens was unsuccessful at protecting fish against subsequent lethal challenges (Evenberg et al., 1984), 2) memory did not develop in survivors of sublethal infections, and 3) diseased fish carried not only A. salmonicida but also other opportunistic pathogens such as A. hydrophila and Pseudomonas ssp. Evenberg also showed that serum proteins and particularly immunoglobulins significantly decreased during A. salmonicida infections. We have started to investigate how A. salmonicida evades or alters the defense system of carp, Cyprinus carpio. These are the first results of the study.

MATERIALS AND METHODS

Fish

Mirror carp, Cyprinus carpio, six months of age and 50 to 60 g in weight, were acclimated for two weeks in laboratory aquaria, supplied with fresh water at 16-18 °C and fed commercial dry pellet (K30, Trouw) daily.

Bacteria

The virulent autoagglutinating strain (V234/81) causative agent of carp erythrodermatitis, the avirulent auto-agglutinating strain (V75/93) and avirulent non-auto-agglutinating strain (126-68) were provided by the Department of Molecular Cell Biology, University of Utrecht, and were cultured as described by Evenberg et al. (1981).

Humoral and cellular immune response

Fish were injected intramuscularly with a suspension of 10^7, and a month later 10^9, sheep red blood cells (SRBC) in PBS. The fish were challenged by an injection under a dorsal scale of 10 ul of A. salmonicida (2 x 10^4 cells/fish) in glycine diluent, 10 days prior to the booster SRBC injection. The diluent consisted of 240 mM glyxine, 30 mM NaCl, 3 mM Na_2HPO_4, 0.004 % sodium oleate and 0.04 % BRIJ 58 (Serva), pH 6.8. Control fish received diluent alone. The number of direct plaque forming cells (PFC) in the pronephros and the serum haemagglutination titer against SRBC were determined using standard techniques.

Groups of 10 fish were injected with a sublethal dose of virulent A. salmonicida (2 x 10^4 cells/fish) in diluent and received first set skin allografts at 5, 8, 11, 14, 17, and 20 days post Aeromonas injection. Controls were injected with diluent and grafted after 11 days. The appearance of the grafts was examined every two days for vascularization, haemorrhage and melanophore destruction. The day at which the grafts showed 100% pigment cell destruction (Median survival time, MST) was recorded for each fish.

RESULTS AND DISCUSSION

Aeromonas salmonicida suppressed the humoral immune response of carp to sheep erythrocytes. Fish sublethally infected with virulent and avirulent strains both showed lower numbers of plaque forming cells in the pronephros (13% and 22% less) than non infected controls (Fig. 1). Infected fish also produced less serum antibodies to sheep cells (38% reduction with the virulent strain and 60% with the avirulent

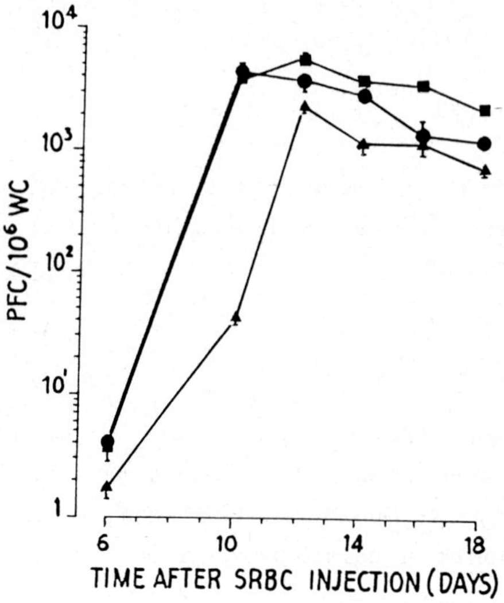

Fig. 1.

Kinetics of the secondary PFC response against 10^9 SRBC in the pronephros of carp at 16-18 °C. Fish were injected under a dorsal scale with PBS (■); $2x10^4$ avirulent (▲); or $2x10^4$ virulent (●). A. salmonicida ten days prior to SRBC. Points represent arithmetic means $\pm$ 1 SE (n=6).

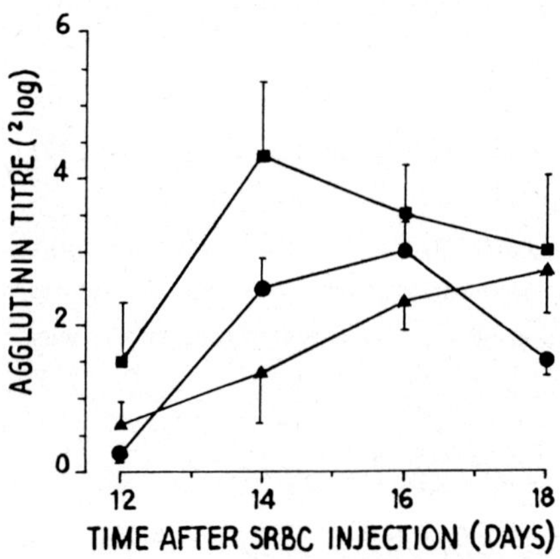

Fig. 2.

Kinetics of the secondary agglutinating antibody response against 10^9 SRBC at 16-18 °C in carp injected under a dorsal scale with PBS (■); $2x10^4$ avirulent (▲); or $2x10^4$ virulent (●). A. salmonicida ten days prior to SRBC. Points represent arithmetic means $\pm$ 1 SE (n=6).

strain 14 days after the booster SRBC injection (Fig. 2). In the case of fish infected with virulent A. salmonicida, this was not a delayed response to the antigen since antibody titers tapered off by 18 days. The same was not seen with fish infected with avirulent A. salmonicida. Antibody titers against formalin killed A. salmonicida cells were not significantly higher than natural antibody levels in sera of non-infected fish after 18 days (natural antibody titers:16-32 and anti-A. salmonicida titers in infected fish: 32-64).

Leucopenia and an increase in large lymphocytes was observed in infected fish. This result agrees with observations made by Klontz et al. (1966). The leucocytolytic factor released by the bacteria in vivo might destroy the mature white blood cells in circulation and lymphoid organs to such an extend as to suppress antibody production. The blood clotting time was also reduced 20-25 days post-infection with both virulent and avirulent A. salmonicida.

Results obtained with skin allografts showed that the rejection was accelerated in infected fish as compared to control. This phenomenon was more pronounced as the disease progressed up to 20 days (Fig. 3). By 14 days after injection of virulent A. salmonicida the MST of grafts was 59% shorter than normal. Since total pigment destruction was used as the criteria for graft rejection, we need to determine if the accelerated reaction was due to an enhanced cellular immune response or a non-specific toxic action of aggressins released by the bacteria on cells of the skin.

Aeromonas -infected fish showed a marked suppression of the inflammatory response to the skin allografts. This result is consistent with observations made by Munro et al. (1980), and Klontz et al. (1966). Klontz suggested that the lack of leucocytic response was due to the destruction of white blood cells by the leucocytolytic factor secreted by A. salmonicida and a depression of hematopoiesis. Above observations suggest that the avirulent strain V75/93 possessed other potential virulence factor(s) besides the A-layer, although it did not induce mortality at a dose of 10^6 CFU/fish.

We are now focusing our attention on the effect of A. salmonicida on complement activity, phagocytosis in vivo and the effect of ECP from cell culture supernatants on immune cells in vitro.

ACKNOWLEDGEMENTS

I thank P. de Graaf (Dept. of Molecular Cell Biology, University of Utrecht) for providing the bacterial strains and technical assistance. We are also grateful to Mr W.J.A. Valen for drawing the figures and to Mrs H. Vertregt for typing the manuscript.

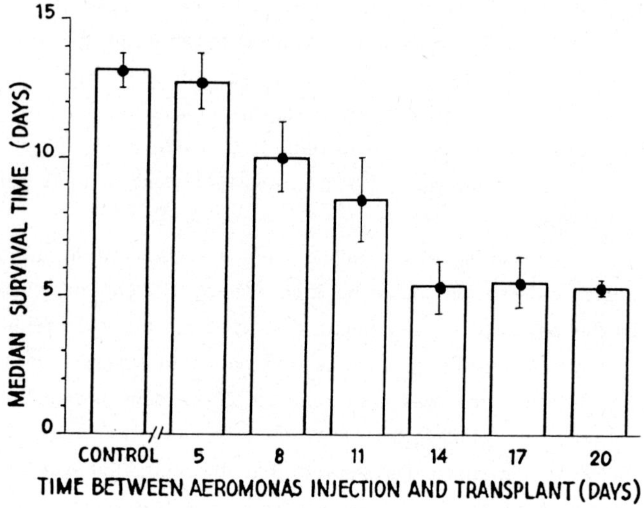

Fig. 3. Median survival time of first set skin allografts in fish grafted 5, 8, 11, 14, 17, and 20 days after sublethal injection of $2x10^4$ virulent (●). A salmonicida per fish. Points represent arithmetic means ± 1 SE (n=10).

REFERENCES

Anderson, D.P. 1974. Fish immunology. Book 4 (239 pp.) in S.F. Snieko and H.R. Axelrod, eds. Diseases of fishes. T.F.H. Pub., Neptune City, N.J.

Anderson, D.P., B.S. Roberson, and D.W. Dixon. 1979. Induction of antibody - producing cells in rainbow trout, Salmo gairdneri Richardson; by flush exposure. J. Fish. Biol. 15: 317-322.

Austin, B., and C.J. Rodgers. 1981. Preliminary observations on Aeromonas salmonicida vaccines. Pages 387-393. in: D.P. Anderson and W. Hennessen, eds. Proceedings of the international symposium on Fish Biologics, Serodiagnosis and Vaccines. Developments in Biological Standardization. S. Karger, Basel.

Cipriano, R.C. 1982. Immunization of brook trout (Salvelinus fontinalis) against Aeromonas salmonicida: immunogenicity of virulent and avirulent isolates and protective ability of different antigens. Can. J. Fish. Aquat. Sci. 39: 218-221.

Cipriano, R.C. 1983. Resistance of salmonids to Aeromonas salmonicida: relation between agglutinins and neutralizing activities. Trans. Am. Fish. Soc. 112: 95-99.

Evenberg, D., R. van Boxtel, B. Lugtenberg, F. Schurer, J. Blommaert, and R. Bootsma. 1982. Cell surface of the fish pathogenic bacterium Aeromonas salmonicida. 1. Relationship between autoagglutination and the presence of a major cell envelop protein. Biochem. Biophys. Acta. 684: 241-248.

Evenberg, D., R. Bootsma and B. Lugtenberg. 1984. Antigens of the fish pathogen Aeromonas salmonicida and their potential as a vaccine candidate. Abstract p. 36-37, 16th. Lunteren Lectures on Molecular Genetics, 'Strategies in vaccine development', October 1984, Lunteren, The Netherlands.

Füller, D.W., K.S. Pilcher, and J.L. Fryer. 1977. A leucocytolytic factor isolated from cultures of Aeromonas salmonicida. J. Fish. Res. Board. Can. 34: 1118-1125.

Herman, R.L. 1968. Fish furunculosis 1952-1966. Trans. Am. Fish. Soc. 97: 221-230.

Karlsson, K.A. 1962. Studies of the haemolysin of Aeromonas salmonicida. Nord Veterinaer medecin 14, suppl. 2.

Klontz, G.W., W.T. Yasutake, and A.J. Ross. 1966. Bacterial diseases in salmonicidae in the western United States: Pathogenesis of furunculosis in rainbow trout. Am. J. Vet. Res. 27: 1455-1480.

Krantz, G.E., J.M. Reddecliffe, and C.E. Heist. 1963. Development of antibodies against Aeromonas salmonicida in trout. J. Immunol. 9: 757-760.

McCarthy, D.H. and R.J. Roberts. 1980. Furunculosis of fish - the present state of our knowledge. Pages 293-341 in M.R. Droop and H.W. Jannasch, eds. Advances in aquatic microbiology, Vol. 2. Academic Press, London.

McCraw, B.M. 1952. Furunculosis of fish. U.S. Fish. Wildl. Serv., Spec. Sci. Rep. Fish. No. 84. 87 pp.

Mellegaard, S. 1983. Purification and characterization of new proteolytic enzymes produced by Aeromonas salmonicida. J. Appl. Bacteriol. 45: 289-294.

Michel, C. 1979. Furunculosis of salmonids: vaccination attempts in rainbow trout (Salmo gairdneri) by formalin-killed germs. Ann. Rech. Vet. 10: 33-40.

Munn, C.B., E.F. Ishiguro, W.W. Kay, and T.J. Trust. 1982. Role of the surface components in serum resistence of virulent Aeromonas salmonicida. Infect. Immun. 36: 1069-1075.

Munro, A.L.S., T.S. Hastings, A.E. Ellis, and J. Liversidge. 1980. Studies on an ichthyotoxic material produced extracellularly by the furunculosis bacterium Aeromonas salmonicida. Pages 98-106 in: W. Ahne, ed. Fish diseases. Third COPARQ-Session. Springer-Verlag, Berlin.

Nomura, S. and H. Saito. 1982. Production of the extracellular hemolytic toxin by an isolated strain of Aeromonas salmonicida. Bull. Jpn. Soc. Sci. Fish. 48: 1589-1597.

Paterson, W.D., and J.L. Fryer. 1974. Effects of temperature and antigen doses on the antibody response of juvenile coho salmon (Oncorynchus kisutch) to Aeromonas salmonicida endotoxin. J. Fish. Res. Board. Can. 31: 1743-1749.

Paterson, W.D. 1981. Aeromonas salmonicida as an immunogen. Pages 375-385 in D.P. Anderson and W. Hennessen, eds. Proceedings of the International Symposium on Fish Biologics: Serodiagnostics and vaccines. Developments in Biological Standardization. S. Karger, Basel.

Sakai, D.K. 1984. The non-specific activation of rainbow trout, Salmo gairdneri Richardson, complement by Aeromonas salmonicida extracellular products and the correlation of complement activity with the inactivation of lethal toxicity products. J. Fish. Dis. 7: 329-338.

Sheeran, B., and P.R. Smith. 1981. A second extracellular proteolytic activity associated with the fish pathogen Aeromonas salmonicida. FEMS Microbiol. Letters 11, 73-76.

Shieh, H.S., and J.R. Mclean. 1975. Purification and properties of an extracellular protease of Aeromonas salmonicida, the causative agent of furuncolosis. Int. J. Biochem. 6: 653-656.

Smith, P.D., D.H. McCarthy, and W.D. Paterson. 1980. Further studies on furunculosis vaccination. Pages 112-119 in: W. Ahne, ed. Fish diseases. Third CO-PRACQ Session. Springer-Verlag, Berlin.

Spence, K.D., J.L. Fryer, and K.S. Pilcher. 1965. Active and passive immunization of certain salmonid fishes against Aeromonas salmonicida. Can. J. Microbiol. 11: 397-402.

Tajima, K., T. Takahashi, Y. Egura, and T. Kimura. 1984. Enzymatic properties of the purified extracellular protease of Aeromonas salmonicida. Ar-4 (EFDL). Bull. Jpn. Soc. Sci. Fish. 50: 145-150.

Titball, R., and C.B. Munn. 1985. Interrelationships extracellular products from Aeromonas salmonicida. in: A.S. Ellis, ed. Recent advances in fish and shell fish pathology. Academic Press, (in press).

Trust, T.J., P.S. Howard, J.B. Chamberlain, E.E. Ishiguro and J.T. Buckley. 1980. Additional surface protein in autoaggregating strains of atypical Aeromonas salmonicida. FEMS Microbiol. Lett. 9, 35-38.
Udey, L.R., and J.L. Fryer. 1978. Immunization of fish with bacterins of Aeromonas salmonicida. Mar. Fish. Rev. 40: 12-17.
Weber, J.M., and B.M. Zwicker. 1979. Aeromonas salmonicida in Atlantic salmon (Salmo salar): occurrence of specific agglutinins to three bacterial pathogens. J. Fish. Res. Bd. Can. 36: 1102-1107.

Veterinary Immunology and Immunopathology, 12 (1986) 339—344
Elsevier Science Publishers B.V., Amsterdam — Printed in The Netherlands

SURFACE ANTIGENS OF VIRULENT STRAINS OF AEROMONAS HYDROPHILA

James S.G. DOOLEY,[1] R. LALLIER,[2] and Trevor J. TRUST[1]

[1]Department of Biochemistry and Microbiology, University of Victoria, Victoria, British Columbia, Canada V8W 2Y2

[2]Department of Pathology and Microbiology, Faculty of Veterinary Medicine, University of Montreal, Saint Hyacinthe, Quebec, Canada

ABSTRACT

Dooley, J.S.G., Lallier, R. and Trust, T.J., 1986. Surface antigens of virulent strains of Aeromonas hydrophila. Vet. Immunol. Immunopathol., 12: 339-344.

Antiserum was raised in rabbits to whole cells of a representative strain from a group of A. hydrophila strains exhibiting enhanced virulence for fish. The major surface antigens of the strain were identified by sodium dodecyl sulfate polyacrylamide gel electrophoresis (SDS-PAGE) and Western blotting. The lipopolysaccharide (LPS) was examined using SDS-PAGE and silver staining. It was found to possess O polysaccharide chains of homogeneous length that were highly immunogenic. The LPS was conserved both morphologically and antigenically throughout the high virulence group. Heat-labile protein antigens were detected after absorption of the antiserum with boiled cells of the homologous strain. Only one major protein antigen, with a molecular weight of approximately 52,000, was present in outer membrane preparations or in whole cell lysates. A representative strain from the high virulence group, strain TF7, was shown by electron microscopy to be covered by a regular surface protein array (S-layer) which was found to be composed primarily of the 52 KD protein antigen. All the other members of the A. hydrophila high virulence group were shown to possess similar S-layers.

INTRODUCTION

Motile Aeromonas species are widespread inhabitants of aquatic environments and are reported to be constituents of the normal gut flora of fish (Neilson, 1978; Trust and Sparrow, 1974). Strains of A. hydrophila are also recognized as fish pathogens causing a form of hemorrhagic septicemia in salmonids (Bullock et al., 1971). In most cases these strains are associated with opportunistic infections. Recently however, a group of highly virulent A. hydrophila strains have been isolated (Mittal et al., 1980). These investigators found that the virulent strains constituted a single serogroup and they suggested that the specificity was determined by the O antigen. The strains also exhibited a number of unique phenotypic properties that were thought to be cell-surface associated. These included autoaggregation during growth in static broth culture and resistance to the bactericidal activity of normal serum. Since the development of a successful vaccine against these pathogenic A. hydrophila

0165-2427/86/$03.50 © 1986 Elsevier Science Publishers B.V.

strains would obviously be desirable, we have initiated a study of the antigenic structure of the cell surface of the high-virulence group. Here we report on the identification of lipopolysaccharide (LPS) and protein antigens unique to this group.

MATERIALS AND METHODS

Bacterial strains and growth conditions

Virulent strains of *A. hydrophila* were isolated as previously described (Mittal et al., 1980) and maintained at -70°C in 15% (vol/vol) glycerol-tryptic soy broth. All strains were grown on Tryptic Soy Agar (TSA) at 37°C for 18 to 48 hours.

Antiserum production

A. hydrophila strain TF7 was grown for 24 hours. The cells were then resuspended in formalin to a density of approximately 10^{10} cells/ml and held overnight at 4°C. They were washed 3 times and resuspended to the same density in phosphate buffered saline (PBS). The initial inoculum was prepared by emulsifying 2 ml of cell suspension in an equal volume of Freund's Complete Adjuvant. Adult New Zealand white rabbits were immunized via both the intramuscular (IM) and subcutaneous (SC) routes. Booster doses, in Incomplete Freund's Adjuvant, were administered SC every 14 days. On day 42 the animals were bled and the serum was collected and stored. Absorption of the antiserum was accomplished by resuspending 10 mg of boiled cells of *A. hydrophila* TF7 in 1.0 ml of serum and incubating the suspension at room temperature for 1 hour. Cells were removed by centrifugation at 12,000 × g for 10 minutes, the supernatant was added to fresh cells and the absorption was repeated.

Sodium dodecyl sulfate polyacrylamide gel electrophoresis (SDS-PAGE)

SDS-PAGE was carried out using the discontinuous buffer system described by Laemmli, 1970. Proteins and LPS were stacked in 4.5% acrylamide at 100 V and separated in 12.5% acrylamide at 200 V. Protein bands were visualized by staining with Coomassie blue. LPS was detected using the silver staining procedure of Tsai and Frasch, 1982. Whole cell lysates were prepared by boiling 1 mg (wet weight) of cells for 10 minutes in 100 µl of solubilization buffer (62.5 mM Tris pH 6.8, 10% glycerol, 3% SDS, 5% β-mercaptoethanol 0.01% bromophenol blue). Outer membranes were isolated by centrifugation following sarkosyl digestion of isolated cell envelopes as described by Filip et al., 1973.

Western blotting

Western blotting was carried out using the Methanol-Tris-Glycine buffer system of Towbin et al., 1979. Proteins and LPS were electrophoretically transferred from SDS-PAGE gels to 0.45 μ nitrocellulose sheets for 18 hours at 60 V. Unreacted binding sites were blocked by incubating the sheets in 30 mM Tris pH 7.3, 0.15 M NaCl and 1% gelatin (TSG) for 1 hour at room temperature. The sheets were then incubated with antiserum, diluted in TSG, for 2 hours. They were washed in 30 mM Tris pH 7.4, 0.15 M NaCl (TS) and reacted with ^{125}I *Staphylococcus aureus* Protein A, at 5×10^5 cpm/ml in TSG for a further 2 hours. After extensive washing in TS and tap water the sheets were dried and subjected to autoradiography.

Electron microscopy

A. hydrophila TF7 was grown for 48 hours and the cells were then resuspended in 30 mM Tris pH 8.0 to a density of 10^{10} cells/ml. They were transferred to 200 mesh copper grids, that had previously been coated with 1% formvar, by floating the grids on drops of the cell suspension. These preparations were negatively stained with either 1% potassium phosphotungstate pH 7.0 or 2% uranyl acetate pH 4.5. The grids were examined in a Philips EM 300 transmission electron microscope at an accelerating voltage of 80 KV.

RESULTS AND DISCUSSION

To determine the major surface antigens of the high virulence group, antiserum was raised in rabbits to whole cells of a representative strain, *A. hydrophila* TF7. The antigens were then identified by SDS-PAGE and Western blotting.

The smooth-type LPS of Gram negative bacteria normally constitutes a major surface antigen. When the LPS of *A. hydrophila* TF7 was analysed by SDS-PAGE and silver staining (Fig. 1, lane 1) it was resolved into two components; a fast migrating component presumably consisting of core oligosaccharide and lipid A and a slower migrating component which resolved into several closely spaced bands composed of core oligosaccharide, lipid A and O polysaccharide. This electrophoretic morphology indicates that the O polysaccharide chains of *A. hydrophila* TF7 are of homogenous chain length. A similar morphology was observed for the LPS of other members of the high virulence group (data not shown). A number of avirulent *A. hydrophila* strains were examined and found to have LPS with heterogeneous chain length O polysaccharides (data not shown). Western blot analysis showed that the whole cell antiserum contained antibodies to LPS (Fig. 1, lane 2) and also showed that the O polysaccharide was the immunodominant region of the LPS molecule since no antibody reactivity was detected with the core-lipid A portion. The whole cell antiserum to *A. hydrophila* TF7 also bound strongly to the O polysaccharides of all the other members of the high virulence group (Fig. 1, lanes 3-7). No reaction was obtained with the heterogeneous chain length O polysaccharides of any other A. hydrophila strains tested (data not shown). With respect to its LPS morphology and antigenicity the A. hydrophila high virulence group is similar to the other important fish pathogen Aeromonas salmonicida, the causative agent of furunculosis. This organism has also been shown to possess highly immunogenic O polysaccharide chains of constant length in its LPS and to exhibit extensive antigenic cross-reactivity among various strains (Chart et al., 1984).

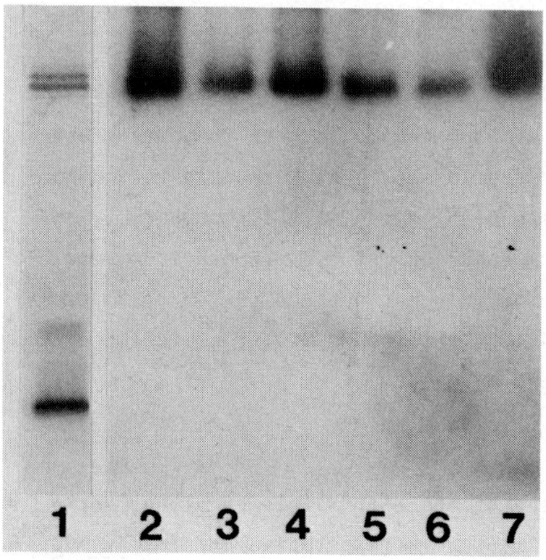

Fig. 1. Structure and immunological cross-reactivity of the LPS of the A. hydrophila high virulence group demonstrated by SDS-PAGE and Western blotting. Proteinase-K digested whole cell lysates were used as a source of LPS. Lane 1, silver stain of A. hydrophila strain TF7 LPS. Lanes 2-7, Western blot analysis with antiserum prepared in rabbits to whole cells of A. hydrophila TF7. (dilution 1:500) reacted with LPS of A. hydrophila strains TF7 (lane), LL1 (lane 3), A80-160 (lane 4), A80-140 (lane 5), P77-115 (lane 6), and A82-256 (lane 7).

The major protein antigens of A. hydrophila TF7 were detected by Western blotting using antiserum absorbed against boiled cells. When reacted against outer membrane preparations (Fig. 2, lane 2) or whole cell lysates (data not shown) after SDS-PAGE separation only one major heat-labile antigen was found to be present. This antigen had an approximate molecular weight of 52,000. Since studies with A. salmonicida had previously shown that virulent strains produced a major surface protein antigen of 49,000 (Phipps et al., 1983), and since this 49,000 M_r protein constituted the major subunit of a tetragonally arranged surface protein array we examined A. hydrophila TF7 by electron microscopy for the presence of a similar structure. Negative staining revealed a regularly arrayed surface layer (S-layer) on this strain (Fig. 3). The S-layer of A. hydrophila TF7 was most easily visualized after it had detached from the cell. The layer appeared to be composed of tetragonally arranged subunits and it completely covered the surface of the cell. Examination of other virulent A. hydrophila strains showed that they all produced similarly arranged S-layers (data not shown). Isolation procedures have provided evidence that the 52,000 M_r protein of A. hydrophila TF7 represents the major S-layer subunit and studies are now underway to further characterize the protein.

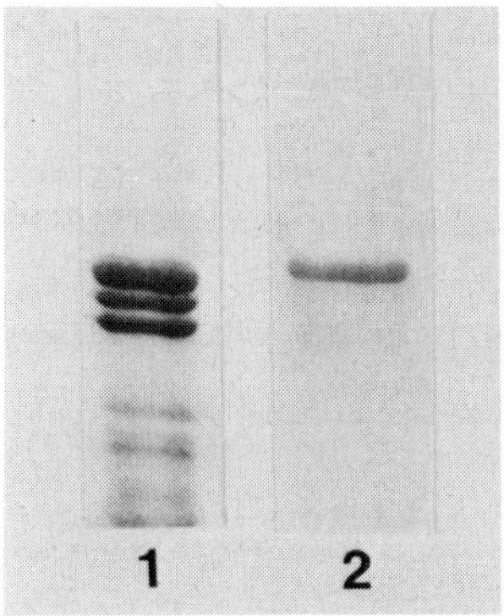

Fig. 2 Identification of the major heat-labile protein antigen in outer membrane preparations of A. hydrophila TF7. Lane 1, outer membrane proteins separated on a 7.5% SDS-PAGE gel and stained by Coomassie blue. Lane 2, Western blot of outer membrane preparation reacted with antisera (dilution 1:500) prepared in rabbits to whole cells of A. hydrophila TF7 and absorbed against boiled cells of TF7. The reaction shown in lane 2 is with a protein of approximate M_r 52,000.

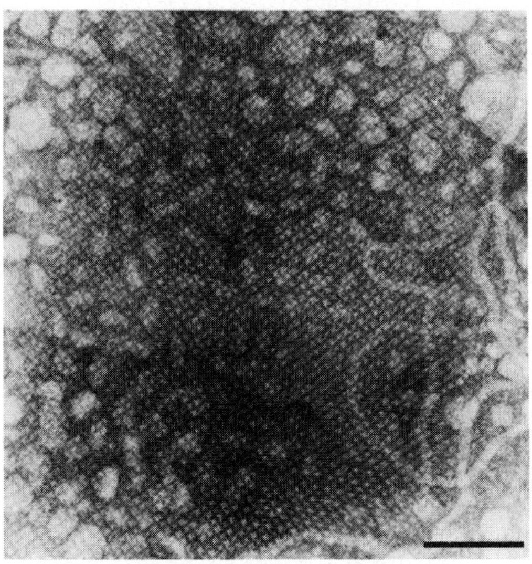

Fig. 3. Regular surface protein array (S-layer) from A. hydrophila TF7 negatively stained with 1% potassium phosphotungstate pH 7. Bar equals 100 nm.

ACKNOWLEDGEMENTS

J.S.G.D. was the recipient of a University of Victoria graduate student fellowship. This study was supported, in part, by the Natural Sciences and Engineering Research Council of Canada. R.G.E. Murray provided valuable advice throughout the course of this study and confirmed the presence of an S-layer on strain TF7.

REFERENCES

Bullock, G.L., Conroy, D.A. and Snieszki, S.F., 1971. In: Snieszki, S.F. and Axelrod, H.R. (Editors), Diseases of Fish, Book 2A, T.F.H. New Jersey, pp. 27-42.

Chart, H., Shaw, D.H., Ishiguro, E.E. and Trust, T.J., 1984. Structural and immunochemical homogeneity of *Aeromonas salmonicida* lipopolysaccharide. J. Bacteriol. 158:16-22.

Filip, C., Fletcher, G., Wulff, J.L. and Earhart, C.F., 1973. Solubilization of the cytoplasmic membrane of *E. coli* by the ionic detergent sodium-lauryl sarcosinate. J. Bacteriol. 115:717-722.

Laemmli, U.K., 1970. Cleavage of structural proteins during the assembly of the head of bacteriophage T4. Nature 227:680-685.

Mittal, K.R., Lalonde, G., Leblanc, D., Olivier, G. and Lallier, R., 1980. *Aeromonas hydrophila* in rainbow trout: relation between virulence and surface characteristics. Can. J. Microbiol. 26:1501-1503.

Neilson, A.H., 1978. The occurrence of Aeromonads in activated sludge: isolation of *Aeromonas sobria* and its possible confusion with *Escherichia coli*. J. Appl. Bacteriol. 44:259-264.

Phipps, B.M., Trust, T.J., Ishiguro, E.E. and Kay, W.W., 1983. Purification and characterization of the cell surface virulent A protein from *Aeromonas salmonicida*. Biochemistry 22:2934-2939.

Towbin, H., Staehelin, T. and Gordon, J., 1979. Electrophoretic transfer of proteins from polyacrylamide gels to nitrocellulose sheets: procedure and some applications. Proc. Natl. Acad. Sci. U.S.A. 76:4350-4354.

Trust, T.J. and Sparrow, R.A.H., 1974. The bacterial flora in the alimentary tract of freshwater salmonid fishes. Can. J. Microbiol. 20:1219-1228.

Tsai, C-M. and Frasch, C.E., 1982. A sensitive silver stain for detecting lipopolysaccharide in polyacrylamide gels. Anal. Biochem. 119:15-19.

Veterinary Immunology and Immunopathology, 12 (1986) 345—350
Elsevier Science Publishers B.V., Amsterdam — Printed in The Netherlands

PROTECTIVE EFFICACY OF AEROMONAS HYDROPHILA VACCINES IN NILE TILAPIA

LILA RUANGPAN[1], T. KITAO[2] and T. YOSHIDA[2]

[1]Brackishwater Fisheries Div., Kasetsart Univ. Campus, Bangkok-10900, Thailand.

[2]Dept. of Fisheries, Faculty of Agriculture, Miyazaki Univ., Miyazaki-880, Japan.

ABSTRACT

Ruangpan, L., Kitao, T. and Yoshida, Y., 1986. Protective efficacy of *Aeromonas hydrophila* vaccines in Nile tilapia. Vet. Immunol. Immunopathol., 12: 345-350.

Protection and serum antibody production against *Aeromonas hydrophila* was examined in nile tilapia, *Tilapia nilotica* (L.). Intraperitoneally injected formalin-killed and Freunds complete adjuvant vaccines were compared using different doses (2.9 x 10^7 and 2.9 x 10^9 cfu/ml). Upon challenge, the protective ability and antibody titers resulting were significantly different between vaccinated and unvaccinated groups. A relative level of protection of 100% was obtained within two-weeks, and a maximum level of 53 - 61% protection was found one-week post-vaccination.

INTRODUCTION

The widespread outbreak of infectious diseases in Thailand during December 1982 to February 1983 resulted in economic loss of over 500 million Baht (Anonymous, 1983). Many species of fishes and varieties of aquatic animals were damaged due to diseases which included parasitic protozoa, bacteria, and fungi (DOF Bangkok, 1983). The most serious cases were found to be infected with *Aeromonas hydrophila* which exhibited 100% incidence of infection in samples reared in farms, and 95.24% in the wild fishes (Boonyaratpalin et al., 1983).

Numerous investigations have been done in order to solve the problems (Boonyaratpalin et al., 1983; Kasornchan and Reungprach, 1983). However, no work has been seriously done on prevention and control aspects. Furthermore, it is evident that studies dealing with fish vaccination in this country are sadly lacking. The present paper aims to investigate protection against *A. hydrophila* induced in *Tilapia nilotica* by intraperitoneal injection of formalin killed cell vaccines, with or without Freunds complete adjuvant.

0165-2427/86/$03.50 © 1986 Elsevier Science Publishers B.V.

MATERIALS AND METHODS

Fish

Nile tilapia, Tilapia nilotica (L.), 12 - 16 cm in total length, were obtained from the Fish Nutrition and Biochemistry Lab., Fac. of Agriculture, Miyazaki Univ. Miyazaki, Japan. Fish were acclimatized in glass aquaria at 18 - 22°C prior to experiment.

Bacterial strains

Eight strains of A. hydrophila isolated from diseased fish sampled during the recent widespread outbreak of diseases in Thailand were provided by the Fac. of Veterinary Science, Chulalongkorn Univ., Bangkok, Thailand. Cultures were maintained in nutrient agar stabs at room temperature until used.

Pathogenicity of Strain Tests

Virulence and lethal doses of each strain were tested employing intraperitoneal injection and hyperosmotic infiltration methods, as described by Antipa et al. (1980). Approximately 10^7 and 10^9 cfu/ml concentrations were used. The number of bacteria were determined by pour plate colony counting.

Vaccine Preparation

A. hydrophila F-639, which proved to be the most virulent isolate, was used in preparation the following vaccines :

a) Formalin killed cells: formaldehyde (37%) was added to 10^7 and 10^9 cfu/ml suspensions of bacterial cells, to a final concentration of 1% (v/v) and left overnight at 4°C. The inactivated cells were harvested and were washed 3-times in saline and then re-suspended.

b) Adjuvant vaccine: Adjuvant vaccine was prepared by removing the saline solution and resuspending the cells at 2-times of the desired concentration. Then the suspension was well mixed with an equal volume of Freunds complete adjuvant (Difco) just before use.

Administration and Challenge

Each test group contained 60 fish. Two groups were vaccinated with 0.1 ml of formalin killed cells, at levels of 10^7 and 10^9 cfu/ml respectively. Two other groups were injected with these doses plus adjuvant. Controls were injected with 0.1 ml of sterile saline solution. All groups were maintained under the same conditions, held at 18 - 22°C and fed with commercial pellets through out the experimental period.

At 1, 2, 3 and 5 weeks after vaccination, each group was injected with 0.1 ml of a 10^9 cfu/ml preparation of A. hydrophila F-639. Mortalities were recorded and removed daily over 15-days. The cause of death was determined by calturing the kidney and liver of dead fish for A. hydrophila The relative level of protection (RLP) in each group was determined using the method of Newman and Majnarichs (1982).

Blood Collection and Antibody Titration

All surviving fish were bled by caudal vein puncture. The serum was removed and used for agglutination test employing a microtiter procedure, and using two-fold dilutions of serum and equal volumes of formalin killed cells of *A. hydrophila* at 10^8 cfu/ml as antigen. The titers were recorded at the last dilution of sera resulting in agglutination.

RESULTS

Eighty percent of the fishes injected with 10^7 and 10^9 cfu/ml of *A. hydrophila* died 3 to 4 days after challenging for pathogenicity tests. No deaths were observed in either group challenged by hyperosmotic infiltration.

Exposure of nile tilapia to *A. hydrophila* at 1-week after vaccination gave mortalities at 33.34 and 40% when vaccinated with 10^7 and 10^9 cfu/ml respectively. No mortalities occurred in the challenged groups 2, 3 or 5-weeks post-vaccination. Unvaccinated groups had high rates of total mortality at 86.66, 73.33, 73.33 and 80% within 3 days (See Table 1, Fig. 1, 2). Presence of *A. hydrophila* was seen in all cultures of liver and kidney samples of dead fish. Mean peak of antibody production in nile tilapia at titres of 65,536 and 130,672 were obtained from groups immunized with 10^7 and 10^9 cfu/ml inocula, four-week post-injection. The mean titers of both groups maintained high titres (2,805 to 49,960) throughout the experiments. Nonimmunized fish maintained constant background titers of between 32 to 64. The titers showed a significant difference between nonimmunized and those immunized groups, at a confidence interval of $P \geqq 0.001$. The titers of the controls remaining after challenge varied from 64 to 65,536.

TABLE 1

Comparison of the relative level of protection (RLP) between unvaccinated control and vaccinated groups receiving different doses of formalin killed and adjuvant vaccines of *A. hydrophila* .

Challenge schedule post-vaccination	Vaccinated groups 10^7 (10^9) cfu/ml		Unvaccinated control (Sterile 0.85% saline)		
	Mortality	RLP	Mortality	RLP	(%)
One-week	33.34 (40.00)	61.60 (53.85)	86.66	0	
Two-week	0	100	73.33	0	
Three-week	0	100	73.33	0	
Five-week	0	100	80.00	0	

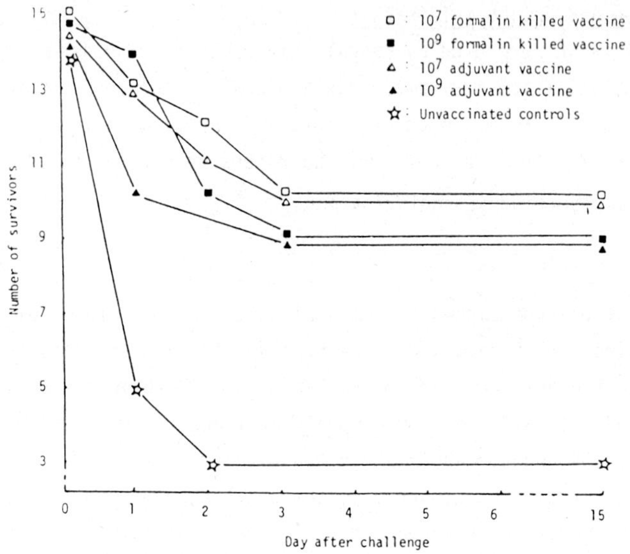

Fig. 1. The number of surviving fishes in unvaccinated control and vaccinated groups injected with different doses of formalin killed and adjuvant vaccines. Challenge was made at one-week post-vaccination.

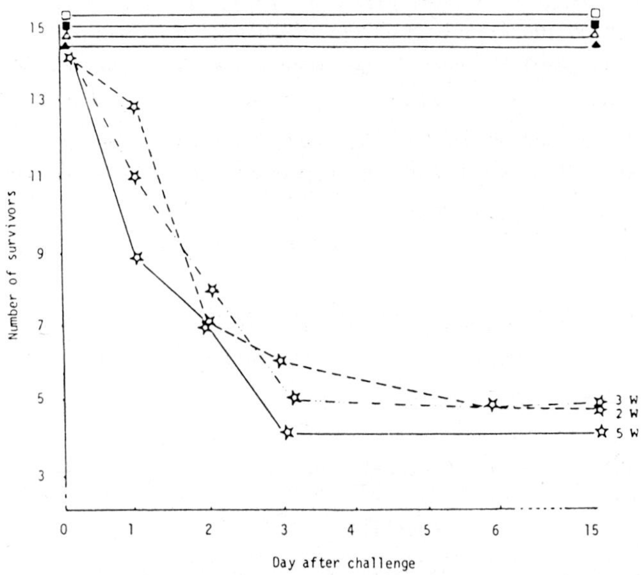

Fig. 2. The number of surviving nile tilapia in unvaccinated control and vaccinated groups injected with different doses of formalin killed and adjuvant vaccines of A. hydrophila. Challenges were made at two, three, and five-week post-vaccination (Legend as for Fig. 1).

DISCUSSION

The results from our tests for the pathogenicity of bacterial strains suggest that the hyperosmotic infiltration challenge technique is ineffective for nile tilapia with A. hydrophila. Consequently, it is reasonable to expect that vaccination by hyperosmotic infiltration may also be ineffective in this situation; although it proved successful for other fishes, with different species of bacteria (Aoki et al., 1982; Croy and Amend, 1977; Johnson and Amend, 1983). Hence, the method of delivery of vaccine as well as the choice of the bacterial strains used for certain species of fish must be taken into consideration. The level of protection in nile tilapia was low during the first week post-vaccination, however, the efficacies of both our vaccines were extremely acceptable when applied two-week before challenging. The conclusion could be made from our results that formalin-killed and adjuvant vaccines did not differ in the degree of protection induced in nile tilapia, as both immunization trials gave remarkably high RLP and high antibody titers. The greater the quantity of antigen inoculated, the higher and longer were the titers maintained. The high titres of antibody production in the controls remaining after challenge may indicate the influences of the genetic factor (Bellanti, 1978).

ACKNOWLEDGEMENTS

We would like to acknowledge financial assistance from the International Foundation for Science, Sweden and the Ministry of Education, Science and Culture of Japan. Thanks are given to Dr. H. TAKEDA who provided nile tilapia for our studies. We also express our sincere thanks to Dr. Douglas P. ANDERSON and Dr. Roselynn M.W. STEVENSON for valuable discussions and reviewing the manuscript.

REFERENCES

Anonymous, 1983. Thairath Newspaper. June 6, 1983, Column 1, P. 1, 16. (in Thai)

Antipa, R., R.W. Gould and D.F. Amend, 1980. Vibrio anguillarum vaccination of sockeye salmon, Oncorhynchus nerka (Walbaum) by direct and hyperosmotic immersion. J. of Fish Diseases. 3: 161-165.

Aoki, T., T. Kitao, M. Fukudome, S. Takahashi and S. Egusa, 1982. Immunization and Challenge of ayu (Plecoglossus altivelis) against vibriosis by the hyperosmotic infiltration method. Bull. Fac. Agri. Miyazaki Univ. 29: 77-85.

Bellanti, Joseph A., 1978. Immunology II. Asian Ed. Press of Igaku Shoin Ltd. Japan. 813 pp.

Boonyaratpalin, S., H. Reuangprach, S. Direkboosarakom, J. Kasornchan and K. Soupamataya, 1983. Bacterial infectious. Thai Fish. Gazette. 36(3): 247-255. (in Thai)

Croy, T.R. and D.F. Amend, 1977. Immunization of sockeye salmon (*Oncorhynchus nerka*) against vibriosis using hyperosmotic infiltration. Aquaculture. 12: 317-325.

DOF Bangkok, Thailand, 1983. Announcement on Fish Diseases. Dept. of Fisheries, Bangkok, Thailand. January 6, 1983. (in Thai)

Jo, Y., 1981. Studies of *Vibrio anguillarum* infection in cultured ayu and its immunological prophylaxis. Shikoku Acta. Medica. 37: 82-110.

Johnson, K.A. and D.F. Amend, 1983. Comparison of efficacy of several delivery methods using *Yersinia ruckeri* bacterin on rainbow trout, *Salmo gairdneri* Richardson. J. of Fish Diseases. 6: 331-336.

Kasornchan, J. and H. Reungprach, 1983. Occurrence of *Aeromonas hydrophila* in natural waters and cultured ponds. Thai Fish. Gazette. 36(3): 257-260.

Newman, S.G. and J.J. Majnarich, 1982. Direct immersion vaccination of juvenile rainbow trout, *Salmo gairdneri* Richardson, and juvenile coho salmon, *Oncorhynchus kisutch (Walbaum)*, with a *Yersinia ruckeri* bacterin. J. of Fish Diseases. 5: 339-341.

Veterinary Immunology and Immunopathology, 12 (1986) 351—357
Elsevier Science Publishers B.V., Amsterdam — Printed in The Netherlands

IMMUNO-RESPONSE IN TILAPIA *Sarotherodon niloticus* VACCINATED WITH *Edwardsiella tarda* BY HYPEROSMOTIC INFILTRATION METHOD

GILDA LIO-PO[1] and HISATSUGU WAKABAYASHI[2]

[1]Aquaculture Department, Southeast Asian Fisheries Development Center
Tigbauan, Iloilo, Philippines

[2]Laboratory of Aquaculture Biology, University of Tokyo
Bunkyo-ku, Tokyo, Japan

ABSTRACT

Lio-Po, G. and Wakabayashi, H., 1986. Immuno-response in Tilapia *Sarotherodon niloticus* vaccinated with *Edwardsiella tarda* by hyperosmotic infiltration method. Vet. Immunol. Immunopathol., 12: 351-357.

Sarotherodon niloticus with average weight of 28.42 $\pm$ 1.87 g were immunized with formalin-killed *Edwardsiella tarda* using the hyperosmotic infiltration method. Test fish maintained in 30 l aquaria were grouped into four treatments. Group 1 and 2 were exposed to a single hyperosmotic treatment on day 0. Group 1 was bled on day 14 and group 2 was bled on day 28. Group 3 was given hyperosmotic treatments twice: on day 0 and day 14 and bled on day 28. Group 4 was an untreated control bled on day 28. All sera were analyzed for agglutinating antibody titer against *E. tarda* flagellar and somatic antigens. Results showed that flagellar and somatic agglutinin titers in all treatments were not statistically significant. Likewise, infection experiments where test fish were challenged with intraperitoneal injection of the test bacterium showed that the vaccination experiment did not effectively protect the test fish from infection by *Edwardsiella tarda*.

INTRODUCTION

The occurrence of *Edwardsiella tarda* as a fish pathogen of cultured fish have been reported earlier among eels (Wakabayashi and Egusa, 1973); Tilapia (Lio-Po *et al.*, 1982; Roberts and Sommerville, 1982); and carp (Sae-Oni *et al.*, 1984). As an important pathogen for fish, research on preventive measures became a natural concern. Among available techniques, vaccination by the hyperosmotic infiltration method of antigen administration showed promising potentials (Antipa and Amend, 1976; Amend and Fender, 1976; Croy and Amend, 1977; Lannan, 1978; Fender and Amend, 1978). Furthermore, booster administration enhanced the efficacy of vaccinations (Kusuda *et al.*, 1978; Antipa and Amend, 1977). Hence, isolates of *E. tarda* obtained from a 1979 *S. niloticus* epizootic in Japan were further studied in a vaccination experiment. The objectives of this study was to determine the humoral antibody response of *S. niloticus* after vaccination with *E. tarda* bacterin in terms of agglutinin production and protection from subsequent challenge.

0165-2427/86/$03.50 © 1986 Elsevier Science Publishers B.V.

METHODS

Experimental fish

Sarotherodon niloticus obtained from Shizuoka Prefecture, Japan were utilized for this study. The average fish weight was 28.42 ± 1.87 g. The fish were acclimatized for no less than two weeks in concrete tanks before the experiments. During acclimation period and the experimental runs, the fish were fed daily a commercially-prepared diet to satiation. Tap water was neutralized with sodium thiosulfate prior to use. Each aquarium was stocked with 15 test fish, provided with aeration and a 30% daily water change.

Preparation of bacteria

Pure cultures of *Edwardsiella tarda* from a 1979 epizootic among *S. niloticus* in Nagaoka, Niigata Prefecture, Japan (Lio-Po *et al.*, 1982) were used. Mass culture of these was made in trypticase soy broth (TSB), incubated at 25°C for 18 h. Approximate cell density was estimated at 2×10^9 cells/ml. The bacterial cells were killed with 0.5% formalin, aseptically washed three times with normal saline solution in a refrigerated centrifuge. The packed bacteria were then resuspended to its original volume with saline to a final pH of 7 and stored at 4°C.

Vaccination procedure

Hyperosmotic infiltration was employed dipping 5 test fish at a time into the bacterin suspension for a 1.5 min dip following the method of Croy and Amend (1977). Control fish were similarly treated except for the substitution of the bacterin with saline. The test fish were grouped into four treatments. Groups 1, 2, and 3 were exposed to the bacterin on day 0 with group 3 fish receiving a second dose of bacterin exposure on day 14. Group 1 fish were bled on day 14, while group 2 and 3 fish were bled on day 28. The fourth group of fish served as control and were bled on day 28. Each treatment including controls consisted of 15 fish. Vaccination was conducted at a temperature of 26 to 32°C.

Collection of fish serum

For group 1, 2 and 3, ten out of 15 fish were randomly removed from their aquaria and bled by severing the caudal artery and filling capillary tubes. Blood was stored at 4°C overnight then individually harvested after centrifugation. Serum was then stored at -20°C. Only 5 fish were bled from the control group.

Agglutination titer determination

E. tarda grown for 24 h on trypticase soy agar tube slants were harvested by dispersion of colonies with saline. Flagellar (H) antigens consisted of bacteria treated with Merthiolate at 1:10,000. Washed cells were diluted with saline to a suspension comparable with the #3 Mc Farland Standard. The somatic (O) antigens were similarly prepared except that the bacterial cell suspension was heated at 100°C for 30 min. Both antigen suspensions were tested for sterility and stored at 4°C until use.

Hyperimmune antisera to *E. tarda* was produced by intravenous injections of rabbits following the method of Carpenter (1975). This specific antiserum was used as positive controls in the subsequent agglutination tests.

The standard microtiter agglutination test was employed using 0.025 ml diluters and droppers. Serial dilutions of the test serum of individual fish were made using phosphate buffered saline (PBS) into disposable plates with "U" wells. After antigens were added and mixed, the plates were covered and incubated for 2 h at 37°C then at 5°C overnight. Negative controls consisted of the PBS and antigen mixture. The results were read macroscopically or confirmed microscopically (20x).

Challenge experiments

The remaining vaccinated fish were injected intraperitoneally with a bacterial dose of 0.1 mg cells per 100 g fish. Five fish of group 1 were challenged on day 14 while a similar number of group 2 and 3 were challenged on day 28 including unvaccinated fish.

Statistical analysis of data

Agglutinin titers to both flagellar and somatic antigens were evaluated statistically applying the analysis of variance at 0.05 level of significance.

RESULTS

The agglutinin titers of vaccinated and unvaccinated fish are shown in Table 1. In three samples, determination of agglutinin titers for H antigen was not performed for insufficient volume of serum obtained. The data showed wide disparity in titers from fish to fish even among fish receiving the same treatment. Agglutinin titers of 16 to as high as 256 among vaccinated fish compared to the sham vaccinated group were detected. The overall means indicated some degree of difference with Group 1 fish yielding the highest agglutinin level 3 to 4 times as much as the control. Statistical tests, however, revealed no significant variation among treatments with those of the unvaccinated fish ($P < 0.05$). In addition, no test fish died through out the duration of the experiments.

TABLE 1

Summary of agglutinin titer of *S. niloticus* immunized with *Edwardsiella tarda*.

Fish no.	Group 1		Group 2		Group 3		Control	
	"H"	"O"	"H"	"O"	"H"	"O"	"H"	"O"
1	4	16	16	16	32	32	16	16
2	256	256	8	16	32	32	16	32
3	8	16	8	8	64	64	8	8
4	4	32	32	32	16	8	16	32
5	128	64	16	32	64	32	4	8
6	64	32	8	16	64	32		
7	64	64	8	-	32	16		
8	4	16	8	-	16	32		
9	8	-	128	64	32	16		
10	4	16	4	16	32	16		
$\bar{x}$	54.40	56.88	23.60	25.00	38.40	28.00	12.00	19.20
$\pm$ s.e.	$\pm$25.97	$\pm$25.73	$\pm$11.87	$\pm$6.31	$\pm$5.94	$\pm$4.95	$\pm$2.53	$\pm$5.42

Group 1, vaccinated on day 0; bled on day 14
Group 2, vaccinated on day 0; bled on day 28
Group 3, vaccinated on day 0 and day 14; bled on day 28
Control, unvaccinated; bled on day 28

Upon challenge with *E. tarda* vaccinated *S.niloticus* manifested total mortalities within 24 to 96 h after intraperitoneal injections (Table 2). Among the sham vaccinated fish, however, mortality appeared relatively faster (24 h to 48 h). Nevertheless, the slight delay in the appearance of mortalities among some of the vaccinated fish, was not statistically significant ($P< 0.05$).

TABLE 2

Results of challenge experiments using *S. niloticus* immunized with *E. tarda* bacterin.

Treatment	Cumulative Mortalities (h)
14 days after single vaccination	5/5 (24-48 h)
28 days after single vaccination	5/5 (24-72 h)
14 days after second vaccination	5/5 (24-96 h)
Control	5/5 (24-48 h)

DISCUSSION

The immunogenicity of *E. tarda* has been demonstrated with eels (Song and Kou, 1981). In the present experiments on *S. niloticus* the agglutinin titer of 256 parallel to those observed among eels was detected in only one of the vaccinated fish. The individual agglutinin levels detected were, in fact, erratic, particularly, the test groups that were exposed to the bacteria only once. Such heterogeniety among individual responses to the same antigen stimulation in fish has been cited as an important factor in fish immunology studies (Dorson, 1984). Moreover, serologic studies of *E. tarda* by Sakazaki (1967) identified 17 O antigens, 11 H antigens and 18 O-H combinations while Edwards and Ewing (1972) reported 49 O antigens, 37 H antigens and 148 O-H combinations. Hence, this great individual variability in immune responses of Tilapia to the test bacteria resulted in statistically insignificant differences among agglutinin titers detected.

Agglutinin levels as a measure of vaccination potency have been reported (Antipa and Amend, 1977; Song and Kou, 1981). Conflicting data, however, are presented by other researchers, reporting protective immunity after vaccination even without detectable antibodies (Rohovec, 1975; Gould *et al.*, 1978; Michel and Faivre, 1982). This protective efficiency of agglutinins when further tested in a challenge experiment in this study, was not demonstrated. Either the use of the two-step hyperosmotic immersion stressed the test fish (Fender and Amend, 1978; Song and Kou, 1981) or the challenge method was too harsh as shown by the differences in mortalities among immunized eels challenged by intraperitoneal injection viz-a-viz by contact (Song and Kou, 1981). The immersion time of the *E. tarda* bacteria of 1.5 min in the present study, although shorter than that used with eels of 3 min (Song and Kou, 1981), is not likely a critical factor as Tatner and Horne (1983) showed that immersion time longer than 10 seconds for *V. anguillarum* vaccine does not increase vaccine uptake.

Although the foregoing results are inconclusive, evidence of immune response are apparent in some fish. Since tilapia culture continues to be adapted worldwide, it is important that the potential of vaccination for disease prevention be explored further. Future experiments should include variables such as antigen variability, the use of adjuvants, less stressful vaccine administration methods and appropriate challenge routes. The possible role of cellular immunity should, likewise, be clarified. In addition, increasing the number of experimental fish and ensuring single parent source should be considered.

*SEAFDEC Contribution no. 173

ACKNOWLEDGEMENTS

Appreciation is due to Dr. Hsu Ta Chuan for technical advice; to Dr. Kishio Hatai, Dr. Syuzo Egusa, the Japan International Cooperation Agency and the Aquaculture Department of the Southeast Asian Fisheries Development Center for making the senior author's training in Japan possible. Likewise, the partial travel support by the organizing committee of the International Meeting on Fish Immunology is appreciated. Thanks, also, to Nicanor Primavera for a critical review of the manuscript.

REFERENCES

Amend, D.F. and Fender, D.C., 1976. Uptake of bovine serum albumin by rainbow trout from hyperosmotic solutions: a model for vaccinating fish. Science, 192: 793-794.

Antipa, R. and Amend, D.F., 1977. Immunization of Pacific Salmon: Comparison of intraperitoneal injection and hyperosmotic infiltration of *Vibrio anguillarum* and *Aeromonas salmonicida* bacteria. J. Fish. Res. Board Can. 34: 203-208.

Carpenter, P.K., 1975. Immunology and Serology. Third Edition, W.B. Saunders Company, Philadelphia/London/Toronto, 345 pp.

Croy, T.R. and Amend, D.F., 1977. Immunization of sockeye salmon (*Oncoryhychus nerka*) against vibriosis using the hyperosmotic infiltration technique. Aquaculture, 12: 317-325.

Dorson, M. 1984. Applied immunology of fish. In: P. de Kinkelin and C. Michel (Editors), Symposium in Fish Vaccination. Theoretical Background and Practical Results on Immunization Against Infectious Diseases. 20-22 February 1984 at Paris, France, Office International des Epizooties, pp. 39-74.

Edwards, P.R. and Ewing, W.H. 1972. Identification of Enterobacteriaceae. Third Edition. Afton Press,362 pp.

Fender, D.C. and Amend, D.F., 1978. Hyperosmotic infiltration: Factors influencing uptake of bovine serum albumin by Rainbow Trout (*Salmo gairdneri*). J. Fish. Res. Board. Can., 35: 871-874.

Gould, R.W., O'Leary, P.J., Garrison, R.L., Rohovec, J.S. and Fryer, J.L., 1978. Spray vaccination a method for the immunization of fish. Fish Pathology, 13: 63-68.

Kusuda, R., Kawai, K., Jo. Y., Akizuki, T., Fukunaga, M. and Kotake, N., 1978. Efficacy of oral vaccination for vibrios in cultured ayu. Bull. Japan Soc. Sci. Fish., 44: 21-25.

Kusuda, R., Toyoshima, T., Iwamura, Y. and Sako, J., 1976. *Edwardsiella tarda* from an epizootic of mullets (*Mugil cephalus*) in Okitsu Bay. Bull. Japan Soc. Sci. Fish., 42: 271-275.

Lannan, J.E., 1978. Vibriosis vaccination of chum salmon by hyperosmotic infiltration. Prog. Fish-Cult., 40: 43-45.

Lio-Po, G.D., Endo, M. and Wakabayashi, H., 1982. A characterization of *Edwardsiella tarda* in *Tilapia nilotica*: biochemical and histopathological analyses. In: Abstracts of papers presented at the eleventh annual meeting of the Philippine Society for Microbiology 7-8 May 1982. University of the Philippines at Los Baños, College, Laguna. Kalikasan, Philipp. J. Biol., 11: 372-278.

Meyer, F.P. and Bullock, G.L.,1973. *Edwardsiella tarda*, a new pathogen of channel catfish (*Ictalurus punctatus*). Appl. Microbiol. 25: 155-156.

Michel, C. and Faivre, B., 1982. Occurrence and significance of agglutinating antibodies in experimental furunculosis of rainbow trout, *Salmo gairdneri* Richardson. J. Fish Dis. 5: 429-432.

Roberts, R.J. and Sommerville, C., 1982. Diseases of Tilapias. In: R.S.V. Pullin and R.H. Lowe-Mc Connell (Editors), The Biology and Culture of Tilapias. Proceeding of the International Conference on the Biology and Culture of Tilapias, 2-5 September 1980, at Bellagio, Italy, pp. 247-262.

Rohovec, J.S., 1975. Oral and parenteral immunization for the control of *Vibrio anguillarum*, the etiological agent of Vibriosis in Salmonid fish. Ph. D. Thesis, Oregon State Univeristy, 82 pp.

Sae-Oni, D., Muroga, K. and Nakai, T., 1984. A case of *Edwardsiella tarda* infection in cultured colored carp *Cyrpinus carpio*. Fish Pathol., 19: 197-199.

Sakazaki, R. 1967. Studies on the Asakusa group of Enterobacteriaceae (*Edwardsiella tarda*). Japan J. Med. Sci. Biol., 20: 205-212.

Song, Y.L. and Kou, G.H., 1981. Immune response of eels (*Anguilla japonica*) against *Aeromonas hydrophila* and *Edwardsiella anguillimortiferum* (*E. tarda*) infection. G.H. Kou, J.F. Fryer and M.L. Landolt (Editors). Proceedings of Republic of China-U.S. Cooperative Science Seminar on Fish Diseases, 23-26 June 1979 at University of Washington, Washington, U.S.A., National Science Council Series No. 3, 107-115.

Tatner, M.F. and Horne, M.T., 1983. Factors influencing uptake of ^{14}C-labelled *Vibrio anguillarum* vaccine in direct immersion experiments with rainbow trout, *Salmo gairdneri* Richardson. J. Fish Biol. 22:585-591.

Wakabayashi, J. and Egusa S., 1973. *Edwardsiella tarda* (*Paracolobactrum anguillimortiferum*) associated with pond-cultured eel disease. Bull. Japan Soc. Sci. Fish., 39: 931-936.

Veterinary Immunology and Immunopathology, 12 (1986) 359—364
Elsevier Science Publishers B.V., Amsterdam — Printed in The Netherlands

THE PERSISTENCE OF INFECTIOUS PANCREATIC NECROSIS VIRUS IN ATLANTIC SALMON

R.M. KNOTT and A.L.S. MUNRO

Marine Laboratory, Victoria Road, P.O. Box 101, Aberdeen AB9 8DB, Scotland

ABSTRACT

Knott, R.M. and Munro, A.L.S., 1986. The persistence of infectious pancreatic necrosis virus in atlantic salmon. Vet. Immunol. Immunopathol., 12: 359-364.

Atlantic salmon leucocytes from Infectious Pancreatic Necrosis Virus (IPNV) carriers showed a suppressed response to phytohemagglutinin stimulation compared with uninfected controls. A significant degree of inhibition of DNA synthesis was observed using ^{3}H-thymidine incorporation. IPNV was isolated from 41% of the stimulated leucocyte cultures supernatants, while only 6% of the unstimulated cultures were found to be positive.

INTRODUCTION

Infectious Pancreatic Necrosis (IPN) is a notifiable disease in Scotland. Restriction of the movement of live fish and eggs has been applied to reduce and contain the transmission of IPNV. Though, only one case of clinical IPN has been found in Atlantic salmon, despite numerous isolations from IPNV carriers, it has not been considered wise to allow the disease to spread.

The isolation of IPNV from many species of fish showing no apparent detriment to fish health (Amend and Pietsche, 1972; Yamamoto, 1975) highlights the importance of examining the relationship that exists between IPNV and Atlantic salmon.

An association of IPNV with leucocytes has previously been noted (Swanson and Gillespie, 1982; Yu et al, 1982). IPNV is not an isolated example of leucotropism by viruses. Measles (Lucas et al, 1978), Cytomegalovirus (St. Jeor and Weisser, 1977), Varicella Zoster Virus (Baba and Shigeta, 1983) and Rubella virus (Van der Loon et al, 1980) have been shown to be associated with the leucocytes of the host in which they are persisting.

In this study, data showing the stimulation of DNA synthesis in leucocytes of Atlantic salmon (*Salmo salar*) with Phytohemagglutinin (PHA) is presented. DNA

0165-2427/86/$03.50 © 1986 Elsevier Science Publishers B.V.

synthesis was monitored by labelling the leucocyte cultures with ^{3}H-thymidine. The apparent suppression of the leucocyte response to the mitogen in a group of IPNV carriers and the subsequent recovery of IPNV from the leucocyte cultures is described. The findings are discussed with respect to the possible effects of infection on the immune response of the salmon, and the diagnosis of the carrier state.

MATERIALS AND METHODS

Fish

The fish used in this study were Atlantic salmon that had been in freshwater for 2 years post hatch. Group 1 were control fish, while Group 2 had been exposed to IPNV and had subsequently become carriers of the virus. The fish were kept in continuously circulating freshwater and were fed on commercial feed pellets (Ewos Baker).

Culture Medium

The Lymphocyte Growth Medium (LGM) used has previously been described (Braun-Nesje et al, 1981). The composition of the Lymphocyte Maintenance Media is identical to LGM, with the omission of the serum. The Tris-MEM-2, contained Eagles minimal essential medium (Gibco 072-110) supplemented with 0.004% 1M tris buffered saline, 2% foetal calf serum, kanamycin 50 μg/ml and fungizone 2.5 μg/ml.

Mitogen

Phytohemagglutinin (PHA) was obtained from the Sigma Chemical Company (28754). It was diluted to 20μg/ml with LGM on the day it was to be used in the leucocyte stimulation assay.

Leucocyte Preparation and Leucocyte Stimulation Assay

Anterior kidney cell suspensions were prepared by gently teasing the tissue sample through a plastic sieve with LMM. Leucocytes were prepared from the cell suspension using lymphocyte separation medium (Flow Laboratories 16-920-54). The leucocytes were then resuspended in LGM.100ul aliquots containing 2 x 10^5 cells received 2μg of PHA. After 2.5 days incubation at 20°C the cells were labelled with ^{3}H-thymidine.

Harvesting procedures and liquid scintillation counting were performed according to Van Dam et al (1978). The results are presented as stimulation indices (SI) where SI = dpm of stimulated leucocytes/dpm for control leucocytes.

Virus Isolation

Aliquots of the supernatants from unstimulated and PHA stimulated leucocytes cultures were collected after 3 days incubation at 20°C. Each sample was inoculated onto Chinook Salmon Embryo cells (CHSE-214). Positive samples were identified from the appearance of cytopathic effect.

RESULTS

The SI values of leucocyte cultures from 20 control salmon (Group 1) were compared with 20 IPNV carrier leucocyte cultures (Group 2). The mean values for the control and IPNV carrier leucocytes were found to be significantly different using the students t-test ($p<0.001$). The control leucocytes were found to give higher SI values, indicating that DNA synthesis was suppressed in leucocytes from IPNV carriers when stimulated with PHA.

Table 1 Suppression of Leucocyte Response to PHA in vitro

	Group 1 (control)	Group 2 (IPNV Carriers)
Mean SI	2.29 ± 0.85	0.63 ± 0.34
Range	1.1 - 4.3	0.2 - 1.59

The results presented in Table II were obtained from 17 of the fish from Group 2. The results indicated are for those samples that were positive after the second pass on CHSE-214 cells.

Table II Activation of IPNV from PHA stimulated leucocytes

	Unstimulated leucocytes	PHA Stimulated leucocytes
% positive	6%	41%

DISCUSSION

The results of the leucocyte stimulation assay with leucocytes from control and persistently infected fish, indicate that leucocytes from the IPNV carriers do not respond to PHA *in vitro*, to the same extent as leucocytes from control salmon.

The apparent suppression of the leucocyte response to the mitogen by IPNV carriers may be indicative of a suppressed immune response in the live animal infected with IPNV. Carriers of IPNV may consequently be more susceptible to other diseases. Indeed, the vaccination of carriers against other fish pathogens may have a reduced efficiency, when compared to the vaccination of control salmon. However, only leucocytes from the anterior kidney were used in this assay and the response of leucocytes from other tissues, and from peripheral blood leucocytes is not known. Overall, the persistent infection may not significantly compromise the host.

A possible explanation for the suppression of DNA synthesis arose on examination of the supernatants of PHA stimulated and non-stimulated leucocyte cultures. The dependence of viruses on host DNA synthesis has previously been established for many viruses including Rous sarcoma virus (Bader, 1964). The enhanced recovery of IPNV from leucocyte cultures that had been stimulated with mitogen (Table II) implies a similar dependence on the genetic machinery of the host for the replication and subsequent release of IPNV. In the leucocyte cultures prepared from IPNV carriers the resting leucocytes may be unable to support viral repliction due to the relative inactivity of host cell genetic machinery. When the cells are stimulated with PHA the cells move from the resting stage and the early events that are initiated in a stimulated leucocyte appear to be utilised by IPNV for its own replication.

Both the controls (Group 1) and the IPNV carriers (Group 2), were tested using standard tissue culture diagnostic techniques. All fish were found to be negative for IPNV. It was only after the leucocytes were stimulated that IPNV could be recovered.

There are likely to be many other factors that are involved in the association of IPNV with Atlantic salmon, including age of fish, seasonal variations, immune status at time of exposure and time of sampling, and the variable assay conditions. The importance of the latter is highlighted by the range and the relatively low SI values for the control fish (Group 1). An improved stimulation assay may facilitate a more reproducible isolation of IPNV.

This data has extensive implications for the diagnosis of IPNV and for the role and effect of the immune response in the establishment and maintenance of the carrier status.

ACKNOWLEDGEMENTS

We thank Mrs L MacFarlane for assistance with cell culture. We wish to thank the Department of Agriculture and Fisheries for Scotland for the provision of research facilities, and the Highlands and Islands Development Board for their financial backing.

REFERENCES

Amend, D.F. and Pietsch, J.P. 1972. An improved Method for Isolating Viruses from Asymptomatic Carrier Fish. Trans. Am. Fish Soc. 101: 267-269.

Baba, M. and Shigeta, S. 1983. Incomplete Growth of Varicella Zoster in Human Monocytes. Microbiol. Immunol. 27.9: 767-778.

Bader, J.P. 1964. The Role of Deoxyribonucleic Acid in the synthesis of Rous Sarcoma Virus. Virol. 16: 436-443.

Braun-Nesje, R., Bertheussen, K., Kaplan, G. and Seljelid, R. 1981. Salmonid Macrophages: Separation in Vitro Culture and Characterisation. J. Fish Dis. 4: 141-151.

Liewes, E.W., Van Dam, R.H., Vos-Maas, R.H. and Bootsma, R. 1978. Optimisation and Kinetics of in Vitro Stimulation of Carp (*Cyprinus carpio*) Leucocytes. Vet. Immunopathol. 3: 325-343.

Lucas, C.J., Ubels-Postma, J.C., Rezee, A. and Galama, J.M.D. 1978. Activation of Measles Virus from Sliently Infected Lymphocytes. J. Exp. Med. 148: 940-952.

St Jeor, S. and Weiser, A. 1977. Resistence of Cytomegalovirus in Human Lymphoblasts and Peripheral Leucocyte Cultures. Infection and Immunity 15: 402-409.

Swanson, R.N. and Gillespie, J.H. 1982. Isolation of Infectious Pancreatic Necrosis Virus from the Blood Components of Experimentally Infected Trout. Can. J. Fish, Aquat, Sci. 39: 225-228.

Van Dam, R.H., Van Kooten, P.T.S. and Van der Donk, J.A. 1978. In Vitro Stimulation of Goat Peripheral Blood Lymphocytes: Optimization and Kinetics of the Response to Mitogens and Allogenic Lymphocytes. J. Immunol. Methods 21: 217-228.

Van der Loon, A.M., Van der Logt, J.T.M. and Van der Veen, J. 1979. Poliovirus Induced Suppression of Lymphocyte Stimulation: A Macrophage Mediated Effect. Imm. 37: 135-143.

Yamamoto, T. 1975. Frequency of Detection and Survival of Infecitous Pancreatic Necrosis Virus in a Carrier Population of Brook Trout (Salvelinus fontinalis) in a lake. J. Fish. Res. Bd Can. 34 (4): 568-570.

Yu, K.K., MacDonald, R.D. and Moore, A.R. 1982. Replication of Infectious Pancreatic Necrosis Virus in Trout Leucocytes and Detection of the Carrier status. J. Fish. dis. 5: 401-410.

Veterinary Immunology and Immunopathology, 12 (1986) 365—372
Elsevier Science Publishers B.V., Amsterdam — Printed in The Netherlands

Experimental Induction of the Carrier State in Yearling Brook Trout: a Model Challenge Protocol for IPNV Immunization

L.M. Bootland, P. Dobos, and R.M.W. Stevenson

Department of Microbiology, College of Biological Science, University of Guelph, Guelph, Ontario, Canada N1G 2W1

ABSTRACT

Bootland, L.M., P. Dobos and R.M.W. Stevenson, 1986. Experimental induction of the carrier state in yearling brook trout: a model challenge protocol for IPNV Immunization. Vet. Immunol. Immunopathol., 12: 365-372.

Brook trout fry (*Salvelinus fontinalis*) were not protected from infectious pancreatic necrosis virus (IPNV) challenge by immersion vaccination with inactivated, purified virus at concentrations of 10^7 to 10^9 pfu/ml. Mortalities in vaccinated groups were higher than for the unvaccinated control group and appeared to be dose-dependent. A challenge protocol for adult brook trout was developed for future vaccine trials. A single intraperitoneal injection of virulent, purified virus was sufficient to make long-lasting carriers of 16 month-old trout. Fish underwent a transient viremia, identified by virus isolation from plasma and leucocytes. Feces were the most reliable samples for identification of IPNV carriers by non-sacrificial testing. Many fish in the remaining infected group were still carriers 12 and 27 weeks post-infection.

INTRODUCTION

Infectious pancreatic necrosis (IPN) epizootics occur widely in salmonid fish culture operations, with fry and fingerlings being especially vulnerable (Hill, 1982). Older fish (5 - 6 months) are resistant to the disease but can become asymptomatic carriers of IPNV, shedding the virus periodically in feces and reproductive products (Wolf et al., 1963; Ghittino et al., 1984). Avoidance is the most effective control measure for IPN, but it is not always possible. Hence, there have been some attempts to develop a vaccine for fry against IPNV, but an effective, practical vaccine has yet to be found.

Injection of young fry with formalin-inactivated IPNV (killed vaccine) did confer protection against subsequent challenge with virulent virus (Dorson, 1977; Hill et al., 1980). However, injection of large numbers of young fry is impractical in a hatchery situation. Hill et al. (1980) found that rainbow trout (*Salmo gairdneri*) fry were moderately protected by a hyperosmotic bath in a killed vaccine. McAllister (personal communication, 1984) was unsuccessful in protecting fry by immersion in a killed virus

0165-2427/86/$03.50 © 1986 Elsevier Science Publishers B.V.

vaccine, but Elahzary (personal communication, 1985) achieved up to 75% protection by bath immersion in high inactivated virus concentrations (10^9 - 10^{10} pfu/ml). Immersion in a live, naturally avirulent flounder IPNV isolate conferred protection on 10 day old brook trout (Salvelinus fontinalis) fry (P.E. McAllister, personal communication, 1984). However, a live, avirulent virus is unlikely to be licensed as a vaccine by regulatory agencies, as it may revert to virulence in salmonids or other species.

While a vaccine could be used to provide immediate protection to fry, it could also be applied to eliminate vertical transmission of IPNV from broodstock to progeny. Adult brook trout and rainbow trout produce neutralizing antibodies when injected with live IPNV (Wolf and Quimby, 1969; Reno, 1976). Sano et al. (1981) demonstrated that adult rainbow trout injected with inactivated virus produced neutralizing antibodies, and upon challenge, were able to eliminate virus from the kidney and spleen if sera ND_{50} were greater that 10^3. However, it was not determined if challenged fish became long-term carriers. This paper reports results obtained in a pilot trial of fry vaccination, and subsequent work on developing a challenge protocol for application in testing vaccination of adult brook trout, a species that is more susceptible to most IPNV isolates than the commonly cultured rainbow trout.

METHODS

Cell Culture:

Monolayer cultures of chinook salmon embryo (CHSE-214) cells were grown at 18°C in Eagles's minimum essential medium with Earle salts (Gibco), supplemented with 6% fetal calf serum, 250 iu/ml pencillin and 200 ug/ml streptomycin (cMEM).

Virus Preparation:

A Quebec IPNV isolate of low passage number in tissue culture, kindly provided by Dr. M. Elazhary, University of Montreal, St. Hyacinthe, Quebec, was used throughout the experiments. Cells were infected, then harvested when complete cytopathogenic effect (CPE) was observed, usually in 3 to 4 days. Virus was concentrated and purified as described by Chang et al. (1978). Briefly, polyethylene glycol precipitated virus was extracted with Freon and purified by isopycnic CsCl gradient centrifugation. The virus band was removed and dialyzed against TNE at 4°C for 3 h. Virus titres were determined using a plaque assay.

Virus Inactivation:

Purified virus was inactivated by a modification of the method of Dixon and Hill (1983). After adding a small amount of phenol red powder to the virus sample, 37% formaldehyde was added to a final concentration of 1/200. The pH was adjusted by adding 1 M Tris until it matched a phenol red standard of pH 7.4. The sample was incubated at 25°C for 7 days, then dialyzed against distilled water for 48 h. To ensure that all virus had been inactivated, an aliquot was inoculated onto a monolayer of CHSE-214 cells. If CPE was absent after 14 days, the preparation was considered inactivated and stored at -70°C until used.

Fry Vaccination:

Brook trout (*Salvelinus fontinalis*) fry were obtained from the Ontario Ministry of Natural Resources hatchery system. At 8.5 weeks of age, fish were divided into 5 groups of 100 fish. For vaccination, each group was immersed in 90 ml of one of the three viral vaccine doses (3.6×10^7, 3.6×10^8 or 3.6×10^9 pfu/ml), in a 1/200 dilution of cMEM, or in water only. All were held for 45 min. at 12°C with oxygenation, then returned to 9 l holding tanks with flowing 10°C well water. Ninety fish in each group, except the vaccination control group, were bath challenged 3 wks post-vaccination at 11.5 weeks of age (av. fish weight 0.15 g). Each group was simultaneously placed into 4 l beakers containing 900 ml of diluted virulent, purified virus (tissue culture pass 5, 1.0×10^6 pfu/ml) at 10°C with oxygenation for 5 h, then returned to holding tanks. Daily mortalities were monitored post-vaccination and for 50 days after challenge.

Adult Challenge:

Brook trout of 16 mo. (250 - 467 g) were obtained from a commercial fish farm. Lethal organ sampling of 23 fish indicated that the stock was IPNV-free. Fish were acclimated for 4 months in 550 l fiberglass tanks with aerated, flowing well water (9 - 13°C). All effluent water was disinfected by chlorination before discharge. Each of 4 test groups contained 20 fish, with approximately equal numbers of males and females. Fish were branded for individual identification using silver nitrate pencils. All the fish in 2 groups were given an intraperitoneal (ip) injection of virulent, purified virus (pass 4, 1.5×10^5 pfu/g body weight), 2 weeks after control sampling. In each of the 2 control groups, half the fish received an ip injection of cMEM.

Non-Lethal Sampling:

Adult fish from all groups were sampled for feces, plasma and peripheral blood leucocytes at 1,3,5, and 8 weeks post-infection (wpi). Fish in two groups were also sampled at 12 wpi and 27 wpi. Each fish was anaesthetized in 100 ppm of MS222 for 1 - 2 min., and a fecal sample taken. A blood sample (15% blood volume) was removed through the dorsal aorta with 22 g 2.5 cm needles on 5 ml plastic syringes. Hematocrit values were measured immediately and the remaining blood added to 100 iu/ml heparin. All samples were refrigerated until processed. Plasma and leucocytes were separated from whole blood using a Percoll (Pharmacia) discontinuous density gradient as described by Yu et al. (1982). Leucocytes samples were stored at 4°C or -20°C, and plasma was kept at -20°C.

Detection of IPNV:

Fecal samples were homogenized and diluted in cMEM (1/20), filter-sterilized, and stored at -20°C. Fecal and plasma samples were tested for IPNV by plating doubling dilutions onto duplicate CHSE-214 monolayers in 96 well plastic microtitre plates. Wells were observed for CPE for 14 days and tested by staphylococcal coagglutination (Kimura et al., 1984). All wells were blind-passaged onto a second microtitre plate, observed for 14 days for CPE, and retested by coagglutination. A sample was considered IPNV-positive if CPE was evident on pass 2 and coagglutination occurred. Leucocytes were tested by leucocyte co-cultivation (Yu et al., 1982), with 0.1 ml and 0.15 ml of each sample plated onto duplicate monolayers. Virus titres in fecal samples were determined using the Spearman-Karber formula. The lowest level of virus detection was 2.30 log $TCID_{50}$/g for feces.

RESULTS

Fry vaccination:

Mortalities from vaccination alone were low (2% - 6% cumulative % mortality after 21 days). At 50 days post-challenge, the vaccinated control group had a low total mortality (8.9%), while the unvaccinated challenged group had a total mortality of 36.7% (Fig. 1). The three challenged groups that had been vaccinated suffered higher mortalities than the unvaccinated-challenged group, in a dose-dependent reponse (Fig. 1).

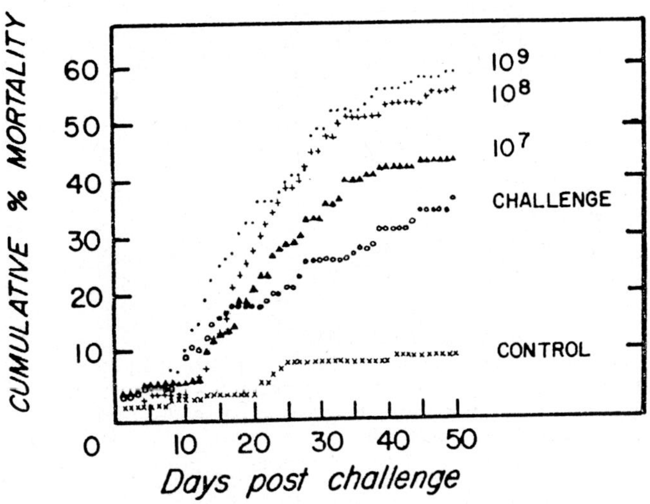

Figure 1. Cumulative percent mortality of 11.5 week-old brook trout fry challenged by immersion for 5 hrs in 10^6 pfu/ml of virulent IPNV. The groups of 90 fish had been vaccinated at 8.5 weeks of age by 45 min. immersion in purified, inactivated IPNV at 10^7 pfu/ml (▲), 10^8 pfu/ml (+) or 10^9 pfu/ml (•). Unvaccinated, challenged control (o); unchallenged control (×).

Adult Carrier State:

At all sampling periods, except 8 wpi, more than 90% of the injected yearling brook trout were shedding viruses in feces (Fig. 2). Although virus incidence in feces showed fluctuations with time, mean virus titres varied only slightly (3.67 - 4.19 log $TCID_{50}$/g). At 27 wpi, 50% of one group of infected fish were still virus shedders (data not shown). Virus levels often fluctuated over a 100 to 7000 $TCID_{50}$ range for successive samples from the same fish, and from fish to fish.

The average yield of leucocytes for the first three bleeds was 10^6 cells/ml. Isolation of virus from leucocytes and plasma fluctuated with time and showed a general decrease over the 12 week sampling period (Fig. 2). Infected fish had viremia, but by 12 wpi, virus had been cleared from the blood. Virus was not isolated from control fish. Hematocrit values were not significantly different (α=0.05) between infected and control groups of fish during 12 wpi. Hematocrits did decrease from the initial bleed (mean 43) to 5 wpi (mean 27), but this was attributed to the fish becoming anemic due to successive blood losses.

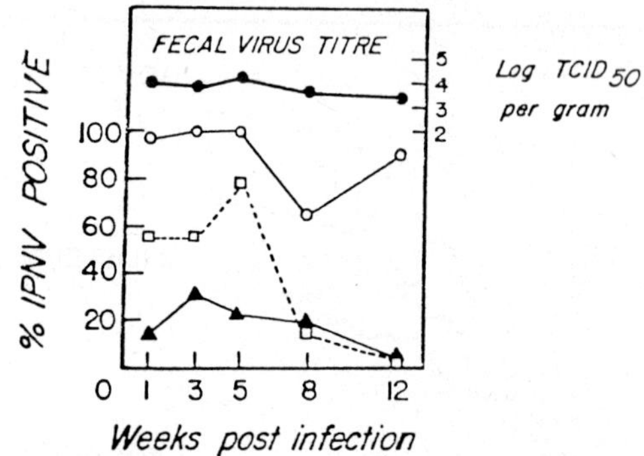

Figure 2. IPNV isolation rates from feces (o), leucocytes (□), and plasma (▲) of 16 month-old brook trout infected by injection of virulent IPNV. Virus titres of feces (•) are shown as log $TCID_{50}$/g. Values shown are the means calculated from 2 groups of 20 fish each, except for the 12 wk sample which is for 1 group only.

DISCUSSION

Brook trout fry vaccinated at 8.5 weeks of age by immersion in an inactivated virus vaccine were not protected from later challenge with IPNV. Indeed, vaccinated groups suffered higher mortalities than unvaccinated controls, with the greatest loss associated with the highest vaccine dose (Fig. 1). One possible explanation for increased susceptibility after exposure to high concentrations of antigen is that fry develop immune tolerance rather than immunity. The recognition of viral antigen as "self" by the neonatal immune system has been suggested as a possible explanation for the long persistence of IPNV in adult trout that are survivors of epizootics (Wolf and Quimby, 1969). The average weight of the fry in our study was 0.15 g at the time of the live virus challenge (11.5 weeks of age). The results of Johnston et al. (1982) suggest that salmonids are not fully immunocompetent at weights of less than 0.5 g. While some recent studies indicate that young fish are protected from tolerigizing doses of antigens (Tatner and Manning, 1985). More information about the response of fry to early exposure to viral antigens is needed before concluding that the results reported here are, in fact, due to tolerance. As brook trout fry of an age susceptible to IPNV are available only once a year, we have not yet investigated the effect of lower antigen doses, immunization at other weights or ages, or any of the other variables that could affect responses.

The immediate concern with these results is their potential implications for development of a successful IPNV vaccine for fry. Although fry vaccinated by injection with inactivated IPNV were protected, administration of IPNV vaccines by other routes have not proved successful (Dorson, 1977; Hill et al., 1980). Successful protection of fry with live-attenuated or naturally avirulent virus preparations (Hill et al., 1980; P.E. McAllister, personal communication, 1984) may have been the result of viral interference - replication of the avirulent virus preventing or limiting growth of virulent virus.

An alternate and perhaps better approach to preventing IPN may be to vaccinate adult fish in order to break the vertical transmission of IPNV. The effect of adult vaccination would need to be tested indirectly, as fish older than 5-6 mo. do not show IPNV mortalities. In this study, we found that a single ip injection of virulent virus was sufficient to establish a long-lasting experimental carrier state.

Feces were the best samples for the non-sacrificial monitoring of carriers. Fluctuating incidence of fecal shedding and comparable virus titres have been observed in natural brook trout carriers and experimentally infected young brook trout (Billi and Wolf, 1969; Yamamoto and Kilistoff, 1979; Hedrick and Fryer, 1982). Isolation of virus from leucocytes is feasible and effective, but presents problems when using repeated blood sampling. Percoll densities used for leucocyte separation had to be adjusted initially for use with brook trout blood, and then altered for each successive bleed as fish became anaemic. Viremia persisted in yearling brook trout for at least 84 days post-infection. This was longer than the 33 days observed for yearling rainbow trout injected with virus (Swanson and Gillespie, 1982). This may well be a species difference, as Yu et al. (1982) were able to detect virus in leucocytes of naturally infected yearling brook trout. At 8 wpi, the 14 infected fish examined were virus carriers, evidenced by the fact that at least 1 of 7 organs was virus-positive (data not shown).

The carriers established in this study were apparently able to transmit IPNV vertically to progeny, based on laboratory spawning and hatching. Progeny from a male infected parent or from two infected parents had typical signs of IPN, although no epizootic resulted. Fry from uninfected parents had low mortality rates and no signs of IPNV (unpublished results). Detection of virus in progeny resulting from laboratory spawning is a tenuous method for evaluating the success of adult vaccination. Reno et al. (1978) and Busch (1984) were not able to demonstrate virus in the progeny of IPNV-infected parents. Mulcahy and Pascho (1985) have discussed similar problems for IHNV (infectious haematopoietic necrosis virus). However, spawning vaccinated fish may provide a means to test for any protection afforded by maternal antibodies transmitted in the eggs.

Acknowledgements

This work was supported by the Strategic Grants Program of the Natural Sciences and Engineering Research Council of Canada. We are grateful for the advice and very practical help of R.A. Johnston, University of Guelph.

REFERENCES

Billi, J.L. and Wolf, K. 1969. Quantitative comparison of peritoneal washes and feces for detecting infectious pancreatic necrosis (IPN) virus in carrier brook trout. J. Fish. Res. Bd. Canada 26(6): 1459-1465.

Busch, R.A. 1984. Virus detection in rainbow trout. FHS/AFS Newsletter 12(1): 6.

Chang, N., Macdonald, R.D. and Yamamoto, T. 1978. Purification of infectious pancreatic necrosis (IPN) virus and comparison of polypeptide composition of different isolates. Can. J. Microbiol. 24: 19-27.

Dixon, P.F. and Hill, B.J. 1983. Inactivation of infectious pancreatic necrosis virus for vaccine use. J. Fish Dis. 6: 399-409.

Dorson, M. 1977. Vaccination trials of rainbow trout fry against infectious pancreatic necrosis. Bull. Off. Int. Epiz. 87: 405-406.

Ghittino, P., Schwedler, H. and de Kinkelin, P. 1984. The principal infectious diseases of fish and their general control methods. In: P. de Kinkelin (editor), Symposium on Fish Vaccination. Office International des Epizooties, Paris, France, pp. 5-38.

Hedrick, R.P. and Fryer, J.L. 1982. Persistent infections of salmonid cell lines with infectious pancreatic necrosis virus (IPNV): A model for the carrier state in trout. Fish Path. 16: 163-172.

Hill, B.J. 1982. Infectious pancreatic necrosis virus and its virulence. In: R.J. Roberts (editor), Microbial Diseases of Fish. Academic Press. pp. 91-114.

Hill, B.J., Dorson, M. and Dixon, P.F. 1980. Studies on immunization of trout against IPN. In: W. Ahne (editor), Fish Diseases. Springer-Verlag, New York, pp. 29-36.

Johnson, X.A., Flynn, J.K. and Amend, D.F. 1982. Onset of immunity in salmonid fry vaccinated by direct immersion in _Virbrio anguillarum_ and _Yersinia ruckeri_ bacterins. J. Fish Dis. 5: 197-206.

Kimura, T., Yoshimizu, M. and Yasuda, H. 1984. Rapid, simple serological diagnosis of infectious pancreatic necrosis by coagglutination test using antibody-sensitized staphylococci. Fish Path. 19: 25-33.

Mulcahy, D., and Pascho, R.J. 1985. Vertical transmission of infectious haematopoietic necrosis virus in sockeye salmon, _Oncorhynchus nerka_ (Walbaum): isolation of virus from dead eggs and fry. J. Fish Dis. 8: 393-396.

Reno, P.W. 1976. Qualitative and quantitative aspects of the infectious pancreatic necrosis virus (IPNV) carrier state in trout. Ph.D. Thesis. University of Guelph, Guelph, Ontario, Canada.

Reno, P.W., Darley, S. and Savan, M. 1978. Infectious pancreatic necrosis: experimental induction of a carrier state in trout. J. Fish. Res. Bd. Canada 35: 1451-1456.

Sano, T., Tanaka, K., and Fukuzaki, S. 1981. Immune response in adult trout against formalin killed concentrated IPNV. Develop. Biol. Standard 49: 63-70.

Swanson, R.N. and Gillespie, J.H. 1982. Isolation of infectious pancreatic necrosis virus from blood and blood components of experimentally infected trout. Can. J. Fish. Aquat. Sci. 39: 225-228.

Tatner, M.F. and Manning, M.J. 1985. The ontogenic development of the reticulo-endothelial system in rainbow trout, _Salmo gairdneri_ Richardson. J. Fish Dis. 8: 189-195.

Wolf, K. and Quimby, M.C. 1969. Infectious pancreatic necrosis: clinical and immune response of adult trouts to inoculation with live virus. J. Fish. Res. Bd. Canada 26: 2511-2516.

Wolf, K., Quimby, M.C. and Bradford, A.D. 1963. Egg-associated transmission of IPN virus of trouts. Virol. 21: 317-321.

Yamamoto, T. and Kilistoff, J. 1979. Infectious pancreatic necrosis virus: quantification of carriers in lake populations during a 6-year period. J. Fish. Res. Bd. Canada 36: 562-567.

Yu, K.K.Y., Macdonald, R.D. and Moore, A.R. 1982. Replication of infectious pancreatic necrosis virus in trout leucocytes and detection of the carrier state. J. Fish Dis. 5: 401-410.

Veterinary Immunology and Immunopathology, 12 (1986) 373—381
Elsevier Science Publishers B.V., Amsterdam — Printed in The Netherlands

MONOCLONAL ANTIBODIES TO THE SP STRAIN OF INFECTIOUS PANCREATIC NECROSIS VIRUS

S. C. WOLSKI, B. S. ROBERSON AND F. M. HETRICK

Microbiology Dept., Univ. Maryland, College Park, MD 20742 USA

ABSTRACT

Wolski, S. C., Roberson, B. S., Hetrick, F. M. 1986. Monoclonal Antibodies to the Sp Strain of Infectious Pancreatic Necrosis Virus. Vet. Immunol. Immunopathol., 12: 373-381.

Twelve hybrids secreting antibody to the Sp serotype of infectious pancreatic necrosis virus (IPNV) were isolated from the fusion of murine myeloma cells and spleen cells from mice immunized with pelleted virus. All of the monoclonal antibodies possessed the kappa (K) light chain isotype. Nine contained the mu (M), two had the gamma 2a (G_{2a}), and one had the gamma 1 (G_1) heavy chain isotype. Using an enzyme-linked immunosorbent assay (ELISA), 10 antibodies were found to be broadly reactive against partially purified representatives of the three serotypes of IPNV, the Sp, Ab, and VR-299 strains. The other two antibodies reacted with the Sp serotype alone. Characterization by immunostaining of viral polypeptides electrophoretically transferred to nitrocellulose sheets was possible only with IgG type antibodies. One of the specific monoclonal antibodies was shown to be directed against the major capsid protein while the other specific monoclonal antibody and the broadly reacting one reacted with the low molecular weight viral polypeptides.

INTRODUCTION

Infectious pancreatic necrosis virus (IPNV) was first isolated by Wolf et al. (1960) from brook trout and is now recognized as a worldwide pathogen of young salmonid fish. Similar viruses have been isolated from a variety of non-salmonid fish and marine molluscs as well (Hill, 1982). The viruses contain a bisegmented, double-stranded RNA genome and are members of the proposed family Birnaviridae (Dobos et al., 1979). The antigenic relationships among the IPN and IPN-like viruses are complex and there is disagreement concerning the number of antigenic types that exist from results of cross-neutralization tests (Okamoto et al., 1983; Nicholson and Pochebit, 1981; Vestergard-Jorgenson and Grauballe, 1971).

Production of monoclonal antibodies to several IPNV serotypes, and their subsequent use in cross-testing with the major Birnavirus isolates, may clarify the antigenic relationships among these viruses. We report here the generation of monoclonal antibodies to the Sp strain of IPNV, one of the two major European serotypes, their characterization, and their reactivity with selected IPNV strains.

MATERIALS AND METHODS

Viruses Employed

The VR-299, Ab, Sp, West Buxton, SB, and GAF strains of IPNV, and the Oregon strain of infectious hematopoietic necrosis virus (IHNV) were obtained from stocks maintained in our laboratory. The SB strain, isolated from striped bass (Schutz et al., 1984), and the GAF strain, isolated from a moribund grey angelfish at the National Aquarium, Baltimore, Maryland, are recent IPNV isolates in our laboratory. The Bonnamy, Reno, Dry Mill, Berlin, Lava Lake, Buhl, Eel virus European (EVE), and d'Honnincthun strains were provided by Dr. Phillip McAllister, National Fish Health Research Laboratory, Leetown, West Virginia. All viruses were plaque purified three times prior to the preparation of stock viruses. Infectious bursal disease virus (IBDV) supplied by Dr. David Snyder, Maryland College of Veterinary Medicine, was a lysate of infected chick embryo fibroblast cells.

Cell cultures employed

The chinook salmon embryo (CHSE-214) cell line was used to propagate and assay the IPNV strains and IHNV. The cells were grown at 15° C in Leibovitz's L-15 medium supplemented with 10% fetal bovine serum (FBS) and 50 ug/ml gentamycin sulfate. The medium used for maintenance of cells during virus propagation or assay was L-15 medium with 2% FBS.

The murine myeloma cell line, X63.Ag 8.653 (653 line), a non-producer of immunoglobulins (Kearney et al., 1978), was obtained from Dr. David Snyder. Cells were grown in a medium consisting of 50% RPMI-1640 and 50% Dulbecco's modified Eagle's Medium supplemented with 3.5 g/l dextrose and 15% serum (RDGS medium). Cells were grown in RDGS containing 10^{-7} M 8-azaguanine and subcultivated at a 1:3 ratio each day for at least three days prior to use in cell fusions.

Partial Purification of Virus

The Sp, Ab, and VR-299 strains of IPNV were partially purified by the method of Snyder et al. (1983). The virus was diluted in TNE buffer (0.01 M Tris-HCl, 0.01 M NaCl, 0.001 M EDTA, pH 7.5) to give a 100X preparation.

Immunization of mice

Fluids from CHSE cultures infected with the Sp strain of IPNV (approximately 10^8 $TCID_{50}$/ml) were harvested, pooled, and centrifuged at 10,000 x g to remove cell debris. The supernatant was collected and centrifuged at 50,000 x g for two hours to pellet the virus. The pellets were resuspended in a volume of TNE buffer to give a 200 fold concentration of the virus, mixed 1:1 with Freund's complete adjuvant, and emulsified. BALB/c mice, two months of age, were injected subcutaneously with 0.3 ml of the emulsion. Eight weeks later, serum was collected and tested for antibody by enzyme-linked immunosorbent assay (ELISA). Four days prior to hybridization, antibody-positive mice were injected intraperitoneally and subcutaneously with 0.3 ml of partially purified virus in TNE buffer.

Enzyme-linked Immunosorbent Assay (ELISA)

Viral antigens used in the assay were gradient purified preparations as described above. Working antigen dilutions were determined by titration against anti-IPN virus, anti-BSA, and normal mouse sera with the dilution chosen being that which gave the highest specific reaction and the lowest background with normal serum. Fluids from uninfected CHSE culture fluids processed in the same manner as the virus-containing fluids, and diluted comparably, served as the control antigen. The ELISA was performed according to the method described by Snyder et al. (1983).

Cell fusion

Equal numbers (2×10^8) of splenic cells and myeloma 653 cells were mixed and co-pelleted at 50 x g for 15 minutes. Fusion of cells with polyethylene glycol (1000) (Goldsby et al., 1977) was followed by resuspension in 120 ml RDGS containing 10^{-4} M hypoxanthine, 2×10^{-6} M aminopterin and 2×10^{-5} M thymidine (HAT medium) and dispensed, 0.1 ml/well, into 96 well plates seeded one day previously with normal mouse spleen cells in HAT medium (2 spleens/100 ml medium). Cells were maintained in 10% CO_2 at 37° C in a humidified incubator. Five days later, half of the medium was removed and replaced with fresh medium. After two weeks, the medium was changed again, and 2-3 days later, culture fluids were tested for the presence of antibody by ELISA.

Cloning of Hybrids

Culture fluids with specific activity against the Sp strain on successive tests were also tested for reactivity against the Ab and VR-299 strains and the CHSE control preparation. All clones reactive with only the Sp serotype and those most highly reactive against all three serotypes were further cloned by limiting dilution, 2-4 times, as necessary. Each clone was expanded by transfer into wells of increasingly larger size, each seeded with a feeder layer one day prior to transplanting. Finally, cells were grown in 75 cm^2 flasks in volumes up to 50 ml, without feeder layers. Antibodies were typed as to heavy and light chain composition with an isotyping kit (Boehringer Mannheim Biochemicals, Indianapolis, IN).

Polyacrylamide Gel Electrophoresis (PAGE) of Proteins

The virus preparations used for PAGE were culture fluids from CHSE monolayers infected with the different IPNV strains. Clarified supernatant from frozen and thawed CHSE monolayer cells was used as a control. Viral proteins were separated by the discontinuous SDS-gel system of Laemmli, (1970) with minor modifications. The final sample buffer contained 0.0625 M Tris-HCl, pH 6.8, 0.5% SDS, 10% glycerol, 5% 2-mercaptoethanol and 0.001% bromphenol blue. Proteins were dissociated by incubation at 37° C for five minutes followed by one minute in a sonic water bath. Low molecular weight markers (Bio-Rad) were treated similarly except that 2% SDS was used and proteins were disrupted by boiling for five minutes. Samples of 25 ul were loaded into a 20 well, 5% stacking gel. The 10% resolving gel was 9 cm long and 0.75 mm thick. Electrophoresis was started at 50 V, and when the tracking dye was concentrated at the interface of the stacking and resolving gels, the voltage was increased to 130 V and allowed to run for four hours.

Western Blot Analysis

Gels were soaked in transfer buffer (25 mM Tris-HCl, pH 8.3, 192 mM glycine, and 20% methanol) for 45 minutes. Likewise, nitrocellulose membranes, filter papers and Scotch pads were pre-saturated in Tris buffer at least one hour. Separated proteins were electrophoretically transferred from the gels to a nitrocellulose membrane at 55 V for 22 hours at 10° C. The molecular weight standards lane was cut out and fixed in 10% acetic acid for ten minutes, stained with Ponceau S and destained with several changes of distilled water. The assay for transferred proteins was that described by Robb et al. (1982) except that protein-antibody complexes were detected with horseradish peroxidase color development reagent (60 mg 4-chloro-naphthol in 20 ml methanol, added to 100 ml TBS with 0.03% H_2O_2).

RESULTS

Monoclonal Antibodies to IPNV

A total of 12 hybridomas secreting antibodies to IPNV were isolated from the fusion of X63.Ag8.653 myeloma cells and spleen cells from mice immunized with the Sp serotype. Cloning of hybrids was done by limiting dilution and continued until all wells tested positive on two successive clonings. Isotypes were determined by an indirect ELISA after the final cloning. All monoclonal antibodies possessed the kappa (K) light chain isotype. Nine of these contained the mu (M) heavy chain isotype, two were IgG_{2a}, and one was an IgG_1. (Table 1).

TABLE 1.
ELISA reactivity patterns of anti-IPNV monoclonals

Clone[a]	Isotype	Virus Sp	Ab	299	IHNV	CHSE	Test Dilution[b]
4-C2-4	IgG_{2a}	100[c,d]	0[e]	0	0	0	64
3-11H2	IgG_1	100	8	15	0	0	65536
4-C4-1	IgG_{2a}	100	58	61	10	0	8
4-1A2	IgM	100	98	99	0	4	512
2-7A7	IgM	100	99	97	0	0	128
2-12F3	IgM	100	93	100	0	0	128
4-3G11	IgM	100	94	98	0	0	1024
3-11G11	IgM	100	91	95	0	2	512
4-11E9	IgM	100	82	85	22	14	64
4-2G11	IgM	57	47	100	20	16	32
3-5D7	IgM	100	81	98	52	37	32
3-5C2	IgM	100	77	95	51	47	64
RDGS	-	0[f]	0	0	0	0	2

[a] First number of each designation represents number of times cloned
[b] Reciprocal of supernatant dilution used in the assays
[c] Normalized values were calculated by the formula:

$$\frac{\text{(observed O. D.)}}{\text{(highest observed O. D.)}} \times 100\%$$

[d] Normalized values represent the average of duplicate readings from two trials.
[e] 0: value was calculated as less than 1%
[f] RDGS: negative control was subtracted from each value before normalizing

ELISA reactivity patterns

Monoclonal antibodies were tested in an ELISA against the three representative serotypes of IPN, along with IHN, an unrelated fish virus, IBDV, an avian virus morphologically and biophysically similar to IPN, and CHSE (host cell) fluid. Table 1 summarizes the results as the average of two separate trials, done in duplicate, against each antigen. Each monoclonal antibody was titrated by serial two-fold dilutions against IPNV Sp to determine the greatest dilution that would produce a high, but non-saturation absorbance value, approximately 0.9 O.D. Two of the IgG antibodies, 4-C2-4 and 3-11H2, reacted specifically with the Sp serotype, while the other IgG cross-reacted with all three serotypes. All of the IgM antibodies were broadly reactive against the three serotypes of IPNV and four of these nine also reacted slightly with the IHNV and CHSE preparations.

Binding of Antibodies to Electrophoretically Separated Polypeptides of IPNV

As shown in Figure 1, whole mouse antiserum against IPNV Sp reacted with viral proteins of all 13 isolates, CHSE fluid, and a few proteins of IBDV. Of the 12 monoclonal antibodies, only the three IgG antibodies were capable of immunologic binding to these disrupted components. Monoclonal antibodies produced by hybridomas 4-C4-1 and 3-11H2 both bound to the same low molecular weight proteins; however, 4-C4-1 antibodies cross-reacted with all isolates, while 3-11H2 antibodies reacted specifically only with those isolates in the Sp serotype, namely, Sp, Bonnamy and d'Honnincthun (Figures 2 and 3). The third hybridoma, 4-C2-4, produced antibodies that were directed against the outer capsid protein and its precursors. It is interesting to note that this monoclonal antibody was serotype specific but did not react with one member, the Bonnamy isolate (Figure 4).

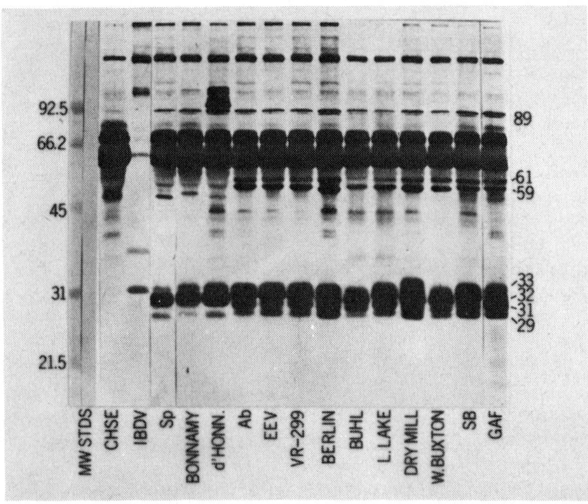

Fig. 1. Western blot analysis of IPNV strains using whole mouse antiserum produced against the SP strain. Virus preparations were lysates of infected CHSE cells.

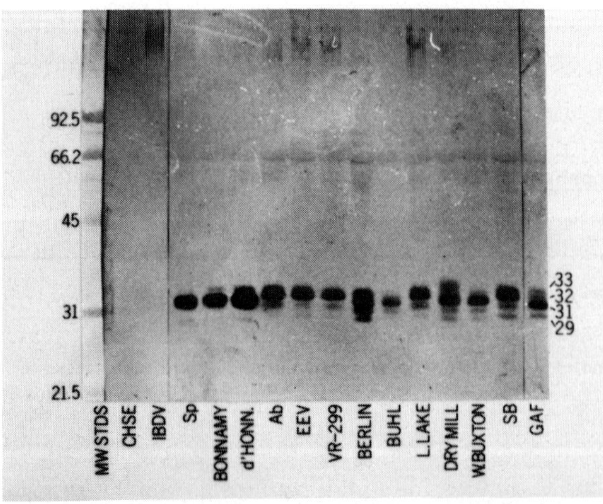

Fig. 2. Western blot analysis of IPNV strains using monoclonal antibody produced by hybridoma 4-C4-1. Virus preparations were lysates of infected CHSE cells.

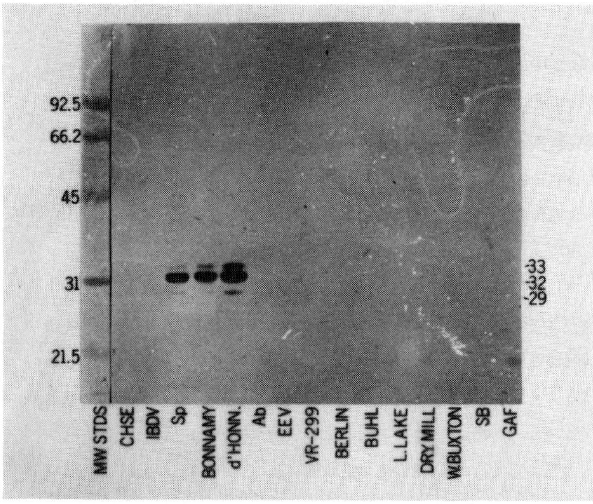

Fig. 3. Western blot analysis of IPNV strains using monoclonal antibody produced by hybridoma 3-11 H2. Virus preparations were lysates of infected CHSE cells

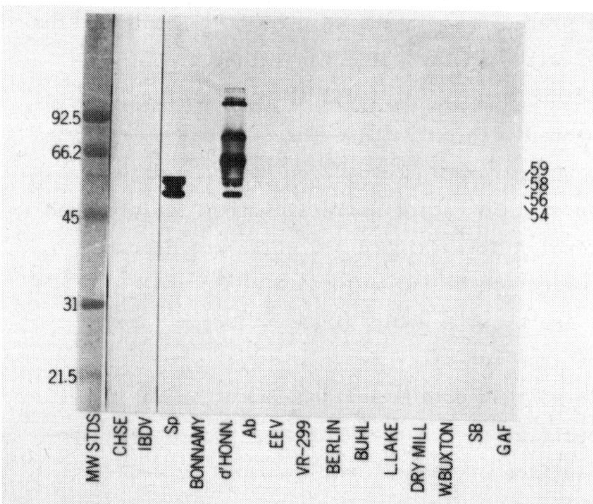

Fig. 4. Western blot analysis of IPNV strains using monoclonal antibody produced by hybridoma 4-C2-4. Virus preparations were lysates of infected CHSE cells.

DISCUSSION

Monoclonal antibodies produced against one serotype of IPNV have been used to study antigenic relationships among various isolates of IPN virus. Mouse serum produced to the whole Sp virus cross-reacts broadly in a Western blot assay with all isolates tested (Figure 1). On the other hand, monoclonal antibodies produced by hybridomas 3-11H2 and 4-C2-4 were more specific, considering not only the target serotype, but also the relatedness of individual viral proteins within the same serotype (Figure 3 and 4). From the protein profiles it is possible to compare molecular weights of the components of different isolates. We observed among the mid-range molecular weight proteins, representing those of the outer capsid, two major proteins per isolate. Ten of thirteen isolates, including VR-299 and Ab possess proteins of equal molecular weights, one protein of 61,000 and one of 59,000. Three isolates, the Sp, Bonnamy and d'Honnincthun, showed a different pattern. These contained a comparable upper band, 59,000, while the lower band of Bonnamy was approximately 57,000 as opposed to 56,000 in the other two. Comparing the low molecular weight proteins, it is obvious that Sp, Bonnamy and d'Honnincthun again are similar to each other, displaying three bands, and different from all other isolates, which exhibit four bands.

There seems to be general agreement that Sp, Ab, and VR-299 represent three distinct serotypes. There is disagreement, however, as to which serotype the remaining isolates should be assigned. The Bonnamy and d'Honnincthun strains have been placed in the same serotype as VR-299 by Macdonald and Gower (1981) while Okamoto et al. (1983) have placed them in the same serotype as Sp. From the reaction of monoclonal 3-11H2 with the low molecular weight proteins (Figure 3), Bonnamy and d'Honnincthun should be placed in the same serotype as Sp. This monoclonal antibody reacted with only these three isolates, and when compared to the immunoblot using whole serum, these three appeared different in that they had only three bands in this region while all other isolates had four. On the other hand, monoclonal 4-C2-4 (Figure 4), which was directed against the mid-range molecular weight proteins, reacted with Sp and d'Honnincthun, but not Bonnamy. Again, with whole virus antiserum, the Bonnamy isolate appears different from the other two.

Ishiguro et al. (1984) speculated that common antigens occur on the inner part of the virion and strain specific ones on the surface. Some strain specific antigen does occur on the surface of the virion, as shown by 4-C2-4 antibodies which reacted against outer capsid proteins. However, antibodies produced by clone 3-11H2 reacted with internal proteins, and they too showed serotype specificity. Monoclonal antibody 4-C4-1 (Figure 2) binds to the same proteins as 3-11H2; however, it cross-reacted with all isolates tested. It is obvious, then, that antigenic relationships are even more complex than previously thought. Ishiguro et al. (1984) showed also that different tests and antibody dilutions can produce conflicting results. For example, the cross-neutralization test showed five strains of IPNV to be serologically quite different, while the immunodiffusion test showed close antigenic relationships. Western blot analyses using a battery of specific monoclonal antibodies to each of the four major proteins of Sp, Ab and VR-299 may be needed to resolve the serotyping controversy definitively.

ACKNOWLEDGMENT

This work was supported by the U.S. Department of Agriculture, Grant No. 82 CRSR-2-1063. We thank Dr. K. Kinchington, Uniformed Services University, Bethesda, MD, for help with photography.

REFERENCES

Dobos, P., Hill, B. J., Hallett, R., Kells, D. T. C., Becht, H., and Teninges, D., 1979. Biophysical and biochemical characterization of five animal viruses with bisegmented double-stranded RNA genomes. J. Virol., 32: 593-605.

Goldsby, R. A., Osborne, B. A., Simpson, E., and Herzenberg, L. A., 1977. Hybrid cell lines with T-cell characteristics. Nature, 267: 707-708.

Hill, B. J., 1982. Infectious pancreatic necrosis virus and its virulence. In: R. J. Roberts (Editor), Microbial Diseases of Fish. Academic Press, London, pp. 91-114.

Ishiguro, S., Izawa, H., Kodama, H., Onuma, M., and Mikami, T., 1984. Serological relationship among five strains of infectious pancreatic necrosis virus. J. Fish Dis., 7: 127-135

Kearney, J. F., Radbruch, A., Liesegang, B., Rajensky, K., 1979. A new mouse myeloma cell line that lost immunoglobulin expression but permits the construction of antibody-secreting hybrid cell lines. J. Immunol., 123: 1548-1550.

Laemmli, U. K., 1970. Cleavage of structural proteins during the assembly of the head of bacteriophage T4. Nature, 227: 680-685.

Macdonald, R. D., and Gower, D. A., 1981. Genomic and phenotypic divergence among three serotypes of aquatic Birnaviruses (Infectious Pancreatic Necrosis Virus). Virology, 95(1): 260-264.

Nicholson, B. L., and Pochebit, S., 1981. Antigenic analysis of infectious pancreatic necrosis viruses (IPNV) by neutralization kinetics. Develop. Biol. Standard., 49: 35-41 (S. Kargel, Basel).

Okamoto, N., Sano, T., Hedrick, R. P., and Fryer, J. L., 1983. Antigenic relationships of selected strains of infectious pancreatic necrosis virus and European eel virus. J. Fish Dis., 6: 19-25.

Robb, M., Nichols, J. C., Whorisky, S. K., and Murphy, J. R., 1982. Isolation of hybridoma cell lines and characterization of monoclonal antibodies against cholera enterotoxin and its subunits. Infection and Immunity, 38: 2567-272.

Schutz, M., May, E. B., Kraeuter, J. N., and Hetrick, F. M., 1984. Isolation of infectious pancreatic necrosis virus from an epizootic occurring in cultured striped bass, _Morone saxatilis_. J. Fish. Dis., 7: 505-507.

Snyder, D. B., Marquardt, W. W., Malinson, E. T., Savage, P. K., and Allen, D. C., 1983. Rapid serological profiling by enzyme-linked immunosorbent assay. III. Simultaneous measurements of antibody titers to infectious bursal disease and Newcastle disease viruses in a single serum dilution. Avian Diseases, 28: 12-24.

Vestegard-Jorgenson, P. E., and Grauballe, P. G., 1971. Problems in the serological typing of IPN virus. Acta Veterinaria Scandinavica, 12: 145-147.

Wolf, K., Snieszko, S. F., Dunbar, C. E., and Pyle, E., 1960. Virus nature of infectious pancreatic necrosis in trout. Proc. Soc. Exper. Biol. Med., 104: 105-108.

Veterinary Immunology and Immunopathology, 12 (1986) 383–386
Elsevier Science Publishers B.V., Amsterdam — Printed in The Netherlands

THE INFLUENCE OF ENVIRONMENTAL TEMPERATURE AND INFECTION ROUTE ON THE IMMUNE RESPONSE OF CARP (CYPRINUS CARPIO) TO SPRING VIREMIA OF CARP VIRUS (SVCV)

W. AHNE

Institute of Zoology and Hydrobiology, University of Munich, Kaulbachstraße 37, D-8000 München 22, Fed.Rep.Germany

ABSTRACT

Ahne, W., 1986. The influence of environmental temperature and infection route on the immune response of carp (Cyprinus carpio) to spring viremia of carp virus (SVCV). Vet. Immunol. Immunopathol., 12: 383-386.

Carp infected by water route and by injection of SVCV developed neutralizing antibodies within 2 - 8 weeks at water temperatures between 10-20°C. At 10°C SVCV persisted 12 weeks in the blood of carp although antibodies were present. Immunized carp showed a solid protective immunity to SVCV.

INTRODUCTION

Spring viremia of carp (SVCV) is a contagious systemic disease of common carp (*Cyprinus carpio* L.) caused by spring viremia of carp virus (SVCV) (Fijan et al., 1971). The infection occurring in most European countries leads either to non, moderate or high mortality rates depending on the condition of the environment. Because little attention has been paid to the immune response of carp to SVCV so far (Sulimanovic, 1973; Fijan et al., 1977; Baudouy, 1978; Fijan and Matasin, 1980) the influence of water temperatures and infection route of SVCV on the immune response in carp has been investigated. This presentation is mostly based on previous studies (Ahne, 1980).

MATERIAL and METHODS

One (50 g) and three year (750 g) old SPF (specific pathogen free) carp were infected with SVCV (Lab-strain 10/5) by

0165-2427/86/$03.50 © 1986 Elsevier Science Publishers B.V.

a) intraperitoneal injection of virus (10^3-10^5 $TCID_{50}$/fish)
b) water bath (2 h, 10^oC, 10^3 PFU of SVCV/ml H_2O)

Infected fish kept at 10, 15 and 20^oC were tested for the presence of virus and antibodies in their blood weekly. Quantification of virus (PFU, $TCID_{50}$) and antibodies (50 % plaque reduction) were carried out according to methods described by Ahne and Wolf (1980).

RESULTS

Intraperitoneal injection of SVCV

Carp (50 g) intraperitoneally infected with 10^3 $TCID_{50}$/fish of SVC showed within 4 weeks mortality rates up to 90% at 10^oC. Multiplication of virus (up to 10^8 $TCID_{50}$/g) could be demonstrated whereas no humoral antibodies were found in the fish 4 weeks after infection. In contrast all infected carp kept at 20^oC survived and showed serum antibody titers up to 1:256.

Carp (750 g) intraperitoneally infected with 10^5 KID_{50} of SVCV were kept at 10^oC for 1 week. Afterwards water temperature was increased to 20^oC. Within two weeks carp developed neutralizing antibodies reaching titers up to 1:1024 at 4 weeks after keeping the fish at 20^oC. Subsequent lowering of the temperature to 10^oC and challenge with 10^6 $TCID_{50}$/fish of SVCV did not influence the immune status of the infected carp. All fish showed a solid protective immunity.

Infection of carp by water bath

Carp (750 g) infected by water bath (10^3 PFU/ml, 2 h, 10^oC) were kept at 10, 15 and 20^oC for more than 4 month. First humoral antibodies appeared 4 weeks at 20^oC, 7 weeks at 15^oC and 8 weeks at 10^oC. At 10^oC SVCV was present in the blood for 12 weeks whereas the virus disappeared after 1 week at 15 and 20^oC. Highest titers of antibodies were found to be 1:256 8 weeks (20^oC) and 9 weeks (15^oC) or 1:128 at 10 weeks (10^oC) after infection. In all fish antibodies persisted for more than 4 months; clinical signs or mortalities were absent and a solid protective immunity to SVCV was evident.

DISCUSSION

The experiments demonstrate that carp are capable of producing humoral antibodies to SVCV even at low temperatures of $10^{o}C$. However, the appearance of neutralizing antibodies was much quicker at $20^{o}C$ than at $10^{o}C$ and the mode of infection influenced the immunresponse also. Carp infected by intraperitoneal injection of SVCV did not produce any antibodies at $10^{o}C$ and infected fish died because of the extended replication of virus in the target organs such as kidney, liver and spleen. In contrast, carp infected by water route with the same amount of virus did not develop any signs of disease but the virus could be demonstrated in the blood of infected carp even 12 weeks after infection. However, 8 weeks p.i. fish showed first neutralizing antibodies, reaching titers up to 1:128 2 weeks later. At this time the spread of virus via blood stream has stopped. It is likely that the extracellular SVCV became neutralized by antiviral antibodies by attachment to the viral G-Proteins, which are responsible for the infectivity of SVCV. A sufficient amount of antibodies to form a noninfectious viral-antibody complex has been produced in 10 weeks after infection at $10^{o}C$.

The results clearly demonstrate that beside the environmental temperature (Avtalion et al., 1973) the route of infection also influences the immune response in carp.

REFERENCES

Ahne, W., 1980. Rhabdovirus carpio-Infektion beim Karpfen (Cyprinus carpio): Untersuchungen über die Reaktionen des Wirtsorganismus.
Fortschr. Vet. Med. 30, 180-183.

Ahne, W. and K. Wolf, 1980. Viruserkrankungen der Fische. In: Krankheiten und Schädigungen der Fische, H.H. Reichenbach-Klinke, ed. pp. 55-105, Gustav Fischer Verlag Stuttgart, New York.

Avtalion, R.R., A. Wojdani, Z. Malik, R. Shahrabani and M. Duczyminer, 1973. Influence of environmental temperature on the immune response in fish.
Curr. Top. Microbiol. 61, 1-35.

Baudouy, A.M., 1978. Virologie animale. - Relation hôte-virus au cours de la Viremie Printanière de la carpe.
C.R. Acad. Sc. Paris, 286, 1225-1228.

Fijan, N., Z. Petrinec, D. Sulimanovic and L.O. Zwillenberg, 1971. Isolation of the viral causative agent from the acute form of infectious dropsy of carp.
Vet. Arhiv, Zagreb, 41, 125-138.

Fijan, N., Z. Petrinec and Z. Stancl, 1977. Hyperimmunization of carp with Rhabdovirus carpio.
Bull. Off. Int. Epiz. 87, 439-440.

Fijan, N. and Z. Matasin, 1980. Spring viraemia of carp: preliminary experiments on vaccination by exposure to virus in water.
Vet. Arhiv, Zagreb, 50, 215-220.

Sulimanović, D., 1973. Immunity of carp to rhabdovirus carpio and determination of antibodies by indirect hemagglutination.
Vet. Arhiv, Zagreb 43, 153-161.

Veterinary Immunology and Immunopathology, 12 (1986) 387—393
Elsevier Science Publishers B.V., Amsterdam — Printed in The Netherlands

THE IMMUNE RESPONSE DURING PROLIFERATIVE KIDNEY DISEASE IN RAINBOW TROUT: A CASE HISTORY

George W. Klontz[1], Arthur W. Rourke[2], and William Eckblad[3]
[1]Dept. of Fish and Wildlife Resources, Univ. of Idaho, Moscow, Idaho 83843
[2]Dept. of Biological Sciences, Univ. of Idaho, Moscow, Idaho 83843
[3]Dept. of Veterinary Science, Univ. of Idaho, Moscow, Idaho 83843 (U.S.A.)

ABSTRACT

Klontz, G.W., Rourke, A.W. and Eckblad, W., 1986. The immune response during proliferative kidney disease in rainbow trout: A case history. Vet. Immunol. Immunopathol., 12: 387-393.

Young-of-the-year rainbow trout clinically affected by proliferative kidney disease (PKD), a systemic protozoan infection, exhibit a massive proliferation of small lymphocytes in the posterior kidney and spleen, a decrease in erythrocyte packed cell volume, hemoglobin, and serum albumins and an increase in beta-globulins. Electronphotomicrographs of the causative agent indicate that it is engulfed within a macrophage which is surrounded by small lymphocytes.

Fish having survived a clinical episode are completely refractory to subsequent infection. Their serum electrophoretic patterns are quite unremarkable.

INTRODUCTION

Proliferative kidney disease (PKD) is a clinically subchronic, self-limiting systemic parasitism of salmonids. Its main clinical features are: anemia, lethargy, enlarged posterior kidney, ascites and bilateral exophthalmia. The morbidity is high (70->90%) but the mortality in uncomplicated cases seldom exceeds 5-7% during a clinical episode (Clifton-Hadley et al., 1984), although there are reports of much higher mortalities (Hedrick et al., 1984).

The causative agent, although unnamed, is currently thought to reside in the Myxozoa (Kent and Hedrick, 1985). Others have placed it in the Haplosporea (Seagrave et al., 1980). Despite these apparent differences of opinion, there is unanimity that the agent is a protozoan.

The incubation period is a matter of weeks, but the nature and source of the infectious stage are unknown. The clinically affected fish apparently do not shed the organism; i.e., there is no demonstrable horizontal transmission. Also, vertical transmission has not been demonstrated (Clifton-Hadley et al., 1984).

There is no known method of chemotherapy or chemoprophylaxis.

The disease is easily diagnosed through demonstrating the causative organism in the kidney tissues. This can be accomplished either through H&E-stained sections or through Leishman-Giemsa-stained imprints of kidney tissue (Klontz and Chacko, 1983).

The purpose of our presenting a case history report in this forum is to bring attention to a possible model for research into the protective immune response in fish. Another purpose is to invite possible collaboration in our continuing efforts to understand the physiological and pathological processes in this disease.

CASE HISTORY

Given the foregoing brief description of PKD, it is somewhat apparent that, although the disease has been recognized since the turn of the century (Plehn, 1924), very little has been documented about the host response to the organism. Our studies during the past three years have been directed to this end with the primary purpose of being able to fulfill Koch's Postulates.

Proliferative kidney disease was first detected in the United States in late 1981 in rainbow trout being raised at the Idaho Department of Fish and Game Hatchery near Hagerman, Idaho (Smith et al., 1981). The episode was characterized as severe; i.e., several thousand under-yearling fish were dying each day. The major etiological agent in the episode was considered to be the organism causing PKD, although there were concurrent infections of infectious hematopoietic necrosis virus and *Sanquinicola klamathensis*, a systemic digenetic trematode. In December, 1981 the facility was depopulated and sterilized with the intent of preventing future episodes of PKD. However, this was not to be. PKD has recurred annually in this facility and at commercial trout farms downstream.

Our prospective epidemiological studies began in early 1982, prior to the appearance of the disease. During the course of sampling the populations or rainbow trout, chinook salmon, coho salmon, steelhead trout and cutthroat trout, the following observations were made:

1. All species of salmonids examined were susceptible to infection and subsequent disease by the causative organism.
2. Horizontal transmission trials were unsuccessful.
3. The incubation period was approximately 40 days.
4. The mortality due to PKD not complicated with superinfections of IHNV and/or *S. klamathensis* was negligible.
5. The causative organism was not limited to the water course supplying the IDFG hatchery. Fish harboring the organism were collected from a

stream in a nearby drainage system.

6. There were very few histopathological changes attributable to the organism noted in clinically ill fish. The major change was the massive hyperplasia of small lymphocytes in the posterior kidney, first, and the anterior kidney, spleen and liver in the latter stages of the clinical course.

7. The clinical course was self-limiting after 60-90 days. At this time no causative organisms could be seen in any of the affected fish.

8. The most striking histopathological feature of the disease was the surrounding of a parasitized macrophage with small lymphocytes (Figs. 1-2).

9. During the peak of the clinical course there were significant decreases in erythrocyte packed cell volume (12-20%) and in the serum proteins (2.5-4.1 g%). Corresponding values for noninfected fish were 35-39% PCV and 5.6-7.0 gm% serum proteins, as measured by optical refractometry.

During the 1983 episode of PKD at the Hagerman IDFG facility, sampling of sentinel populations began in mid-January and continued on a monthly basis until the organism was detected. The following conclusions were made from these efforts:

1. The heretofore reported susceptibility of the organism to water temperatures less than 12°C was rendered equivocal. Although exposing clinically affected fish for 12 hours to water temperatures in the 6-10°C range did shorten the clinical course somewhat (40-50 days as opposed to 60-90 days), the results did not agree with those reported previously (Ferguson, 1981).

2. The observations recorded during the 1982 episode were recorded also during the 1983 episode.

3. A relationship of prevalence of the organism and fish condition factor (length [mm]:weight [g] relationship) was noted. Those fish exhibiting a poor nutritional status; i.e., having an average condition factor $<1.0 \times 10\text{-}5$, had a much lower prevalence of infection than did those fish exhibiting a high nutritional status; i.e., having an average condition factor $>1.3 \times 10\text{-}5$. Also the fish having the high condition factors exhibited few, if any, clinical signs; e.g., anemia, lethargy, or sensitivity to handling.

4. All attempts to detect the reservoir of infection were unsuccessful as were attempts to transmit the organism from clinically affected fish to susceptible sentinel fish.

The studies conducted during the 1984 episode merely confirmed observations made during the 1982 and 1983 episodes. The possibility of an avian vector was investigated and was proven to be spurious.

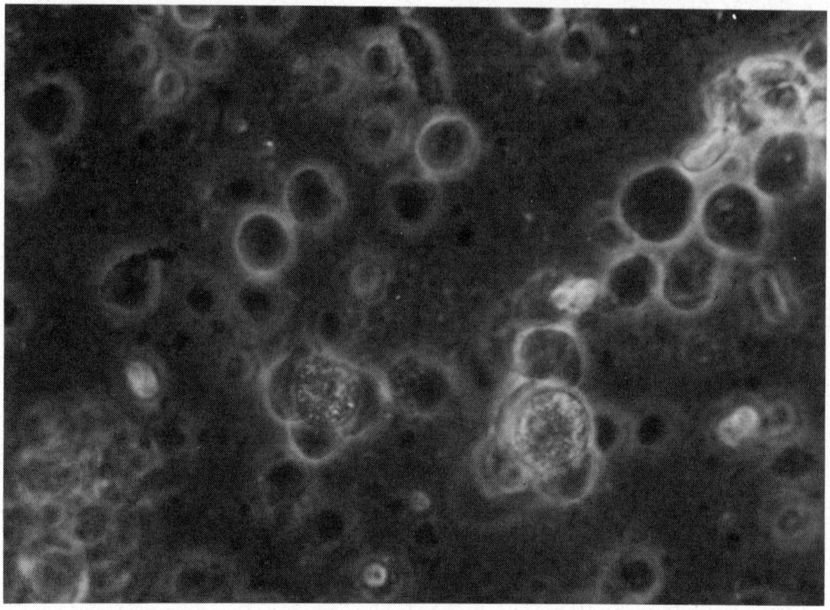

Fig. 1. Phase contrast photomicrograph of the PKD-causing organism in a fresh preparation of rainbow trout kidney. Note small lymphocytes surrounding the two parasitized macrophages.

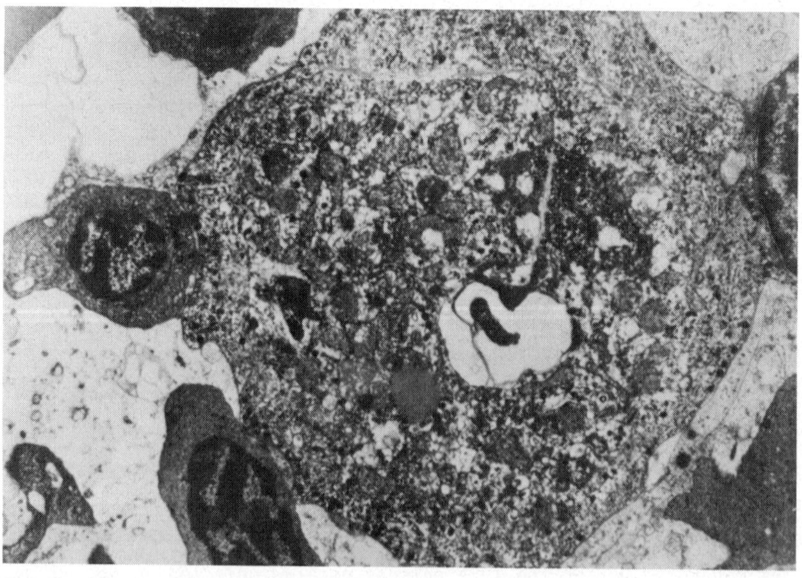

Fig. 2. Electronphotomicrograph of a macrophage parasitized by a PKD-causing cell. Note the small lymphocytes attached to the macrophage cell wall.

The just completed studies of the 1985 episode have been very insightful. So far, at this writing, the following observations have been recorded:

1. During the clinical phase of the disease there was a progressive increase in the beta-globulin portion of the serum proteins. The major increase was in the 600 kiloDalton range - the range of IGm in the salmonid. The levels often were more than 40% of the total serum protein fractions (Table 1). These values were determined by densitometric scanning of several hundred clinical and nonclinical serum samples subjected to gel electrophoresis.

2. Also during the clinical phase there was a progressive decrease in serum albumin until the recovery phase of the disease commenced. Serum albumin levels in clinically healthy trout ranged from 40-60% of the total serum protein fractions. In clinically affected animals the range decreased to 14-40%.

TABLE 1.
Serum electrophoresis data from fish in the clinical phases of Proliferative Kidney Disease and uninfected fish.

	Clinical Stage of the Disease[1]			
	Uninfected	Early	Middle	Late
Number	54	6	11	14
	(% of Total Serum Proteins)			
beta Globulins				
(Range)	14.3-41.7	21.7-44.4	22.1-38.9	23.8-48.9
(Mean)	28.01	36.07	30.33	34.77
(Std. Dev.)	7.90248	10.4209	5.64625	7.49373
Albumins				
(Range)	22.9-64.3	24.4-60-9	16.7-50.0	14.9-57.1
(Mean)	37.07	35.42	28.53	29.44
(Std. Dev.)	10.6622	12.9978	11.8306	9.48105

[1]Uninfected: Rainbow trout from a non-PKD system.
Early: 30-35 days post-exposure. Organisms detectible in the posterior kidney and spleen.
Middle: 60-70 days post-exposure. Organisms contain "daughter" cells.
Late: 90+ days post-exposure. Organisms beginning to undergo deterioration.

3. In the lower intestinal tracts of >2-year trout free-living in the water supply to the Hagerman facility there was a 30-50% prevalence of an amoeboid organism which has not been seen in any under-yearling, free-living or hatchery fish harboring the PKD-causing organism.

This finding gave rise to the speculation that the >2-year fish were refractory to systemic infection by the PKD-causing organism but not to intestinal infection. The antigenic identity of this amoeboid organism is to be determined using convalescent serum in the indirect immunofluorescent technique.

4. The incubation period was found to be consistently 28-32 days. At this time very few phagocytized organisms were noted. During the ensuing 6-8 weeks the numbers of organisms increased many-fold and began to decline to the point of there being none detected after 16-20 weeks post-exposure. There was no mortality during each of the 9 induced clinical episodes from which samples were taken.

CONCLUSIONS

It is our collective opinion that, from the foregoing observations on some of the epidemiological facets of PKD, the following can be said - somewhat safely:

1. The organism causing PKD is highly antigenic and stimulates a cell-mediated immunity.
2. The disease is not a threat to confined or free-living salmonid populations.
3. Those of us investigating the immunological nuances of the disease need help from the fish immunology community.

With respect to the conclusion that the organism is highly antigenic, this is not a new revelation about systemic parasitisms in fish. The metacercaria of *Diplostomum spathaceum*, a systemic digenetic trematode, also are quite antigenic in their host (Bortz et al., 1984). Even external protozoa, such as *Ichthyophthirius multifiliis* have been shown to be antigenic in their subcuticular parasitic phase (Beckert, 1975). However, in none of these cases has the resultant response been to the degree as that seen in PKD. To our knowledge, there are no reports of any systemic infection - regardless of causes - generating the massive lymphocytic hyperplasia seen in this disease. It is speculated currently that this hyperplasia directly contributes to the mortality attributed to PKD. If there is no or only moderate lymphoid hyperplasia, the host exhibits only a moderate anemia from which recovery is uneventful with the disappearance of the organism in the kidney and spleen.

In summary, this disease, in our opinion, represents a potential model for increasing our understanding of cell-mediated immunity in the salmonid. The data which could be acquired from in-depth immunological investigations of this disease should be applicable to studies of protective immunity against other pathogens - particularly the important viral and bacterial pathogens which for years have geen great causes for concern amongst public and private agencies.

ACKNOWLEDGMENTS

These studies were supported by funding from the Idaho Department of Fish and Game, the National Marine Fisheries Service (P.L. 88-309) and the Animal Health and Disease Program of the U.S.D.A.

REFERENCES

Beckert, H., 1975. Observations on the biology of *Ichthyophthirius multifiliis* (Fouquet, 1876), its susceptibility to Ethyoxyquin, and some immunological responses of channel catfish, *Ictalurus punctatus*, to this parasite. Ph.D. dissertation, Univ. Southeast. La., 198 p.

Bortz, B.M., Kenny, G.E., Pauley, G.B., Garcia-Ortigoza, E. and Anderson, D.P., 1984. The immune response to immunized and naturally infected rainbow trout (*Salmo gairdneri*) to *Diplostomum spathaceum* as detected by enzyme-linked immunosorbant assey (ELISA). Dev. Comp. Immunol., 8:813-822.

Clifton-Hadley, R.S., Bucke, D. and Richards, R.H., 1984. Proliferative kidney disease of salmonid fish: A review. J. Fish. Dis., 7:363-378.

Ferguson, H.W., 1981. The effects of water temperature on the development of proliferative kidney disease in rainbow trout (*Salmo gairdneri* Richardson). J. Fish Dis. 4(2):175-177.

Hedrick, R.P., Kent, M.L., Rosemark, R. and Manzer, D., 1984. Proliferative kidney disease (PKD) among Pacific salmon and steelhead trout. Bull. Eur. Ass. Fish Path., 4(3):34-37.

Kent, M.L. and Hedrick, R.P., 1985. PKX, the causative agent of proliferative kidney disease in Pacific salmonid fishes and its affinities with the Myxozoa. J. Protozool., 32(2):254-260.

Klontz, G.W. and Chacko, A.J., 1983. Methods to detect the organism causing proliferative kidney disease in salmonids. Bull. Eur. Ass. Fish Pathol., 3(3):33-36.

Plehn, M., 1924. Praktikum der Fischkrankheiten. E. Schweizerbartsche Verlagsbuchhandlung, Stuttgart. pp. 423-424.

Seagrave, C.P., Bucke, D. and Alderman, D.J., 1980. Ultrastructure of a haplosporean-like organism: The probable causative agent of proliferative kidney disease in rainbow trout. J. Fish Biol., 16(4): 453-459.

Smith, C.E., Morrison, J.K. and Ramsey, H.W., 1981. Proliferative kidney disease (PKD): First outbreak in North America. Fish Health News, 10(1):iii-iv.

Veterinary Immunology and Immunopathology, 12 (1986) 395—402
Elsevier Science Publishers B.V., Amsterdam — Printed in The Netherlands

THE SEASONAL ANTIBODY RESPONSE IN JUVENILE SUMMER FLOUNDER (*PARALICHTHYS DENTATUS*) TO THE HEMOFLAGELLATE *TRYPANOPLASMA BULLOCKI*

E.M. BURRESON and L.J. FRIZZELL

Virginia Institute of Marine Science and School of Marine Science, College of William and Mary, Gloucester Point, Virginia 23062 USA

ABSTRACT

Burreson, E. M. and Frizzell, L. J., 1986. The seasonal antibody response in juvenile summer flounder (*Paralichthys dentatus*) to the hemoflagellate *Trypanoplasma bullocki*. Vet. Immunol. Immunopathol., 12: 395-402.

An immuno-blot assay was used to investigate the serum antibody response in flounder injected with formalin-killed flagellates (immunized) and those injected with saline (control) and challenged with live *T. bullocki* after 21 days. Fish were held at 20°C and at ambient temperature from October through June. At 20°C immunized fish had significantly higher antibody titers than control fish, but immunized fish were not protected from infection with *T. bullocki*. At ambient temperature, after initial flagellate growth phase, antibody titer varied directly with temperature (2-25°C) and *T. bullocki* intensity varied inversely with titer. Flagellates were eliminated from the peripheral circulation in both immunized and control fish when antibody titer peaked in May. Recovered fish were immune to homologous challenge for at least one year.

INTRODUCTION

The hemoflagellate *Trypanoplasma bullocki* (Strout, 1965) parasitizes a wide variety of marine and estuarine demersal fishes along the Atlantic coast of North America (Laird and Bullock, 1969; Becker and Overstreet, 1979; Burreson and Zwerner, 1982). The biology of *T. bullocki* in juvenile summer flounder, *Paralichthys dentatus*, in Chesapeake Bay has been studied intensively (Burreson, 1982; Burreson and Zwerner, 1982; 1984). Juvenile flounder become infected in the fall and remain infected through the winter and early spring, but no infected flounder occur after early summer. This observation led Burreson and Zwerner (1982) to hypothesize that the rapid decrease in prevalence of *T. bullocki* in late spring was a result of either mortality of infected fish or activation of the immune response as water temperature increased and subsequent elimination of the flagellate. Further research revealed that mortality of *T. bullocki* infected flounder did occur during winter, but also revealed that many infected fish survived (Burreson and Zwerner, 1984). Preliminary studies on the immune response to *T. bullocki* in flounder showed that trypanoplasmacidal lysis activity increased

0165-2427/86/$03.50 © 1986 Elsevier Science Publishers B.V.

as water temperature increased in the spring (Sypek and Burreson, 1983). This observation suggests that the host's humoral immune response is responsible for the elimination of *T. bullocki* during spring.

The purpose of this paper is to investigate the production of *T. bullocki*-specific antibodies in immunized and non-immunized juvenile summer flounder held at ambient temperature through the normal infection period.

METHODS

Collection and Maintenance of Fish

Juvenile summer flounder (150-230 mm) were collected by otter trawl from the lower York River during September 1984. Fish were divided into two groups of 20, tagged with numbered spaghetti tags, and bled and checked for *T. bullocki* infections. Fish in group 1 were immunized (see below) and fish in group 2 were controls (non-immunized). Fifteen fish from each group were held in an indoor, shallow, rectangular tank (0.6 x 3.2 m) with flowing York River water at ambient temperature; the remaining five fish from each group were placed into a 0.6 x 1.6 m tank with recirculating water (20 ppt) maintained at 20 ± 1°C. A third group of eight tagged fish was held similarly at 20°C and was used to determine if fish that resolved *T. bullocki* infections were immune to homologous challenge. Fish were fed live shrimp (*Paleomonetes pugio* and *Crangon septemspinosa*) or sliced squid daily.

Immunization and Infection

On 17 October 1984 all fish in groups 1 and 2 were bled from the caudal hemal arch with needle and syringe. Blood was allowed to clot for 1 h at room temperature, refrigerated overnight, centrifuged for 5 min and serum collected and stored at -18°C in microcentrifuge tubes. Immediately after bleeding, each fish in group 1 was injected with 1.5×10^6 formalin killed *T. bullocki* from stock cultures. Ten fish (7 at ambient and 3 at 20°C) were injected IM with 0.2 ml of a 1:1 mixture of Freund's complete adjuvant and *T. bullocki* in PBS. The remaining ten fish were injected IP with 0.1 ml *T. bullocki* in PBS. The fish in group 2 were injected IP with 0.2 ml PBS. On 22 October 1984 fish in group 1 were boosted with an IM or IP injection of 1.5×10^6 killed *T. bullocki* without adjuvant. On 8 November 1984, 21 days after initial immunization, most fish in groups 1, 2 and 3 were injected IP with 0.1 ml live *T. bullocki* culture (1.3×10^5 flagellates in MEM + 20% FCS). Five fish each from the ambient temperature regime in groups 1 and 2 were challenged by allowing *T. bullocki* infected leeches to feed on the fish. After challenge all fish in groups 1 and 2 were bled weekly through December, then monthly through March and bimonthly through June. Fish in group 3 were bled weekly for 11 weeks and then bimonthly until termination of the experiment. During week 12 four of the eight fish in group 3 were each challenged with 1.3 x 10^5 live flagellates injected IP.

A single summer flounder remaining from experiments conducted during 1983 and held at ambient temperature was also bled monthly from October 1984 through March 1985. This fish had been infected with *T. bullocki* during the winter of 1983/84 and had eliminated the infection during May 1894. On March 26, 1985 (T = 9.4°C) this fish was challenged with 4.5 x 10^5 live *T. bullocki* and bled bimonthly.

Sera were collected as previously described. At each bleeding a drop of blood from each fish was mixed with a drop of 0.6% saline on a glass slide, covered with a coverglass and observed at 100X for *T. bullocki*. Infection intensity was scored subjectively as very light, light, moderate or heavy and converted to a no./mm^3 as described by Burreson and Zwerner (1984).

Enzyme Immunoassay

Antibody titers to *T. bullocki* in flounder sera were measured by immunoblot EIA (BioRad). Best results in preliminary assays were achieved with an initial 1:100 dilution of flounder sera in 1% gelatin-tris buffer solution (antibody buffer), a 1:2000 dilution of rabbit anti-summer flounder Ig serum (RASF) in antibody buffer and a 1:3000 dilution of goat anti-rabbit IgG-horseradish peroxidase conjugate (GAR-HRP, BioRad) in antibody buffer. Summer flounder Ig was purified by J. S. Stolen, National Marine Fisheries Service, Sandy Hook, New Jersey. Rabbit anti-flounder Ig was prepared by D. P. Anderson, National Fish Health Research Laboratory, Kearneysville, West Virginia. Each flounder serum sample was initially analyzed at a dilution of 1:100. Titer of sera that tested positively (contained antibody) was determined by a two-fold dilution series from 1:100 to 1:6400. All assays were done at room temperature (22-24°C). Titer is expressed as the reciprocal of the dilution.

All assays were performed using numbered 5 mm squares of nitrocellulose membrane soaked in tris buffered saline (TBS, 20 mM tris, 500 mM NaCl, pH 7.5) for 5 minutes and air dried. A 3 ul drop of *T. bullocki* culture (2.5 - 3.5 x 10^6 flagellates/ml) was applied to each membrane and air dried. Membranes were placed in 40 ml blocking solution (3% gelatin-TBS) and gently agitated on a laboratory rotator for 45 min. Membranes were individually transferred to snap-cap vials containing 3.0 ml of diluted flounder serum, and incubated for 2 h with gentle agitation. Membranes were rinsed and washed as previously described, transferred to a petri dish containing 30 ml RASF and incubated for 1 h with agitation. Membranes were rinsed, washed, and placed in 30 ml of GAR-HRP for 1 h with agitation. Membranes were rinsed, washed and placed in HRP substrate/color development solution (10 ml of 0.3% 3,3′-diamino benzidine tetrahydrochloride in ice cold methanol added to 50 ml of 0.06% ice cold H_2O_2 {30%} in TBS) for 20 min. Color development was stopped by immersing membranes in DH_2O for 10 min. A blue dot indicated a positive reaction.

Positive and negative controls were run with each assay. The positive control was rabbit anti- *T. bullocki* serum prepared by the authors by injecting a rabbit IM with 1.0 ml PBS-washed live flagellates (1.45×10^7) from stock cultures every other day for 3 days. Freund′s complete adjuvant was used 1:1 for the first two injections. Twelve days after the last injection, the rabbit was boosted SC with 1.45×10^7 PBS-washed live flagellates. The rabbit was bled by cardiac puncture 7 d later. The negative control was pre-injection serum collected from the same rabbit.

Differences in antibody titer and flagellate intensity means were tested for statistical significance with a one-way ANOVA.

RESULTS

Inspection of titer values indicated no difference between fish immunized IM with Freund′s adjuvant and those immunized IP without adjuvant. Thus, data from all immunized fish within each temperature regime were combined for analyses. Some fish challenged via very lightly infected leeches and held at ambient temperature did not become infected and were eliminated from the analyses, i.e. four fish from the immunized group and two fish from the control group.

Fish held at 20°C

Juvenile flounder responded to formalin-killed *T. bullocki* and were producing low levels of antibody three weeks after immunization (Fig. 1). Two weeks after challenge with live flagellates mean titer of immunized fish had increased dramatically and was significantly greater ($P<0.05$) than titer of control fish. All fish became infected with *T. bullocki* after challenge, but intensity remained very low (Fig. 2). Infections were no longer detectable in most fish five weeks post-challenge (week 8) and antibody titers decreased in each subsequent sample.

Antibody titer and flagellate intensity in Group 3 fish (Figs. 3 and 4) followed a pattern similar to Group 2 (control) fish except that one of the 8 fish had an antibody titer of 1,600 at weeks 11 and 13 and those values increased the mean considerably. The average titer of the four fish reinjected with live flagellates on week 11 increased greatly over the next two

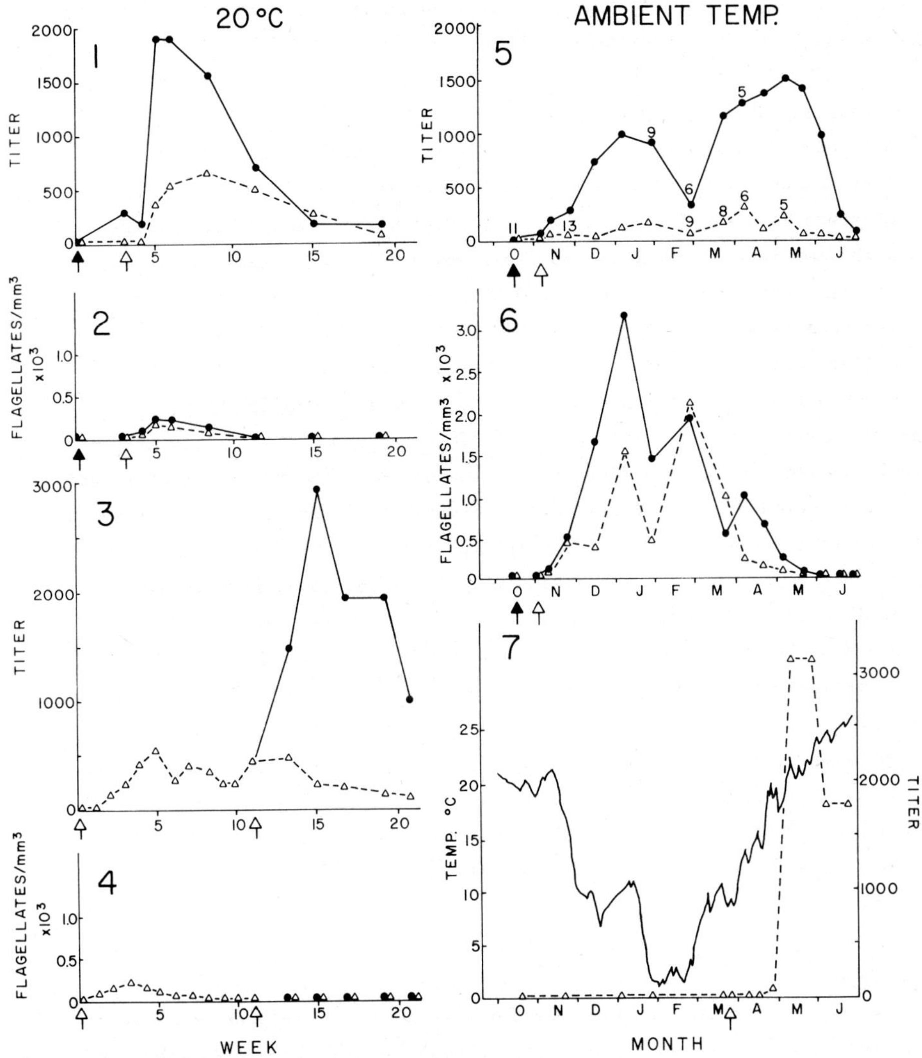

Figures 1-7. Results of experimental studies. Solid arrow is date immunized, open arrow is date challenged. Figs. 1-2. Mean antibody titer and flagellate intensity of immunized (solid line) and control (dashed line) fish held at 20°C. Figs. 3-4. Mean antibody titer and flagellate intensity of fish inoculated with live *T. bullocki* at week 0. Solid line and closed circles represent fish reinoculated at week 11. Figs. 5-6. Mean antibody titer and flagellate intensity of immunized (solid line) and control fish (dashed line) held at ambient temperature. Number of fish sampled (surviving) is shown above data points. Fig. 7. Mean daily temperature (solid line) in ambient holding tank and titer of single fish challenged one year after recovery from previous infection (dashed line).

weeks (Fig. 3); no flagellates were observed in the blood of these fish for the remainder of the experiment.

Fish held at ambient temperature

Antibody titer and flagellate intensity of immunized and control fish held at ambient temperature are shown in Figures 5 and 6. Holding tank temperature is shown in Figure 7. Antibody titer and flagellate intensity in both immunized and control fish followed a similar seasonal pattern, but titer was significantly greater ($P<0.05$) in immunized fish. Intensity differences between the two groups were not significant ($P>0.05$). Flagellate intensity increased rapidly through December as did antibody titer even though temperature declined to below 10°C during the period. By late January *T. bullocki* intensity had decreased sharply, possibly as a result of elevated antibody titer. At the end of February, temperature had been well below 5°C for over a month and antibody titer was greatly reduced. Flagellate intensity increased sharply at this time. As water temperature increased to near 10°C in March, antibody titer increased rapidly and flagellate density decreased rapidly. Infections were resolved by early June and antibody titers had declined to very low levels by early July.

Mortality was high in both immunized (55%) and control (62%) fish held at ambient temperature as a result of *T. bullocki* infections (Fig. 5).

The single, previously infected fish remaining from 1983 experiments had no serum antibodies to *T. bullocki* on the six bleedings prior to live flagellate challenge (Fig. 7). Six weeks after challenge titer increased rapidly to 3,200. No *T. bullocki* were observed in this fish after challenge.

DISCUSSION

The immune response in summer flounder is a complex interaction between temperature and *T. bullocki* intensity. From November through December as numbers of *T. bullocki* increased rapidly, antibody titer also increased even though the temperature decreased from 20°C to about 9°C; however, during this initial phase, titer response in ambient fish was slow and did not approach maximum values attained by fish treated similarly and held at 20°C. From January through early May antibody production in ambient fish appeared to be directly related to temperature, and flagellate intensity appeared inversely related to titer.

The role of temperature in the immune response in fish is well documented (Avtalion, 1981). Stolen et al. (1984a, b) reported that summer flounder can produce antibody at environmental temperatures as low as 7.5°C. In the present study antibody was present at temperatures near 3°C but it was ineffective in regulating levels of *T. bullocki* since the intensity of infection increased considerably during the winter. Wishkovsky and Avtalion (1982) suggest that fish may be able to survive pathogenic infections during cold periods if memory had been established at high temperatures. This does not appear to be true at the very low (1-5°C) temperatures encountered by summer flounder infected with *T. bullocki*, at least during the first winter after infection. However, by early March antibody titer had increased greatly as the temperature reached 8 or 9°C and flagellate intensity had decreased. It is interesting that the host's immune response cannot resolve the flagellate infection in the fall since temperature is above 10°C for about two months and antibody titer is relatively high. The log phase growth of the flagellate may overpower the immune response and by the time it begins to finally reduce flagellate levels, the extremely cold period of late January and February allows the flagellate to increase in numbers again. Temperatures near 2°C are common for long periods each winter in the Chesapeake Bay and it is during this period that mortality of infected juvenile flounder occurs (Fig. 5) (Burreson and Zwerner, 1984).

Even though a live flagellate challenge three weeks after immunization elicited a secondary immune response at both 20°C and at ambient temperature, the antibody was not protective and had no effect on parasitemia. Similar results were reported by Lom (1979) using irradiated flagellates as the immunogen. A delayed *Trypanosoma* parasitemia was observed in goldfish after immunization, but immunization had no effect on subsequent *Trypanoplasma* infections. However, in one part of the present study, recovered flounder were protected when challenged 11 weeks after initial inoculation. A typical secondary response was observed. These results suggest that 3 weeks post-immunization may be insufficient time for protection to develop in the fish. However, a more likely explanation for lack of protection is that formalin fixation altered the surface coat antigens responsible for inducing protection. Thus, antigens may have been recognized but did not elicit protection, or antigens other than those that induce protection may have been recognized since whole flagellates were used in the assay.

The most interesting result of this study may be the classic secondary response and protective memory observed after challenge of the previously infected fish held in the laboratory for over one year. The long delay after challenge before response may have been a result of the low temperature (9°C) at challenge. Stolen et al. (1984b) reported that the anamnestic character of the secondary response in summer flounder was lost at 8°C. The absence of *T. bullocki*-specific antibody in this previously infected fish for six months prior to challenge suggests that the immunity is sterile, in contrast to evidence presented by Woo (1981) that immunity in goldfish to *Trypanosoma danilewskyi* is non-sterile.

The results of this study suggest that increased antibody production during early spring is reponsible for the elimination of *T. bullocki* infections in summer flounder and also that recovered fish are immune for at least one year, even if challenged at temperatures as low as 9°C.

ACKNOWLEDGEMENTS

We thank Heidi K. Byrne for maintaining and bleeding the experimental fish and for maintaining *T. bullocki* cultures, and Drs. Douglas P. Anderson and Joanne S. Stolen for preparing the rabbit anti-summer flounder Ig serum. This research was supported in part by the Office of Sea Grant, NOAA, under Grant No. NA80AA-D-00021 and the Virginia Sea Grant Program through Project No. R/MP-1. Virginia Institute of Marine Science Contribution No. 1278.

REFERENCES

Avtalion, R. A., 1981. Environmental control of the immune response in fish. Crit. Rev. Environm. Contr., 11:163-188.

Becker, C. D. and Overstreet, R. M., 1979. Haematozoa of marine fishes from the northern Gulf of Mexico. J. Fish Dis., 2:469-479.

Burreson, E. M., 1982. The life cycle of *Trypanoplasma bullocki* (Zoomastigophorea:Kinetoplastida). J. Protozool., 29:72-77.

Burreson, E. M. and Zwerner, D. E., 1982. The role of host biology, vector biology, and temperature in the distribution of *Trypanoplasma bullocki* infections in the lower Chesapeake Bay. J. Parasitol., 68(2):306-313.

Burreson, E. M. and Zwerner, D. E., 1984. Juvenile summer flounder, *Paralichthys dentatus*, mortalities in the western Atlantic Ocean caused by the hemoflagellate *Trypanoplasma bullocki*: evidence from field and experimental studies. Helgolander Meeresunters., 37:343-352.

Laird, M. and Bullock, W. L., 1969. Marine fish hematozoa from New Brunswick and New England. J. Fish. Res. Bd. Canada, 26:1075-1102.

Lom, J., 1979. Biology of trypanosomes and trypanoplasms of fish. In: W. H. R. Lumsden and D. A. Evans (Editors), Biology of Kinetoplastida, 2. Academic Press, London/New York/San Francisco, pp. 269-337.

Stolen, J. S., Draxler, S. and Nagle, J., 1984a. A comparison of temperature mediated immunodulation between two species of flounder. Immunol. Commun., 13:245-253.

Stolen, J. S., Gahn, T., Kasper, V. and Nagle, J. J., 1984b. The effect of environmental temperature on the immune response of a marine teleost (*Paralichthys dentatus*). Dev. Comp. Immunol., 8:89-98.

Sypek, J. P. and Burreson, E. M., 1983. Influence of temperature on the immune response of juvenile summer flounder, *Paralichthys dentatus*, and its role in the elimination of *Trypanoplasma bullocki* infections. Dev. Comp. Immunol., 7:277-286.

Wishkovsky, A. and Avtalion, R. R., 1982. Induction of helper and suppressor functions in carp (*Cyprinus carpio*) and their possible implication in seasonal disease in fish. Dev. Comp. Immunol. Suppl. 2, pp. 83-91.

Woo, P. T. K., 1981. Acquired immunity against *Trypanosoma danilewskyi* in goldfish, *Carassius auratus*. Parasitol., 83:343-346.

Veterinary Immunology and Immunopathology, 12 (1986) 403–412
Elsevier Science Publishers B.V., Amsterdam — Printed in The Netherlands

THE IMMUNE RESPONSE OF A MARINE TELEOST, *PSEUDOPLEURONECTES AMERICANUS*, (WINTER FLOUNDER) TO THE PROTOZOAN PARASITE *GLUGEA STEPHANI*

R. LAUDAN [1], J.S. STOLEN [2], and A. CALI [1]

[1] Department of Zoology and Physiology., Rutgers University, Newark, New Jersey 07107 (USA)
[2] Sandy Hook Laboratory., Highlands, New Jersey 07732 (USA)

ABSTRACT

Laudan, R., Stolen, J.S. and Cali, A., 1986. The immune response of a marine teleost, *Pseudopleuronectes americanus*, (Winter flounder) to the protozoan parasite, *Glugea stephani*. Vet. Immunol. Immunopathol., 12: 403-412.

G. stephani is an intracellular cyst-forming microsporidan parasite that is found in the intestine of winter flounder (WF) *Pseudopleuronectes americanus*. No detectable humoral response was seen in parasitized fish or in fish injected with either spores or spore homogenate from this parasite. Quantification of total immunoglobulin (Ig) levels showed a decrease in Ig levels rather than enhancement, 21 days after intramuscular (IM) injections of spores ($3x10^6$/ml). When a second injection of spores was administered on day 21 and tested 3 weeks later, a further decrease in total serum Ig's occurred. A decrease in total IgM levels also occurred in WF that were simultaneously injected with *G. stephani* and the antigens, horse red blood cells (HRBC) or formalin-killed *Klebsiella pneumonia* (KP). The total Ig levels of fish injected with an antigen plus spores was not as low as those injected with the parasite alone. The Ig levels, as well as antibody titers to HRBC and KP were however, lower when compared to fish injected only with the HRBC or bacteria. Disrupted spore homogenate injected into winter flounder, showed a less marked decrease in Ig levels when compared with whole spores. When a single IM injection of spores was given, followed by two weekly injections of indomethacin (a drug that inhibits prostaglandin activity), no decrease in Ig levels occurred and levels were comparable to control (saline injected) fish.

INTRODUCTION

The microsporidan parasite, *Glugea stephani*, parasitizes some economically important flatfish in North America and in several European countries (Sprague, 1977). This intracellular organism can be recognized by the white cysts (1-2mm) that are formed anywhere along the intestine (Stunkard and Lux, 1965;Olson, 1976;

Cali and Olson, 1978; Takvorian and Cali, 1981, 1984). These infections can debilitate and cause mass martality by placing a metabolic strain on the host or by occluding the digestive tract (McVicar, 1975; Weidner, 1976; Takvorian and Cali, 1981).

The parasite may be injected directly by the host or may infect the host via a crustacean vector which it has consumed (Stunkard and Lux, 1965; McVicar, 1975).

The infection is temperature dependent and established in 24 hours. Winter flounder, Pseudopleuronectes americanus, are susceptible to parasitism when the temperatures reach 16°C or above. If the winter flounder remains in warmer water, the infected cells will hypertrophy and the parasite will proliferate, leading to the development of a cyst. Host mortality can occur within 6-8 weeks. If the host returns to colder waters, the proliferation will be curtailed (Olson, 1976, 1981).

Three types of host responses may occur in an intracellular parasitic infection: encapsulation, inflammation, or specific immune responsiveness. Suppression of many of these responses is not uncommon in fish (Dykova and Lom, 1978; Dykova et al., 1980; Weissenberg, 1968; McVicar, 1974) or mammals (Niederkorn and Shaddock,1983; Cox, 1984).

These experiments examine the host response in winter flounder to the parasite. The results indicate suppression rather than enhancement. Instead of increased immunoglobulin levels after injection of G. stephani, a decrease was seen. The effect of prostaglandins on this response was also examined.

MATERIALS AND METHODS

Fish

Winter flounder 24-34 cm in length were caught by otter trawl in Sandy Hook Bay, N.J., U.S.A. They were maintained in 200 gallon flow-through salt water tanks at 19°C and acclimated for at least one week before being used in experiments.

Injections:

Parasite

The parasite G. stephani (GS) was collected by dissecting out the cysts from infected winter flounder intestine. They were disrupted with a tissue grinder to separate the spores. The spore suspension was then filtered, the spores washed 6 times in saline and suspended to $3x10^6$/ml. One half ml of this suspension was injected into specific groups of WF.

Other antigens

Horse Red Blood Cells (HRBC); a 20% suspension in sterile saline.

Klebsiella pneumonia (KP); a 5% suspension of formalin-killed bacteria.

Spore homogenate, a 10% solution of disrupted GS spores using a Braun homogenizer.

Indomethacin

Indomethacin (IDM, donated by Merck Inst. Rahway, N.J.) was dissolved in ethyl alcohol to a concentration of 7.5 mg/ml and diluted with a 15% gelatin solution. The dosage administered was 100 ug/100g body weight.

Collection of serum

Fish were bled from the caudal vein, the serum separated, heat inactivated at 56°C for 30 min. and stored at -20°C until tests were performed.

Quantitation of antibody levels

Agglutination titers were determined using the microtitration method, and total immunoglobulin levels by single radial immunodiffusion assays (SRID) (Fahey and McKelvey, 1965). Agarose contained 4% rabbit anti-winter flounder IgM. 5 microliters of sera was added to each well along with standards. The diameter of the precipitate was measured to the nearest 0.1mm.

Experiment 1

Fish were divided into 5 groups of 7 or 8 fish, all receiving 1/2 ml intramuscular (IM) injections of antigens or sterile saline on day 0 and day 21. The groups were injected as follows: 1. HRBC, 2. HRBC+spores, 3. disrupted spores, 4. KP, 5. KP+spores

6. spores, 7. saline. Fish were bled on days 0, 21, and 42 after the initial injection. The serum was heat-inactivated at 56°C for 30 min. and stored at -20°C until tests were performed.

Experiment 2

Fish were divided into 3 groups of 8 fish/group and injected with 1/2 ml IM injections. The groups were : 1. GS on day 0, and IDM twice weekly beginning on day 1 for 3 weeks, 2. GS on day 0 and 15% gelatin twice weekly, beginning on day 1 for 3 weeks, and 3. saline twice weekly beginning on day 1 for 3 weeks. Fish were bled weekly for serum.

RESULTS

Preliminary experiments showed a decrease in total immunoglobulin (Ig) levels 21 days following IM injections of *G. stephani* spores, with a further decrease observed three weeks later following a second injection of spores on day 21.

By comparison winter flounder injected with the antigens HRBC or *K. pneumonia*, showed an increase in Ig levels and high titers to the antigens by day 21 and day 42. Fish injected with *G. stephani* spores together with the antigens HRBC and *K. pneumonia*, showed a significant decrease in both total Ig levels (Figs. 1 and 2) and titers to the antigens. The WF injected with the spores only showed an even greater decrease in the total Ig levels, with a standard deviation of ± 1.5 mm of the precipitin ring.

Similar tests were conducted using spore homogenate (Langley, 1981) instead of whole spores. A decrease in total Ig levels was detected but was not as marked as in fish injected with 1/2 ml of intact spores. The decrease was however greater by day 42 than that seen in WF injected with the erythrocyte antigen and whole spores simultaneously (Fig. 1).

Winter flounder were given injections of indomethacin (a drug that inhibits prostaglandin acitivity) two/times, following a single 1/2 ml injection of *G. stephani* spores ($3x10^6$/ml). The

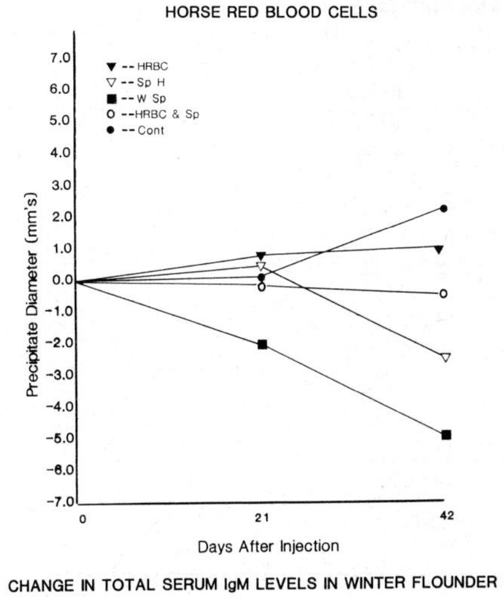

Fig. 1. Total immunoglobulin levels determined by the SRID assay in winter flounder. A comparison between fish injected with horse red blood cells (HRBC), Glugea stephani spore homogenate (Sp H), whole spore (W Sp), HRBC & Sp, and Cont. (Saline). The points represent the difference in the mean diameter of the precipitate ring after injection.

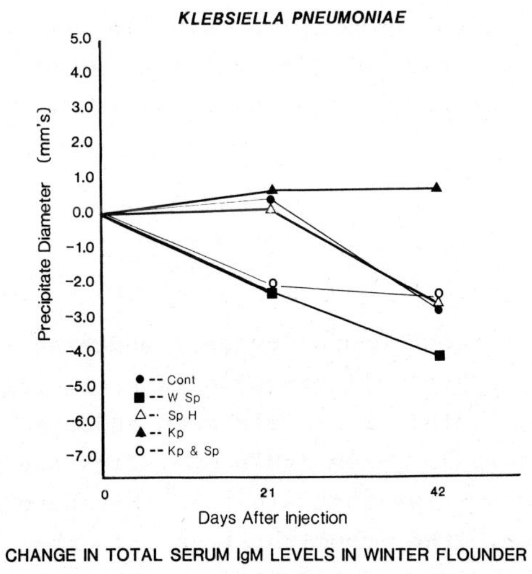

Fig. 2. Total immunoglobulin levels determined by the SRID assay in winter flounder. A comparison between control saline-injected fish, Glugea stephani whole spores (W Sp), spores homogenate (Sp H), a 5% suspension of bacteria Klebsiella pneumonia (Kp), and Kp & Sp. The points represent the difference in the mean diameter of the precipitate ring after injection.

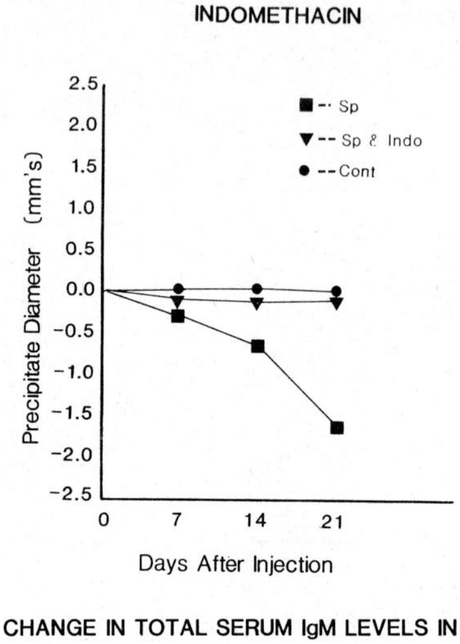

Fig. 3. The effect of indomethacin on the total immunoglobulin levels of Glugea stephani spore injected winter flounder. Fish were injected with spores (Sp), spores and 1/2 ml of indomethacin twice weekly (Sp & Indo), or saline control (Cont). The points represent the difference in the mean diameter after injection.

total Ig levels detected were similar to those found in control fish that were injected only with sterile saline. The WF injected with spores and a 15% gelatin solution showed a significant decrease ($p<0.001$) in the total Ig levels by day 21 (Fig. 3).

DISCUSSION

Attempts made to detect humoral or cell mediated responses to injections of spores, have all proved negative. Glugea stephani caused a decrease in total IgM levels when injected into winter flounder. This decrease in serum IgM's may allow the parasite to spread further throughout the host. In fish that have returned to colder waters however, the proliferation of the parasite in naturally infected fish is arrested (Olson, 1981). When comparing Ig levels of WF in which the infection has been arrested, to those of uninfected fish, no significant difference was observed.

This seemed to indicate that the immune system of WF can recover from an earlier parasitic infection. Other investigators have also shown that temperature directly affects the parasite and the hosts response to the parasite (Sypek and Burreson, 1983; Clem et al., 1984, Stolen et al., 1984a,b; van Muiswinkel, 1984).

There has been other evidence of suppression of host responses. This was demonstrated by Dykova and Lom (1978) and Dykova et al. (1980) with Glugea anomala in the three-spined stickleback and Glugea plecoglossi in Plecoglossus altivelis. Both suppressed the inflammatory response of their host. Similar findings were also documented by Weissenberg (1968) and McVicar (1975). In mammals the humoral and cell-mediated response was reduced by 5-10% accompanied by an increase in the number of suppressor cells, after infection by the parasite Trypanosoma brucei. There is however, little evidence that the parasite affects T and B cells directly. It is more likely that the suppression occurs at the macrophage level with the release of mediators (Cox, 1984).

Injections of the WF with spore homogenate (Fig. 1) showed a decrease in the total Ig levels although not as great as the decrease seen with whole spores. This implies that a substance within the spore or the spore coat may be affecting the Ig levels directly or may stimulate macrophages to release immunosuppressive factors such as prostaglandins. The spores do not seem to inhibit Ig production by blockading the reticuloendothelial system within the spleen or anterior kidney of the WF.

The suppressive or catabolic affect caused by the parasite is further demonstrated by the decreased IgM found in WF injected with the whole spores or spore homogenate, together with the antigens HRBC or K. pneumonia. A similar decrease in IgM levels was also observed after injecting WF simultaneously with HRBC, K. pneumonia and G. stephani. Winter flounder injected only with the bacterial and erythrocyte antigens showed an increase in IgM levels. This would imply that antigenic competition was not the cause of the suppression and that the suppression was caused by the interference of the parasite with the host's normal response to foreign antigens. All winter flounder injected with a mixture of spores and antigens had the same proportional decrease of serum IgM's (±0.1mm).

Winter flounder injected with G. stephani, and also injected with indomethacin 2 time/week, showed no decrease in serum IgM levels. Similar results were found when IDM was injected 3 times a week. However when IDM was injected once weekly, a decrease in the Ig levels was seen, which was equivalent to the fish injected only with the spores (unpubl. results). It may be that prostaglandins were involved in the suppression by the parasite. Immunosuppression of T and B cells by prostaglandins has been well documented (Quagliata et al. 1973; Melmon et al., 1974; Mihas et al., 1975; and Pelus, 1977). The decrease of Ig levels seen following weekly injections of indomethacin in spore-injected fish showed that smaller doses of the drug may not be sufficient to neutralize the prostaglandins released. Spores phagocytosed by macrophages may trigger the release of prostaglandins by the macrophage, which in turn caused a suppression of the response

The explanation for the decrease in serum IgM in the fish may in part be attributed to the half-life of the IgM molecule and/or some catabolic process triggered by the spores or by mediators released in the presence of the spores.

ACKNOWLEDGMENTS

Our thanks to Doug Anderson for the rabbit anti-winter flounder serum, Helen Strausser for her suggestions and guidance, Fritz Farwell for his help with the fish and in the laboratory, Sue Draxler for her laboratory assistance and to the Sandy Hook Laboratory for the use of the facilities.This is contribution number 4 from the Department of Zoology, Rutgers-Newark.

REFERENCES

Cali, A. and Olson, R.E., 1978. The ultrastructure of *Glugea stephani* (Hagenmuller) development in *Parophrys vetulus*, In Symposium on Ultrastructure of the Developmental Stages of Microsporidia. International Colloquim on Invertebrate Pathology. Prague,Czech.

Clem, L.W., Faulman, E., Miller, N.W., Ellsaesser, C., Lobb, C.J., Cuchens, M.A., 1984. Temperature-mediated process in teleost immunity: differential effects of in-vitro and in vivo temperatures on mitogenic responses of channel catfish lymphocytes. Dev. Comp. Immunol., 8:313-322.

Cox, F.E.G., 1984. How parasites evade the immune response. Immunol. Today., 5:32-34.

Dykova, I. and Lom. J., 1978. Tissue reaction of the three-spined stickleback Gastenosteus aculeatus L. to infection with G. anomala, J. Fish Dis., 1:83-90.

Dykova, I., Lom, J., and Egusa, S., 1980. Tissue reaction to Glugea plecoglossi infection in its natural host Plecoglossus altivelis. Folia Parasit., 27:213-216.

Fahey, J.L. and McKelvey, E.M., 1965. Quantitative determination of serum immunoglobulins in antibody-agar plates. J. Immunol., 94:84-90.

Langley, R., 1983. Two-dimensional electrophoretic analysis of microsporidan spore proteins. in Ph.D. Dissertation, Rutgers University, Newark, N.J., pp. 13-17.

McVicar, A.H., 1975. Infection of plaice Pleuronectes platessa L. with Glugea stephani in a fish farm under experimental conditions. J. Fish Biol., 7:611-619.

Melmon, K.L., Bourne, H.R., Weinstein, Y., Shearer, G., Kram, J., and Bauminger, S., 1974. Hemolytic plaque formation by leukocytes in vitro. J. Clin. Invest., 53:13-21.

Mihas, A.A., Gibson, R., Hirschowitz, B., 1975. Suppression of lymphocytes transformation by 16, dimethyl PgE_2 and unsaturated fatty acids. Proc. Soc. Exp. Biol. Med., 149:1026-1028.

Niederkorn, J.Y. and Shadduck, J.A., 1980. Role of antibody and complement in the control of Encephalitozoan cuniculi infections by rabbit macrophages. Infec. Immun., 27:995-1002.

Olson, R.E., 1976. Laboratory and field studies on Glugea stephani (Hagenmuller), a microsporidan parasite of pleuronectid flatfishs. J. Protozool., 23:158-164.

Olson, R.E., 1981. The effect of low temperature on the development of microsporidan Glugea stephani in English sole (Parophrys vetulus). J. Wild Dis., 17:559-562.

Pelus, L.M., 1977. Prostaglandin production in tumor-bearing mice: their role in immune suppression. in Ph.D. Dissertation, Rutgers University, Newark, N.J., pp. 19-54.

Quagliata, F., Lawrence, V.J.W., Phillips-Quagliata, J.M., 1973. Prostaglandin E. as a regulator of lymphocyte function. Selective action on B lymphocytes and synergy with procarbazine in depression of immune responses. Cell Biol., 6:457-465.

Sprague, V., 1977. Annoted lists of species of microsporidian In: L. Bella and T.C. Cheng (Eds.) Systematics of the Microsporida, Plenum Press, New York. pp. 31-334.

Stolen, J.S., Gahn, T., Kasper, V., and Nagle, J.J., 1984a. The effect of the environmental temperature on the immune response of a marine teleost (Paralichythys dentatus). Dev. Comp. Immunol., 8:89-98.

Stolen, J.S., Draxler, S., Nagle, J.J., 1984b. A comparison of temperature-mediated immunomodulation between two species of flounder. Immunol. Commun., 13:245-253.

Stunkard, H. and Lux, F., 1965. A microsporidan infection of the digestive tract of the winter flounder Pseudopleuronectes americanus. Biol. Bull., 129:371-387.

Sypek, J.P., and Burreson, E.M., 1983. Influence of temperature on the immune response of juvenile summer flounder, Paralichthys dentatus, and its role in the elimination of T. bullocki infections. Dev. Comp. Immunol., 7:277-286.

Takvorian, P.M. and Cali, A., 1981. The occurrence of Glugea stephani in American winter flounder, Pseudopleuronectes americanus from the New York-New Jersey lower bay complex. J. Fish Biol., 18:491-501.

van Muiswinkel, W.B. and Jagt, L.P., 1984. Host-parasite relationships in fish and other ectothermic vertebrates. Dev. Comp. Immunol., suppl. 3:105-208.

Weidner, E., 1976. Ultrastructure of the peripheral zone of Glugea induced xenoma. J. Protozool., 23:234-238.

Weissenberg, R., 1968. Intracellular development of the microsporidian Glugea anomala in hypertrophying migratory cells of the fish Gasterosteus aculeatus: an example of the formation of xenoma tumors. J. Protozool., 15:44-57.

Veterinary Immunology and Immunopathology, 12 (1986) 413–419
Elsevier Science Publishers B.V., Amsterdam — Printed in The Netherlands

IMMUNOSUPPRESSION OF CARP (CYPRINUS CARPIO L.) TO ICHTHYOPHTHIRIASIS USING THE CORTICOSTEROID TRIAMCINOLONE ACETONIDE

G. HOUGHTON and R.A. MATTHEWS

Dept. of Biological Sciences, Plymouth Polytechnic, Plymouth, Devon, PL4 8AA, England

ABSTRACT

Houghton, G. and Matthews, R.A., 1986. Immunosuppression of carp (Cyprinus carpio L.) to ichthyophthiriasis using the corticosteroid triamcinolone acetonide. Vet. Immunol. Immunopathol., 12: 413-419.

The immune response of juvenile mirror carp (Cyprinus carpio L.) has been investigated in relation to protective immunity and immunosuppression to the disease ichthyophthiriasis. Protective immunity was induced by exposing juvenile carp to approximately 2,000 theronts per fish for 3 hours at a concentration of approximately 80 theronts cm^{-3} in dechlorinated water pH 7.0 - 7.2, 20 ± 2°C in the dark, on three separate occasions of 14 day intervals. Following each exposure, re-infection was prevented by transferring fish to clean aquaria twice daily from day 5-10. Fish were challenged 4 weeks following exposure to the third immunising infection with a potentially lethal dose of approximately 8,000 theronts per fish for 3 hours at a concentration of approximately 320 theronts cm^{-3}. All immunised fish survived although 19% showed initial signs of invasion, the parasites in these instances being confined to periphery of fins. Mortalities of 100% were recorded in non-immunised controls, first deaths occurring 5 days after challenge. Fourteen days following challenge, immune fish received one of the following treatments; intraperitoneal injection of the corticosteroid triamcinolone acetonide at a dose of 200 $\mu g\ g^{-1}$ body weight, intraperitoneal injection of 0.85% saline or left untreated; non-immunised fish were subjected to similar procedures. On challenge 6 days later, all fish developed heavy infection with up to 100% mortalities with the exception of immunised fish administered saline or left untreated. Repeat experiments gave comparable results. The results indicate that immunosuppression can be induced by administration of high levels of synthetic corticosteroid. The possibility of elevated levels of adrenocorticotrophic hormones occurring in fish populations subjected to stress could be significant in lowering resistance to disease even following programmes of vaccination.

INTRODUCTION

Ichthyophthiriasis or 'white spot' is a major disease of freshwater fish and occurs worldwide leading to great economic loss (Paperna, 1972; Hines and Spira, 1973; Nigrelli, Pokorny and Ruggieri, 1976). The causative agent, Ichthyophthirius multifiliis Fouquet, 1876 (Protozoa: Ciliophora) 'Ich',

0165-2427/86/$03.50 © 1986 Elsevier Science Publishers B.V.

invades the epithelium of skin and gills, where after a period of growth, of a duration dependant upon temperature, it enters the aquatic environment undergoing a cycle of multiplication with the production of new infective stages, the theronts

That fish can acquire protective immunity to 'Ich' has been shown by Bauer (1953), Beckert and Allison (1964) and Hines and Spira (1974). Goven, Dawe and Gratzek (1980) have successfully protected channel catfish against the disease by immunisation with cilia isolated from *Ichthyophthirius multifiliis* and a related species *Tetrahymena pyriformis*. It is possible that other materials of parasitic origin in addition to cilia and including secretory products, may serve also as protective antigen.

The aim of the present study was to determine whether the protective immune response could be suppressed following administration of a corticosteroid. Such investigations of immunosuppression are considered highly pertinent to the development of effective programmes of vaccination in fish farms (documented in the discussion section). Selection of juvenile carp (*Cyprinus carpio* L.) 10-12 weeks of age for experiments was considered relevant as fish are more prone to damage by the disease when young and thus would gain maximum benefit from protection at this stage. Previous immunological studies have been chiefly confined to the response of adult fish (Beckert and Allison, 1964; Hines and Spira, 1974).

MATERIALS AND METHODS

Fish

Juvenile *C. carpio* were used in all experiments and for the routine maintenance of *I. multifiliis*. Those used for experiments were bred from stock at Plymouth Polytechnic or were obtained as fry from The Hampshire College of Agriculture, Sparsholt, Hants. Prior to experiments, fish from both sources were maintained free from exposure to *I. multifiliis.*

Fish were maintained in perspex aquaria of 12 litre capacity. Aquaria were aerated and kept at a temperature of 20 $\pm$ 2°C with pH range of 7.0 - 7.5. In addition, water quality was maintained by biological filtration using sub gravel filters; partial changes of water being undertaken at 2-3 week intervals. Stocking densities in experimental aquaria were established at 5-10 fish of 10-12 weeks of age (mean weight 650 mg). Fish were fed twice daily a mix of No. 2 trout pellets (Ewos Baker, Bathgate, West Lothian) and goldfish flake (King British, Bradford, West Yorkshire).

Parasite

I. multifiliis was established from 2 trophonts isolated from a single goldfish imported from Japan. This parasite strain was maintained for up to 9 months after which period there was a loss of viability although there was no change in infection procedures.

Experimental procedures

Experimental infection of fish was undertaken by transferring susceptible carp to small perspex tanks (capacity of 2 litres) and containing theronts. Theronts were used 5-10 hours following emergence from the reproductive cysts. For immunisation experiments, fish were exposed to theronts for 3 hours in the dark. Particular care was taken to ensure a pH of 7.0 - 7.2 as relatively small fluctuations from these values was known to effect the viability of theronts. Aeration was restricted to a period of 2 hours, starting 30 minutes after introduction of the fish to ensure non turbulent periods for the theronts. For quantitative studies, numbers of theronts were estimated cm^{-3} with the aid of a Sedgewick Rafter Counting Cell (Dickerson et al., 1981).

Immunisation

Fish were immunised by exposure to theronts at approximate doses of 80 cm^{-3}, 2,000 per fish on 3 separate occasions at 14 day intervals. From days 5-10 following each exposure, reinfection was prevented by transferring fish to clean aquaria at 10-14 hour intervals. By day 10 all trophozoites had completed their development and were removed from aquaria during fish transfer and before further infective stages were produced. Twenty eight days after the final antigen exposure fish were challenged with a potentially lethal dose of approximately 8,000 theronts per fish at a concentration of approximately 320 cm^{-3}. Following challenge, in contrast to immunisation procedures, fish were returned to holding tanks and any infection allowed to continue. Uninfected controls were used to confirm lethal dose on challege and to check viability of theronts during immunisation. In addition some were maintained free from 'Ich' until the termination of the experiment.

Immunosuppression

Immunosuppression of ichthyophthiriasis was investigated following stress induced by the synthetic corticosteroid, Triamcinolone acetonide (Sigma, U.K.). Fourteen days after challenge, immunised fish were administered approximately 200 $\mu g\ g^{-1}$ body weight of Triamcinolone acetonide suspension in 0.85% saline by intraperitoneal injection. Additional fish were injected with 0.85% saline or left untreated. Non-immunised control fish were also subjected to the same procedures. Six days after administration of the corticosteroid, half of the immunised fish and half of the non-immunised controls, with representatives from each treatment, were challenged using the procedure previously described.

RESULTS

Immunisation

The results (Table 1) show that after immunisation with controlled infections of 'Ich', all immunised fish survived on challenge. Although infections developed in 19% of the challenged, immunised fish, these were light, restricted to periphery of fins, and caused no deaths. Non-immunised controls subjected to challenge infections, suffered 100% mortalities, first deaths occurred after 5 days.

Immunosuppression

After injection of corticosteroid (Table 2), all immunised and non-immunised fish developed heavy infections of 'Ich' with 100% mortalities. Deaths also occurred in saline and untreated controls, but not in immunised fish injected with saline or left untreated.

TABLE 1

The effect of a potentially lethal challenge of *I. multifiliis* after immunisation with three serial infections of the parasite.
Data represent pooled results from two separate experiments.

Group and no. of fish	% Infected	Degree of Infection	% Mortality
immunised (120)	19	very light, periphery of fins	0
control (30)	100	very heavy, entire body	100

DISCUSSION

The results indicate first that juvenile carp less than 12 weeks of age can respond to antigenic stimulus from the parasite *I. multifiliis* by eliciting an immune response which protects against lethal challenge. Secondly, protection thus elicited can be suppressed when a high dose of a synthetic corticosteroid is administered.

Triamcinolone acetonide has previously been used to investigate the immune response of fish to other pathogens. Anderson *et al.* (1982) have found that it can affect the immune response in fish immunised to *Yersinia ruckeri*; this leads to a reduction in splenic antibody producing cells, circulating antibody titres, and numbers of splenic lymphocytes. Although the mechanisms

TABLE 2

The effect of the corticosteroid Triamcinolone acetonide on the immune response of 10-12 week old carp to <u>I. multifiliis</u>. Each group was comprised of 10 fish. Results of a repeat experiment are shown in parenthesis.

Group	Treatment	Re-challenged	% Infected	Degree of Infection dose and area	% Mortality *
Immunised	0	0	0 (0)	None	0 (0)
Immunised	Saline	0	0 (0)		0 (0)
Immunised	Corticosteroid	0	0 (0)		0 (0)
Control	0	0	0 (0)		0 (0)
Control	Saline	0	0 (0)		0 (0)
Control	Corticosteroid	0	0 (0)		0 (0)
Immunised	0	'Ich'	30 (0)	None or very light, periphery of fins	0 (0)
Immunised	Saline	'Ich'	30 (0)		0 (0)
Immunised	Corticosteroid	'Ich'	100 (100)	Very heavy, entire body	100 (100)
Control	0	'Ich'	100 (100)		100 (50)
Control	Saline	'Ich'	100 (100)		100 (50)
Control	Corticosteroid	'Ich'	100 (100)		100 (100)

* All mortalities occurred within 6 days of experiment 1 and 11 days in experiment 2 (results shown in parenthesis).

of suppression have not been examined here, the results do suggest that immune protection against I. multifiliis might not necessarily be maintained following administration of immunosuppressant drugs or exposure of the host to any other factors inducing physiological stress.

The effects of stress on fish defence mechanisms has been extensively reviewed by Ellis (1981). That stress can lower resistance of fish to disease has already been established (Wedemeyer and Wood, 1974; Pickering and Duston, 1983). Donaldson (1981) described how the physiological response to stress leads to increase in circulating corticosteroids. However, interpretation of the results in the present study must be viewed with some degree of caution in view of the use of the synthetic product triamcinolone acetonide and the high dose used. Nevertheless, it might be concluded that any factors in a fish farming situation leading to elevated corticosteroid levels could interfere with protective immunity to ichthyophthiriasis. Such factors include netting, transportation, water quality and crowding. Consideration of these should be taken into account in the development of vaccine programmes for fish.

ACKNOWLEDGEMENTS

This research was supported by an Instant Award Studentship from the Science and Engineering Research Council awarded to G. Houghton.

REFERENCES

Anderson, D.P., Roberson, B.S. and Dixon, O.W., 1982. Immunosuppression induced by a corticosteroid or an alkylating agent in Rainbow trout (Salmo gairdneri) administered a Yersinia ruckeri bacterin. Developmental and Comparative Immunology. Supplement 2, 197-204.

Bauer, O.N., 1953. Immunity of fish occurring in infection with Ichthyophthirius multifiliis Fouquet. Doklady Akademii Nauk. SSSR. 93: 377-379 (In Russian).

Beckert, H. and Allison, R., 1964. Some host responses of white catfish to Ichthyopthirius multifiliis Fouquet. Proceedings of the 18th Annual Conference of the South Eastern Association of Game Commissioners, 18: 438-441.

Dickerson, H.W., Dawe, D.L., Gratzek, J.B., Brown, J. and Pyle, S.W., 1981. Induction of Ichthyophthirius multifiliis Fouquet infections in channel catfish Ictalurus punctatus Rafinesque : Standardization of the procedure. In : International Symposium of Fish Biologies: Serodiagnostics and Vaccines. Proceedings of a Symposium, 26 - 30 April, 1981, at Leetown, West Virginia, U.S.A. S. Karger, Basel. Developments of Biological Standardization, 49, pp. 331-336.

Donaldson, E.M., 1981. The pituitary-interrenal axis as an indicator of stress in fish. In : A.D. Pickering (Editor), Stress and Fish. Proceedings of a Symposium, 9-12 September, 1980, at University of East Anglia, Norwich, England. Academic Press, London and New York, pp. 11-47.

Ellis, A.E., 1980. Stress and the modulation of defence mechanisms in fish. In : A.D. Pickering (Editor), Stress and fish. Proceedings of a Symposium, 9-12 September, 1980, at University of East Anglia, Norwich, England.

Academic Press, London and New York. pp. 147-165.
Goven, B.A., Dawe, D.L. and Gratzek, J.B., 1980. Protection of channel catfish, Ictalurus punctatus Rafinesque, against Ichthyophthirius multifiliis Fouquet by immunization. Journal of Fish Biology, 17: 311-316.
Hines, R.S. and Spira, D.T., 1973. Ichthyophthirius multifiliis (Fouquet) in the mirror carp Cyprinus carpio L. I. Course of infection. Journal of Fish Biology, 5: 385-392.
Hines, R.S. and Spira, D.T., 1974. Ichthyophthiriasis in the mirror carp, Cyprinus carpio (L.) V. Acquired immunity. Journal of Fish Biology, 6: 373-378.
Nigrelli, R.F. Pokorny, K.S. and Ruggieri, G.D., 1976. Notes on Ichthyophthirius multifiliis. A ciliate parasitic on freshwater fishes, with some remarks on possible physiological races and species. Transactions of the American Microscopical Society , 95, 607-613.
Paperna, I., 1972. Infection by Ichthyophthirius multifiliis on fish in Uganda. The Progressive Fish Culturist, 34: 162-164.
Pickering, A.D. and Duston, J., 1983. Administration of cortisol to brown trout, Salmo trutta L., and its effects on the susceptibility of Saprolegnia infection and furunculosis. Journal of Fish Biology 23: 163-175.
Wedemeyer, G.A. and Wood, J., 1974. Stress as a predisposing factor in fish diseases. U.S. Department of the Interior. Leaflet No. 38, 1-7.

Veterinary Immunology and Immunopathology, 12 (1986) 421—430
Elsevier Science Publishers B.V., Amsterdam — Printed in The Netherlands

IMMUNOLOGICAL CLASSIFICATION OF A PIKE LYMPHOMA

J.S. THOMPSON[1] and A.A.I. KOSTIALA[2]

[1]Department of Limnology, University of Helsinki, Helsinki (Finland)

[2]Department of Bacteriology and Immunology, University of Helsinki

ABSTRACT

Thompson, J.S. and Kostiala, A.A.I., 1986. Immunological classification of a pike lymphoma. Vet. Immunol. Immunopathol., 12: 421-430.

Monoclonal and polyclonal antibodies against mammalian intermediate filament (IF) proteins were used to demonstrate IF expression in tissues and lymphoma tumors of northern pikes, Esox lucius L., from the Åland Islands of Finland by indirect immunofluorescence microscopy. Frozen sections of pike tissues demonstrated IFs in a manner confirming their evolutionary conservation and subclass specificity. Tumor cells showed morphological resemblance to head kidney cells and were positive for vimentin while negative for cytokeratin, desmin, neurofilament proteins, and glial fibrillary acidic protein. The results show that the neoplasm is a mesenchymal as opposed to an epithelial, muscle, neural, or glial tumor, and is probably hemic cell derived.

A rabbit anti-pike IgM antiserum showed that up to 90% of mononuclear (MN) cells isolated on Ficoll-Isopaque gradients from peripheral blood, spleen and head kidney were surface- and cytoplasmic-immunoglobulin positive by indirect immunofluorescence, while a maximum of 5% of tumor cells were positive. A maximum of 5% of MN cells from hemic tissues exhibited rosettes when incubated with AET-treated sheep red blood cells; however, only 1% of cells in the tumor formed rosettes.

Lymphocyte proliferation assays were performed on MN cells from hemic tissues and tumor using phytohemagglutinin P, concanavalin A, tuberculin purified protein derivative and lipopolysaccharide W in medium supplemented with fetal calf serum or autologous pike plasma. Proliferation indices in hemic tissues were similar in the groups. However, all proliferation indices in tissues were significantly higher than corresponding values in the tumor. These assays show that pike MN cells respond when stimulated by T and B cell mitogens, but that this reactivity is lacking in the tumor.

INTRODUCTION

An epizootic of lymphoma occurs in the northern pike, Esox lucius L., from the Åland Islands of Finland (Thompson, 1982). It consists of cutaneous tumors varying in size and number. The neoplastic cells are mononuclear and may infiltrate to the muscle tissue beneath. On the basis of hematoxylin and eosin-stained light microscopic sections they have been tentatively identified as lymphoblasts or stem cells and are morphologically similar to esocid lymphomas reported from other parts of the world.

The cytoplasm of virtually all eukaryotic cells is filled with systems of filaments termed the cytoskeleton. They perform structural and other tasks and

0165-2427/86/$03.50 © 1986 Elsevier Science Publishers B.V.

consist of microtubules and microfilaments. Further investigations have revealed a third major system of filaments 100 Å in diameter, termed intermediate filaments. These are composed of chemically and immunologically heterogeneous subunits and can be divided into five major subclasses: (a) cytokeratin, in epithelial cells and cells of epithelial origin, (b) desmin, in smooth, skeletal and cardiac muscle cells and some nonmuscle cells, (c) vimentin, in mesenchymal cells, (d) glial fibrillary acidic protein (GFAP), in glial cells and cells of glial origin, and (e) neurofilament, in neurons (Lazarides, 1982).

In mammals, immune responses are known to be based on complex interactions between several types of lymphoid cells. Fish are also known to possess an immune system consisting of lymphocytes and immunoglobulins. That there are equivalents to mammalian T and B cells in fish is suggested e.g. by the hapten-carrier effect found in antibody responses (Stølen and Mäkelä, 1975), by lymphocyte proliferation in the presence of known T and B cell mitogens (Olson, 1967; Lopez et al., 1974; Etlinger et al., 1976; DeLuca et al., 1983), as well as by demonstration of surface markers on lymphocytes (Ellis and Parkhouse, 1975; Lewis et al., 1979; Lobb and Clem, 1982; DeLuca et al., 1983).

Recent investigations on normal and diseased cells of other species link types of tissues to certain structural proteins. Research into the cellular nature of the present esocid neoplasm has not previously gone beyond morphological examination. In the present studies efforts are undertaken to examine the origin and type of the tumor more closely by immunological methods.

MATERIALS AND METHODS

Northern pikes

Living tumorous pikes of both sexes were transported by air from Mariehamn, Åland, to Helsinki in cold natural seawater. They were housed in 0.5 m^3 tanks at the Department of Limnology in natural seawater or in a commercial artificial seawater mix at $+4^o$ C.

Demonstration of intermediate filaments

Polyclonal antibodies were raised in rabbits as described earlier (Virtanen et al., 1981) against human cytokeratin polypeptides of epidermal type and against cytoskeletons of cultured human fibroblasts. Rabbit antibodies to desmin were a gift of Dr. R.A. Badley (Unilever Research, Bedford, UK) and rabbit antibodies to neurofilament triplet polypeptides were kindly provided by Dr. Doris Dahl (Harvard University, Cambridge, MA, USA).

Monoclonal antibodies were prepared at the Department of Pathology, University of Helsinki, using the technique of Köhler and Milstein (1975). BALB/c mice were immunized, single cell suspensions were prepared from the spleens, and for fusion the myeloma cell line P3/NS-1/1-AgH-1 was used. The specificities of the antibodies raised were as follows: anti-cytokeratin antibodies PKK 1, 2 and 3, anti-vimentin antibodies 4B5 and 24BA6, anti-neurofilament protein antibody 14BA8, and anti-GFAP antibody (Virtanen et al., 1985; Thompson et al., 1985).

Tumors were excised from pike skin and necrotic tissue removed. They were wrapped in gauze moistened with Ca- and Mg-free Dulbecco's PBS, stored briefly at $+4^{0}$ C and frozen at -20^{0} C. Small pieces of pike intestine, body wall skeletal muscle, heart, liver, testis, head-, mid-, and posterior kidneys, and brain were treated similarly. Frozen sections were fixed in -20^{0} C methanol, washed in PBS and incubated with the respective antibodies for 30 min at $+20^{0}$ C. After washing they were incubated with fluorescein isothiocyanate (FITC)-coupled rabbit anti-mouse IgG, or goat anti-rabbit IgG antibodies (Cappel Laboratories, PA) for 30 min and mounted in glycerol. A Zeiss Standard microscope with an epi-illuminator IIIRS was used.

Media and mononuclear cell suspensions

Cell medium consisted of RPMI 1640 containing 100 µg/ml of penicillin and streptomycin, 0.3 mg/ml of L(+)-glutamine and 20 mM HEPES. For lymphoid cell cultures, the medium was supplemented with either fetal calf serum (FCS) or with autologous tumor pike plasma (APP) at a final concentration of 10% . Digestion fluid (DF) for tumors was prepared fresh each time by addition to RPMI of DNase-1 type III and collagenase type IA (both at 0.2 mg/ml, Sigma), and HEPES. A stock solution of Ficoll-Isopaque (FIP, Pharmacia Fine Chemicals) was prepared and used for separation of mononuclear (MN) cells, as described by Bøyum (1968). For best separation of cells, it was first diluted 9:1 with Dulbecco's Ca- and Mg-free PBS.

Cell suspensions were prepared from peripheral blood, head kidney, spleen, and tumor of one or two pikes at a time. A living pike was bled from the ventral aorta into a heparinized syringe. Head kidneys and spleens were removed, teased apart in cell medium and the cell suspensions filtered through sterile gauze. Tumors were removed, teased apart, immersed in DF for 30 min at $+4^{0}$ C with a magnetic stirrer, and filtered through gauze. After washing, cell medium was added. Undiluted blood, lymphoid or tumor cell suspensions were layered over FIP, centrifuged at 1500 rpm for 40 min at $+20^{0}$ C, MN cells collected at the interface, and the cells were washed.

Lymphocyte proliferation assay

Phytohemagglutinin P (PHA, Difco) was reconstituted in distilled water at a concentration of 2 mg/ml and concanavalin A (Con A, Pharmacia) at 1 mg/ml. Preservative-free tuberculin purified protein derivative (PPD, State Serum Institute, Copenhagen) at 1 mg/ml in PBS was used. Lipopolysaccharide W (LPS,

Eschericia coli 055:B5, Difco) was reconstituted in distilled water at a concentration of 4 mg/ml, sonicated and sterilized by membrane filtration. The mitogens were further diluted in cell medium to give final concentrations as follows: PHA 2.5, 25 and 250 µg/ml; Con A 1.25, 12.5, and 125 µg/ml; PPD 1, 10, and 100 µg/ml; and LPS 5, 50, and 500 µg/ml.

The response of MN cells to mitogens was tested in 0.2 ml of culture medium containing either FCS or APP. Triplicate cultures of 10^5 cells/well were set up in round bottomed microtiter plates which were tightly sealed and incubated at $+20^{\circ}$ C for a total of 4 or 5 days. Twentyfour hours before harvest, 1 µCi of ^{3}H-thymidine (5 Ci/mM, Amersham) was added to each well. The cells were harvested on a glass fiber filter, and counts per minute measured in a liquid scintillation counter. The proliferation index is the ratio of radioactivity in mitogen-stimulated cultures to that in the absence of stimulants.

Surface marker studies

Rabbit anti-pike IgM antiserum was kindly provided by Dr. Willem B. van Muiswinkel, Agricultural University Zodiac, Wageningen, The Netherlands. It was heat inactivated at $+56^{\circ}$ C for 30 min.

For cytoplasmic immunoglobulin (CIg), cytocentrifuge preparations of FIP-banded MN cells were fixed in paraformaldehyde, then transferred to -20° C acetone for 10 min. They were incubated in a 1:4000 dilution in PBS of rabbit anti-pike IgM, with 0.5% human (HSA) or bovine (BSA) serum albumin added to reduce nonspecific binding. After 40 min in a moist chamber at $+20^{\circ}$ C, they were washed in PBS and further incubated for 30 min in a 1:40 dilution of FITC-conjugated swine anti-rabbit Ig (Dako, Copenhagen), washed again and mounted in PBS-glycerol.

For surface immunoglobulin (SIg), MN cells were suspended in a 1:4000 dilution in PBS of rabbit anti-pike IgM with 0.5% BSA or HSA, and incubated for 30 min on ice. The cells were washed twice in PBS and incubated in 1:40 FITC swine anti-rabbit Ig for 30 min on ice. After washing twice, the supernates were removed and the cells gently suspended. A drop each of cell suspension and PBS-glycerol were placed on glass slides and fluorescence was visualized under a Leitz Ortholux UV microscope. Controls for CIg and Sig were cells incubated in normal rabbit serum or nonFITC-conjugated swine anti-rabbit Ig. For sheep red blood cell (SRBC) rosettes, the cells were treated with 2-aminoethyl-isothiouronium bromide hydrobromide (AET, Sigma) according to the method of Pellegrino et al. (1975). MN cells in RPMI were added to a suspension of SRBC and incubated at $+20^{\circ}$ C for 15 min with gentle agitation every 5 min. They were spun at 450 rpm for 3 min at $+4^{\circ}$ C and incubated for 30 min on ice. The tubes were gently rotated until the pellets were suspended and RPMI added down the sides of the tubes. A drop of the suspension was placed on a Bürker chamber with a Pasteur pipette without a bulb. After a few minutes, a coverslip was gently applied and rosettes counted. Lymphocytes binding three or more SRBC were regarded as positive; the percentage of rosette-forming cells in 200-300 leukocytes was noted.

Statistical analysis

Differences in lymphocyte proliferation assays between tissues and tumors of pikes were assessed by the Mann-Whitney U-test.

RESULTS

Demonstration of intermediate filaments by indirect immunofluorescence microscopy

As can be seen in Table 1, skin staining with monoclonal and polyclonal anti-cytokeratin antibodies was seen in the epidermis and with anti-vimentin antibodies in the dermis. Desmin was found in skeletal muscle and in the muscle layer of the intestine. Vimentin was present in blood vessels of the skeletal muscle. Intestinal epithelial cells were positive when treated for cytokeratin. Liver hepatocytes were keratin-, vimentin-, and desmin negative, although muscular blood vessel elements did exhibit vimentin and desmin activity. Heart muscle was keratin negative, but did exhibit a weakly positive vimentin reactivity in the connective tissue component, as well as desmin positivity in the muscle component in both the atrial and ventricular areas. In head kidney scattered vimentin positive cells were noted but no keratin positivity was seen. Mid- and posterior kidneys showed variable glandular-like staining when incubated with anti-keratin monoclonals and were also positive for vimentin (not shown). Testis showed some cytokeratin and vimentin reactivity and in myoid elements desmin-like material was observed, whereas sperm exhibited vimentin positivity when incubated with polyclonal anti-vimentin antibodies. Brain, but no other tissue, was positive when treated with anti-GFAP and anti-neurofilament protein polyclonal and monoclonal antibodies. Tumor cells were negative for keratin, desmin, neurofilament protein, and GFAP, but exhibited staining with anti-vimentin antibodies.

Expression of surface markers

FIP-banded MNs from blood, spleen, head kidney, and tumor were tested for surface and cytoplasmic Ig by indirect immunofluorescence using a polyclonal anti-pike IgM antiserum (Table 2). Even at a high dilution virtually all head kidney cells and a great majority of those from blood and spleen demonstrated Ig, whereas tumor cells were only occasionally positive. The proportion of cells forming SRBC rosettes was low in all tissues and tumor.

TABLE 1

Demonstration of intermediate filaments in tissues and cutaneous tumors of pikes by indirect immunofluorescence using monoclonal and polyclonal antibodies

Organ	Antibody against							
	Cytokeratin		vimentin		desmin	neurofilament		GFAP
	mc	pc	mc	pc	pc	mc	pc	pc
SKIN								
epidermis	+/-	+	-	-	-	-	-	-
dermis	-	-	+	+	-	-	-	-
SKELETAL MUSCLE								
myofibers	-	-	nd	-	+	-	-	-
vessels	-	-	nd	+	-	-	-	-
INTESTINE								
epithelium	+	-	-	-	-	-	-	-
muscle	-	-	-	-	+	-	-	-
connective tissue	-	-	+	+	-	-	-	-
LIVER								
hepatocytes	-	-	-	-	-	-	-	-
vessels	-	-	+	+	+	-	-	-
HEART								
ventricle	-	-	-	+	+	-	-	-
atrium	-	-	-	+	+	-	-	-
MID KIDNEY								
tubules	+	-	nd	-	-	-	-	-
HEAD KIDNEY	-	-	nd	+	-	-	-	-
POSTERIOR KIDNEY	+	-	nd	-	-	-	-	-
TESTIS								
tubules	-	w	nd	-	-	-	-	-
myoid layer	-	-	nd	-	+	-	-	-
sperm	-	-	nd	+	-	-	-	-
BRAIN								
neurons	-	-	-	-	-	+	+	-
glia	-	-	-	-	-	-	-	+
TUMOR	-	-	+/-	+	-	-	-	-

GFAP = glial fibrillary acidic protein
mc = monoclonal
pc = polyclonal
nd = not done
w = weak fluorescence

Mitogenic responses of mononuclear cells

MNs from blood, spleen, head kidney, and tumor were cultured in medium supplemented with FCS or APP in the presence of mitogens. It was found that the concentrations of mitogens most often inducing maximal cell proliferations were 2.5 μg/ml for PHA, 12.5 μg/ml for Con A, 100 μg/ml for PPD, and 50 μg/ml for LPS. For each organ, an optimal proliferation index was calculated whether from day 4 or day 5 culture and regardless of mitogen concentration. The results are seen in Table 3 and show that the mean indices were significantly higher in all the lymphoid organs than in the tumor which did not respond by cell proliferation at all. The optimal proliferation indices of cells from the various lymphoid organs did not differ significantly from each other nor was there any significant difference in mitogenic responses in the presence of FCS or APP.

TABLE 2

Expression of surface and cytoplasmic Ig and receptors for SRBC by mononuclear cells from tissues and tumors of pikes

Organ	Percentage positive		
	Surface Ig	Cytoplasmic Ig	SRBC rosettes
Blood	90	90	≤5
Spleen	90	90	≤5
Head kidney	95	95	≤5
Tumor	1-5	1-5	0-1

TABLE 3

Mononuclear cell proliferation indices of pike tissues and tumor in fetal calf serum and in autologous pike plasma

Organ	Mitogen	Fetal calf serum		Autologous plasma	
		number of pikes	mean index ± SE	number of pikes	mean index ± SE
Blood	PHA	21	2.4 ± 0.5 [a]	20	2.5 ± 0.3 [b]
	Con A	21	3.5 ± 0.5 [a]	19	2.8 ± 0.4 [a]
	PPD	21	3.5 ± 0.5 [a]	20	5.1 ± 0.9 [a]
	LPS	20	2.6 ± 0.3 [a]	19	3.5 ± 0.8 [a]
Spleen	PHA	19	2.3 ± 0.3 [a]	22	3.1 ± 0.3 [a]
	Con A	19	2.8 ± 0.4 [a]	22	3.8 ± 0.4 [a]
	PPD	20	3.4 ± 0.6 [a]	22	5.5 ± 0.9 [a]
	LPS	20	2.9 ± 0.6 [a]	22	3.3 ± 0.5 [a]
Head kidney	PHA	20	2.5 ± 0.6 [a]	28	2.3 ± 0.1 [a]
	Con A	20	3.7 ± 0.5 [a]	28	2.6 ± 0.3 [a]
	PPD	20	2.6 ± 0.3 [a]	28	4.4 ± 0.4 [a]
	LPS	20	2.9 ± 0.4 [a]	28	2.9 ± 0.3 [a]
Tumor	PHA	18	0.9 ± 0.1	20	1.6 ± 0.2
	Con A	17	1.5 ± 0.3	20	1.6 ± 0.2
	PPD	17	1.2 ± 0.1	21	1.7 ± 0.2
	LPS	18	1.1 ± 0.1	21	1.2 ± 0.1

[a] $p \leq 0.001$ when compared with tumor cell responses
[b] $p \leq 0.01$ when compared with tumor cell responses

DISCUSSION

Davison (1981) found evidence that the various subclasses of intermediate filaments are more or less conserved throughout the vertebrates and in some invertebrates. In the present study, indirect immunofluorescence of pike tissues revealed a tissue type specific expression of IFs that is highly reminiscent of that seen in mammalian and avian species. The presence of desmin and keratin in intestine is expected for an organ containing smooth muscle and epithelium. The staining seen in skeletal and cardiac muscles was likewise expected. Vimentin positive activity in these organs is most probably attributable to fibroblasts, macrophages, and endothelial cells. Desmin activity in liver blood vessel walls indicates their muscle nature, while that in testis would indicate muscle needed for expulsion of sperm during spawning. Keratin found in testis probably represents epithelium associated with the membrane surrounding it. Keratin activity in mid- and posterior kidneys is localized mostly in tubules and glomeruli, and indicates their renal nature. The lack of keratin and presence of vimentin in head kidney would be expected for an organ which is almost entirely hemopoietic, as would the positive activities for neurofilament protein and GFAP in the brain. In the tumor, lack of cytokeratin, desmin, GFAP, and neurofilament protein activities was not suggestive of an epithelial, muscle, glial, or nerve cell origin. It is significant, therefore, that the only IF protein noted in the pike tumor was vimentin, which is a mesenchymal marker.

The results using a polyclonal anti-pike IgM antiserum are in agreement with findings in other species of fish that practically all lymphocytes show a positive membrane fluorescence (Lobb and Clem, 1982; DeLuca et al., 1983). In fact, pike MNs from lymphoid tissues were also found to possess cytoplasmic Ig. This is in contrast to the tumor which was negative; the low numbers of Ig positive cells associated with the tumor were probably derived from the peripheral blood. Lewis et al. (1979) described the presence of up to 17% of SRBC rosette-forming cells in the blood of channel catfish, Ictalurus punctatus Rafinesque. In the present pikes, the number of SRBC rosetting cells was much lower in all tissues and tumor. The mitogenic responses of MNs from the lymphoid organs of the present tumorous pikes were significantly higher than that of the tumor cells themselves.

In cytocentrifuge preparations, pike tumor cells resemble those seen in head kidney, the chief hemopoietic organ in teleost fish, suggesting that head kidney and tumor are related tissues. Their vimentin positivity further leads us to conclude that the Åland pike cutaneous tumor is of mesenchymal origin and is probably hemic cell derived. However, the tumor cells lack membrane and cytoplasmic Ig as well as the ability to respond to polyclonal stimulation by several mitogens. They might have lost these markers during malignant transformation. Equally as likely, however, are the possibilities that they may be a lymphoid cell population which does not demonstrate typical T and B cell markers or that they may represent a cell type which is not lymphoid derived.

ACKNOWLEDGEMENTS

The technical assistance of Ms. Raili Taavela, Ms. Pipsa Kaipainen, Ms. Anna-Maria Siivonen, and Ms. Paula Rahikainen is acknowledged. This study was supported by grants from the Finnish Cancer Research Fund, Finnish Medical Research Council, the Sigrid Jusélius Foundation, the Finnish Natural Resources Research Foundation, the University of Helsinki, and the Finnish Cultural Foundation.

REFERENCES

Bøyum, A., 1968. Isolation of mononuclear cells and granulocytes from peripheral blood. Scand. J. Clin. Lab. Invest., 21 (Suppl. 97): 77-89.

Davison, P.F., 1981. Intermediate filaments: intracellular diversities and interspecies homologies. In: H. G. Schweiger (Editor), International Cell Biology 1980-1981. Springer-Verlag, Berlin, Heidelberg, New York, pp. 286-292.

DeLuca, D., Wilson, M., and Warr, G. W., 1983. Lymphocyte heterogeneity in the trout, Salmo gairdneri, defined with monoclonal antibodies to IgM. Eur. J. Immunol. 13: 546-551.

Ellis, A. E. and Parkhouse, R. M., 1975. Surface immunoglobulins on the lymphocytes of the skate, Raja naevus. Eur. J. Immunol. 5: 726-728.

Etlinger, H. M., Hodgins, H. O., and Chiller, J. M., 1976. Evolution of the lymphoid system. I. Evidence for lymphocyte heterogeneity in rainbow trout revealed by the organ distribution of mitogenic responses. J. Immunol. 116: 1547-1553.

Köhler, G. and Milstein, C., 1975. Continuous cultures of fused cells secreting antibody of predefined specificity. Nature 256: 495-496.

Lazarides, E., 1982. Intermediate filaments: A chemically heterogeneous developmentally regulated class of proteins. Ann. Rev. Biochem. 51: 219-250.

Lewis, D. H., Eurell, T. E., Cannon, M. S., and Grumbles, L. C., 1979. T and B cell analogues from peripheral blood of immune channel catfish, Ictalurus punctatus. J. Fish Biol. 14: 31-37.

Lobb, C. J. and Clem, L. W., 1982. Fish lymphocytes differ in the expression of surface immunoglobulin. Dev. Comp. Immunol. 6: 473-479.

Lopez, D. M., Sigel, M. M., and Lee, J. C., 1974. Phylogenetic studies on T cells. I. Lymphocytes of the shark with differential response to phytohemagglutinin and Concanavalin A. Cell. Immunol. 10: 287-293.

Pellegrino, M. A., Ferone, S., Dierich, M. P., and Reisfeld, R. A., 1975. Enhancement of sheep red blood cell human lymphocyte rosette formation by the sulfhydryl compound 2-aminoethylisothiouronium bromide. Clin. Immunol. Immunopathol. 3: 324-333.

Olson, G. B., 1967. Nonspecific and specific lymphoid blastogenesis in leukocyte cultures from Polyodon spathula and Dasyatis americana. Fed. Proc. 62: 357.

Stølen, J. S. and Mäkelä, O., 1975. Carrier preimmunization in the anti-hapten response of a marine fish. Nature 254: 718-719.

Thompson, J. S., 1982. An epizootic of lymphoma in northern pike, Esox lucius L., from the Åland Islands of Finland. J. Fish Dis. 5: 1-11.

Thompson, J. S., Virtanen, I., and Lehto, V.-P., 1985. Intermediate filaments in normal tissues and lymphomas of northern pike, Esox lucius L., from the Åland Islands of Finland. J. Comp. Pathol., submitted.

Virtanen, I., Lehto, V.-P., Lehtonen, E., Vartio, T., Stenman, S., Kurki, P., Wager, O., Small, J. V., Dahl, D., and Badley, R. A. 1981. Expression of intermediate filaments in cultured cells. J. Cell. Sci. 50: 45-63.
Virtanen, I., Miettinen, M., Lehto, V.-P., Kariniemi, A.-L., and Paasivuo, R., 1985. Diagnostic application of monoclonal antibodies to intermediate filaments. Ann. NY Acad. Sci., in press.

AUTHOR INDEX

SUBJECT INDEX